Qualitinomics

Celebrating
30 Years of Publishing
in India

Qualitinomics

Healthcare Quality Simplified

Sangita Reddy | Dr K. Hari Prasad
Dr Anupam Sibal | Gaurav Loria

Apollo

HarperCollins *Publishers* India

First published in India by HarperCollins *Publishers* 2023
4th Floor, Tower A, Building No. 10, DLF Cyber City,
DLF Phase II, Gurugram, Haryana – 122002
www.harpercollins.co.in

2 4 6 8 10 9 7 5 3 1

P-ISBN: 978-93-5699-801-8
E-ISBN: 978-93-5699-800-1

None of the content in this book is intended to be a substitute for professional medical advice and should not be relied on as health or medical advice, diagnosis or treatment. Always seek the guidance of your doctor or other qualified health professional with any questions you may have regarding your health or a medical condition.

Typeset in 11/15.2 Adobe Caslon Pro at
Manipal Technologies Limited, Manipal

Printed and bound at
Thomson Press (India) Ltd

MIX
Paper
FSC FSC® C010615

This book is produced from independently certified FSC® paper
to ensure responsible forest management.

To our patients—who deserve the best quality care

Acknowledgements

TREMENDOUS COLLECTIVE EFFORT has gone into the making of this book that is aimed at promoting a high-quality healthcare ecosystem.

Our foremost debt of gratitude to Dr Prathap C. Reddy, Chairman, Apollo Hospitals Group, for being the inspiration in our continued quest for excellence. Thank you for being our guiding light.

Without the support of our peers and team at Apollo Hospitals Group, this book would not exist. Thousands of unsung heroes of medicine—doctors, nurses, technicians, maintenance, biomedical, housekeeping, food and beverages, transport, administration and front office staff who came together to learn, create and adopt a new way of working that was patient-centric, process-driven, transparent and evidence-based—we thank and acknowledge all of you. Quality is a team sport and you have won the match every time. Special thanks go out to the leadership at Apollo, especially Dr Preetha Reddy, Ms Shobana Kamineni, Ms Suneeta Reddy, all unit and functional heads, contributing authors and the ground teams at

Apollo, for providing the invaluable insights that have gone into this book.

Additionally, we would also like to thank organizations like ISQua, NABH, JCI, Ministry of Health and Family Welfare (Union and State Health Ministries), NPSIF and other renowned institutes that have been tirelessly working towards patient safety.

Our patients are the single greatest source of motivation for us to improve in every sphere, and this acknowledgement would be incomplete without recognizing their role in the creation of this book.

We gratefully acknowledge the publishers HarperCollins, especially Rakesh Chander and Hina Khajuria, for giving this work its final shape and bringing it to fruition.

Last but not the least, we would like to thank our cherished readers. We hope you find value and wisdom within these pages.

Sangita Reddy
Dr K. Hari Prasad
Dr Anupam Sibal
Gaurav Loria

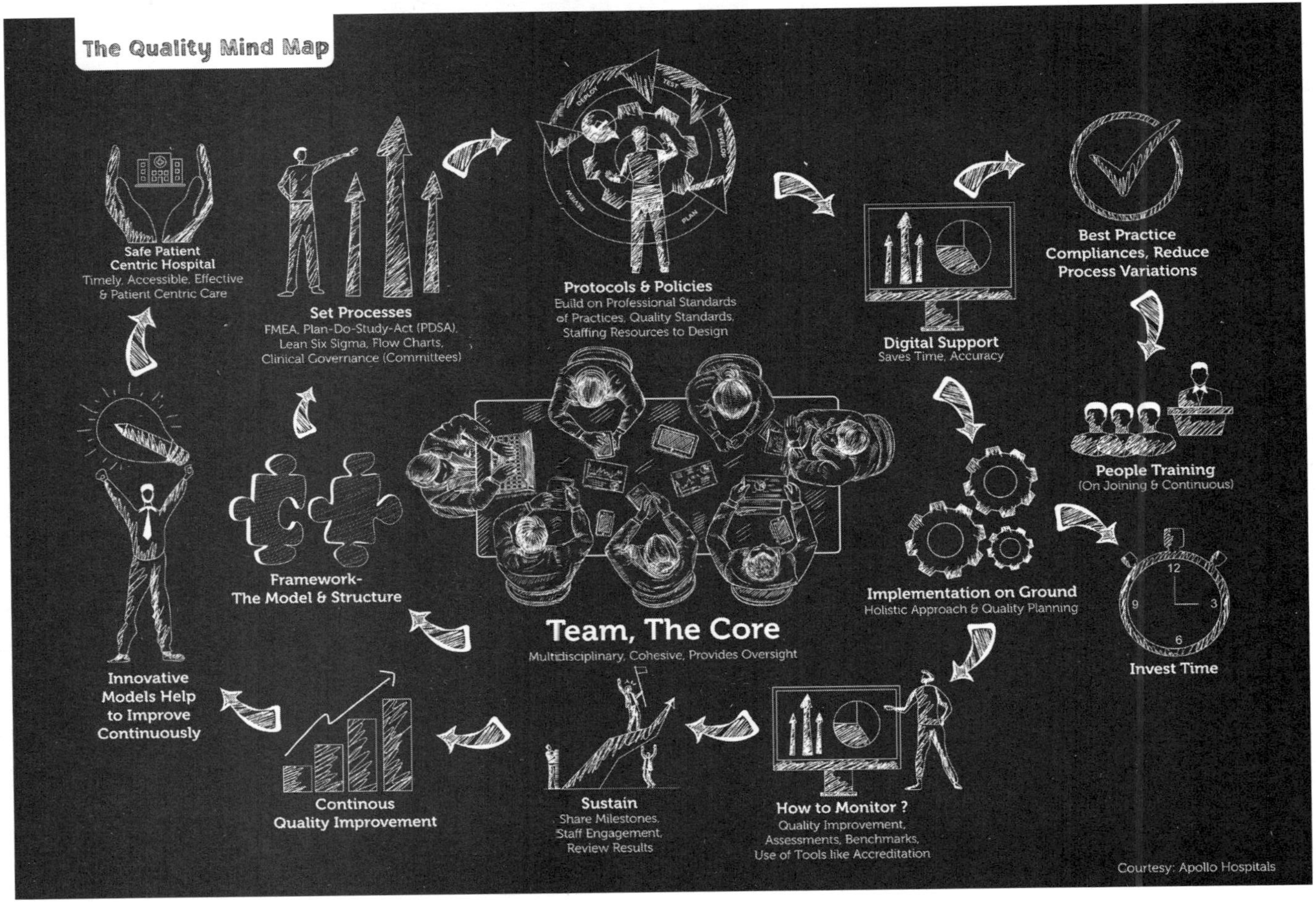
The Quality Mind Map
Safe Patient Centric Hospital
Timely, Accessible, Effective & Patient Centric Care
Set Processes
FMEA, Plan-Do-Study-Act (PDSA), Lean Six Sigma, Flow Charts, Clinical Governance (Committees)
DEPLOY
TEST
DEVELOP
PLAN
REVIEW
Protocols & Policies
Build on Professional Standards of Practices, Quality Standards, Staffing Resources to Design
Digital Support
Saves Time, Accuracy
Best Practice Compliances, Reduce Process Variations
People Training
(On Joining & Continuous)
Implementation on Ground
Holistic Approach & Quality Planning
12
3
6
9
Invest Time
Team, The Core
Multidisciplinary, Cohesive, Provides Oversight
Framework- The Model & Structure
Innovative Models Help to Improve Continuously
Continous Quality Improvement
Sustain
Share Milestones, Staff Engagement, Review Results
How to Monitor ?
Quality Improvement, Assessments, Benchmarks, Use of Tools like Accreditation
Courtesy: Apollo Hospitals

Contents

India: The Healthcare Destination of the World xiii

Quality in Healthcare Is Non-Negotiable xvii

Apollo's Laser Focus on Patient Safety xxiii

1. The Right Structure Is the Only Key to Success 1
2. Hospital Accreditation: Our Journey 19
3. Quality Improvement Essentials: First Step of Improvement 45
4. The Right Plan Is the Base for the Right Execution 59
5. Team Engagement: A Silent Driver of Quality Patient Care and Safety 81
6. Risk Management 97
7. Importance of Surveys and How to Conduct Them 123
8. Clinical Pathways 141
9. Quality Indicators: What Gets Measured Gets Improved 165
10. Incident Reporting: Report It to Stop It 181

11. Collaborative Governance in Hospitals 199

12. Measuring Reliability in Healthcare: Think–Plan–Act Differently 221

13. The Right Culture Drives Safety 247

14. IT in Healthcare Quality: An Optimistic Outlook 267

CASE STUDIES

Case Study 1: Medical Record Completion 285

Case Study 2: Patient Falls 296

Case Study 3: Surgical Safety 314

Case Study 4: Medication Error Analysis 326

Case Study 5: Employee Health and Safety 351

Case Study 6: Anaesthesia and Surgical Care 366

Case Study 7: Surgical Site Infections 376

Case Study 8: Pause the Pressure Injury 403

Case Study 9: Apollo Safety Development Model: Building a Culture of Safety at Apollo Specialty Hospitals 420

Case Study 10: The Quality for Excellence (Q4E) Programme 436

In Gratitude 451

Chapter Contributors 453

Foreword

India: The Healthcare Destination of the World

THE PROFESSION OF medicine has always been admired, valued and held in high regard. Doctors across the globe are deemed to be no less than gods, as they can save or change lives. Medicine is a very serious profession which comes with great responsibility. Even the slightest of mistakes or misjudgement by a medical professional could cost a person their life.

Today, India has become one of the world's most cost-effective healthcare destinations with the latest technology tools deployed across care delivery. In recent years, our country has emerged as a major hub for medical tourism. It is considered among the top six medical value travel destinations in the world, with a market that is expected to reach $50 billion by 2025.

When I came back to India to start Apollo, it was my dream and resolve to help provide high quality healthcare at par with the best in the world.

Today, I look back with pride at what we have achieved in the last forty years. Besides cutting-edge technology and state-of-the-art facilities, we have created a close-knit family of doctors and staff dedicated to one single mission: top-notch healthcare with a human touch.

Apollo Hospitals Group, the first corporate healthcare in India, has been a driving force in strengthening the engagement between the healthcare industry, academia and government.

Our unrivalled knowledge base, top-notch doctors, extensive experience, affordable treatment and premier hospitals have enabled us to lead the medical tourism market. We have pioneered open heart surgeries and cardiac catheterization in the early '80s, simultaneous kidney–pancreas transplant, the first en-bloc combined heart and liver transplant and more life-saving procedures.

Our numerous hospitals have been among the first in India to receive international healthcare accreditation by the America-based Joint Commission International (JCI) and NABH.

Furthermore, to give a boost to skilled manpower in India, we have collaborated with the Ministry of Rural Development, Ministry of Skill Development and Entrepreneurship, Government of India and the National Skill Development Corporation (NSDC), and state government entities and corporates, to make healthcare education more practically relevant. We have propagated a paradigm shift from the traditional teaching approach to one that elicits interest, nurtures curiosity and encourages questioning.

We offer various up-skilling courses for healthcare professionals, and skilling courses for school and college students. The focus is on imparting job-specific skills that will make the Indian healthcare professional a part of the much sought-after global workforce.

Ensuring world-class medical facilities to every individual in India has been our mission. We are committed to achieving and maintaining excellence in healthcare for the benefit of humanity.

'Tender Loving Care' is a way of life at Apollo Hospitals and the values and vision of Apollo Hospitals Group have transformed the Indian healthcare landscape.

Purity, patience and persistence have fuelled the success of Apollo Hospitals in meeting the changing healthcare needs in India.

The quality of healthcare and its direct impact on patient well-being is a deep concern. Our mantra is to identify the need of India and fill the lacuna using the trio of innovation, technology and commitment. The best of doctors and facilities—and most critically, the human touch make Apollo Hospitals Group one of the most sought multispecialty hospitals in India.

This book is yet another important step in our continued quest for excellence. In these pages, we explore an integrated approach to achieving even higher levels of quality, while always being anchored deeply in empathy and compassion. I personally believe that it is our humane approach to healing that makes us the most trusted name in healthcare.

I hope this book will serve as a useful reference for those working tirelessly towards building a robust healthcare ecosystem. Above all, my wish is for this book to inspire the next generations of the Apollo family so that our successors can be just as proud of our legacy as we are today.

Dr Prathap C. Reddy
Founder–Chairman, Apollo Hospitals Group

Quality in Healthcare Is Non-Negotiable

I BELIEVE IT would be fair to say that enhancing the quality of care rendered to patients has been like a rule, since the time of Hippocrates. Subsequently, innumerable iconic individuals have contributed to the quality improvement movement and catalysed positive change for humanity at large.

The nineteenth-century obstetrician Ignaz Semmelweis, renowned as the 'Father of Hand Hygiene', championed hand-washing for physicians; the embodiment of care Florence Nightingale instilled Listerean principles of infection control in hospitals. There is a long list of such innovators who have all been instrumental in making quality a non-negotiable aspect of healthcare. In 1951, in USA, a firm set up the Joint Commission on Accreditation of Healthcare Organizations (JCAHO) for the accreditation of quality in healthcare.

There are considerable evidences highlighting that accreditation programs improve clinical outcomes and these programs should be supported as a tool to enhance the quality of healthcare services.

Accreditation involves the trained external peer reviewers to evaluate a healthcare organization's compliance and compare it with pre-established performance standards.

In India, concerted efforts towards it began only at the turn of the millennium. A needle-eye focus on quality in healthcare is hugely pertinent in India, as there are vast discrepancies in the standards of health infrastructure, human resources, care protocols and even regulations, with public health continuing to be a state subject in the country.

Earning a patient's trust is paramount in medicine, and accreditation provides a recognizable hallmark of quality. Yet, even in early 2000s, a plan to achieve quality accreditation was considered audacious for an Indian hospital, especially the hallowed distinction of being recognized by the Joint Commission International (JCI), the global 'Gold Standard' of healthcare accreditation.

It was an inherent pioneering culture that motivated us in Apollo to start thinking about an accreditation from JCI. Personally, this seemingly uphill endeavour proved to be a defining moment of my career in healthcare. Supported by the founding family and the senior teams of Apollo, in 2003, I travelled to Oakbrook, Illinois, USA.

In a strange turn of events, in the neighbourhood that I was staying in Oakbrook, I met Karen Timmons, who at that time was president and CEO of JCI. I would be remiss if I did not acknowledge her encouragement, which helped me return home to India with the resolve to make sure that one of our hospitals would soon be accredited with this 'Gold Standard' in quality.

My father and founder–chairman of Apollo Hospitals, Dr Prathap C. Reddy, chose Indraprastha Apollo Hospitals, Delhi to be the first in our Group that would prepare itself for the JCI accreditation. For an Indian hospital, getting ready to achieve JCI accreditation was no easy matter. It was an unprecedented initiative, and no one knew what JCI's requirements were. My sister Suneeta who helped Indraprastha Apollo at that time had always wanted an international accreditation. Dr Reddy put Late Dr Mehrotra in charge, who then put together a team, which took off in full steam from day one. Supporting him, Dr Anupam Sibal, Apollo's Group Medical Director, ensured that all the requisite 'best practices' were put in place.

The JCI Standards Manual was dissected, and a set of crisp but detailed policies was created. A lot of documentation was introduced by way of plans, medical records and standard operating procedures. The infrastructure was revamped. Every day was arduous, but our end goal—of accreditation—made it worth the while.

It was landmark day, when after twenty-four months of preparation, on 13 June 2005, a team of three JCI surveyors reached India to carry out the first-ever JCI survey for a hospital in India. Five days of feverish activity ensued: every inch of the facility was covered and all systems and processes were studied. On 18 June 2005, a preliminary report was handed over to Indraprastha Apollo Hospital, with a recommendation for the hospital to be accredited based on an assessment of 1,033 measurable elements. They say the first step is always the hardest, and it was no different with our first JCI accreditation. Since then, eight hospitals in the Apollo network have been accredited by the JCI, and India has forty-one JCI accredited facilities as on date. Any thought process must be translated and without the efforts of Hari, Anupam, and Gaurav, we would not have achieved what we have in quality at Apollo. On the behalf of the healthcare sector, I thank you all along with other stalwarts like Dr Giridhar Gyani, Dr Atul Mohan Kochchar, Dr Jonathan Perlin, Dr Vijay Aggarwal, Dr Narottam Puri, Dr Naresh Trehan, Dr Ashutosh Raghuvanshi, Dr Devi Shetty and many more of you who make this possible every day.

Over the years, the Medical and Quality Team led the creation of The Apollo Standards of Clinical Care (TASCC) to establish standards of clinical care that ensure that every Apollo Hospital delivers safe and quality clinical care to its patients, irrespective of the location and size of the hospital. TASCC embodies sets of process requirements and outcome measures that underlie the Apollo Hospitals' approach to clinical care. In this manner TASCC makes up the double helix of the Apollo Group's clinical fabric.

Apollo's success with the JCI accreditation forged an all-new charter for Indian healthcare. Sangita, Dr Trehan and many others visited Thailand to study their Quality Council and had many deliberations before they presented a document to the Government and Quality Council of India. The Quality Council of India established the National Accreditation Board for Hospitals and Healthcare Providers (NABH). A think tank was assembled from within the healthcare industry, comprising the brightest minds. The first set of 509 objective elements were announced in 2006.

The NABH accreditation system is a graded model, with progressive levels of accreditation—starting from pre-entry to full accreditation. This gives even smaller hospitals an opportunity to apply for accreditation and work towards improving the quality of care, irrespective of the size of the hospital or the resources available.

Currently, there are more than 900 healthcare facilities accredited by NABH. In addition, NABH is accredited by the International Society for Quality in Healthcare (ISQua)—which implies that these standards are at par with global standards.

At this juncture, I would also mention that the quality journey provided immense clarity in raising the bar in clinical excellence. It certainly held us in good stead while combatting the COVID-19 pandemic: when the Indian Council of Medical Research (ICMR) started authorizing labs to perform RTPCR, the NABH accreditation was an essential criterion.

Also, to fortify India's fight during this unprecedented crisis, the Apollo Hospitals Group harnessed its accreditation experience, spanning a decade and half, to standardize testing, infection control protocols, isolation, augmentation of capacity, human resource deployment and treatment protocols. The accreditation requirement of epidemic preparedness came in handy. This expertise helped the quality team led by Gaurav Loria in developing the 'Red Book', a compilation of standardized treatment protocols for COVID-19, which was updated over fifty-two times and continuously shared with healthcare organizations across India.

Personally, I have always believed that healthcare is the business of caring; it is a service, beyond being an integral element of the infrastructure. Therefore, it is vital that leaders in healthcare lead with empathy and persevere to transform access, experience and outcomes by putting people at the heart of all that they do. Hence, high tech must always be accompanied by high touch.

Healthcare is rapidly becoming digital first. There are huge investments being made into advanced technologies that will soon bridge gaps and make high quality care truly accessible to all in need. Nevertheless, an aspect of utmost importance to the successful adoption of digital health initiatives is the integration of patient voice into decisions to ensure a human-centric care experience. I must acknowledge our Medical, Quality, Nursing and IT Team for their dedicated work and futuristic thinking.

In the present day, across most parts of the world, a critical element considered while developing health policies is the quality of care in health services. Therefore, it has also been identified as essential towards achieving the health-related goals and targets outlined under the Sustainable Development Goals (SDGs).

Today's quality is tomorrow's sustainability. In view of this, I firmly believe that each of us must be committed to meticulously addressing aspects of our performance that have an opportunity for improvement, and contribute to building healthier ecosystems and communities.

Dr Preetha Reddy

Executive Vice-chairperson, Apollo Hospitals

References:

1. P. Gupte, *Healer: Dr Prathap Chandra Reddy and the Transformation of India* (Delhi: Penguin Books, 2013).

Apollo's Laser Focus on Patient Safety

THE FOUNDING FATHER of medicine, Hippocrates, knew what science later proved through clinical studies—the mind and the body are intimately linked and one cannot be healthy without the other, which is why, no matter how evolved the physical aspect of treatment, it is the physician's healing touch that makes all the difference.

We are fortunate to live in these times when cutting-edge technology—Proton therapy, robotic surgeries, artificial intelligence and more—enable us to save lives with a promise of good quality living for years to come. Simultaneously and equally, enhancing the quality of care rendered to patients while they are under medical care is of prime importance.

With the incredible advances in medical science, the world of healthcare is growing increasingly complex. Naturally, this carries with it some potential adverse events such as errors and risks.

Therefore, a cornerstone of patient safety is continuous improvement aimed at minimizing errors and learning from adverse events.

For instance, take the simple case of mix-ups in medication. From the doctor writing a prescription to the purchase of medicines from the pharmacy and their administration to the patient by the nurses, one error at any step of the process can lead to grave consequences.

Of course, to err is human, and errors are almost inevitable in the high-pressure environment of healthcare systems. However, the onus to achieve near-perfection in this crucial field is upon the leadership, and while the task is arduous, it is by no means unachievable.

The primary step towards ensuring seamless performance is to create an environment that is open and transparent. Safety-first should be a declared motto, and systems and policies must not only be put into place, but also implemented to the letter.

Personally, I have always believed in taking a holistic but systematic approach to any task at hand. And the field of patient safety is no different. The challenges are multi-pronged.

Besides medication errors, the potential risk factors include diagnostic errors, hospital infection risk, surgical care and injection safety, transfusion and radiation quality, to name only a few. Mistakes, overexposure, lack of hygiene in some or all of these can cause severe harm and need to be avoided at all costs.

Speaking of costs, let there be no compromise on the personal safety of a patient under our care. We make absolutely no room for even the slightest let up on our part, lest a precious life be harmed or lost. All of this is possible only when the collective mantra is 'healing with a human touch'.

So real is the challenge of improving patient safety that the World Health Organization (WHO) has dedicated an annual day to it. In 2019, the World Health Assembly (WHA) adopted a resolution to observe World Patient Safety Day on 17 September. Let us support the worldwide mission to abolish healthcare risks and errors with all our hearts and might.

For the past several years, the healthcare system across the world has been challenged by pandemics and the large increase in non-communicable diseases.

Our best defence is the ability to create and nurture strong resilient patient processes. Understanding that every life is precious and what we can do together will be a force multiplier for the healthcare in every region.

Suneeta Reddy
Managing Director, Apollo Hospitals Group

1

The Right Structure Is the Only Key to Success

It is pertinent to identify opportunities to enhance the healthcare organizations' operations for improving patient care by synergizing with others and promoting patient involvement as partners in the care delivery process.

To minimize harm and maximize benefits, the healthcare system must suitably implement a reliable competency framework to build motivation among staff and offer world-class services in a consistent manner.

This chapter mentions how a well-structured and well-defined competency framework plays a pivotal role in achieving an organization's goals in line with its mission and vision. It also focuses on empowering the staff of an organization to drive a culture of quality and patient safety across all levels of the organization.

'Quality is free. It's not a gift, but it's free. The "inequality" things are what cost money.'

—Philip Crosby

Introduction

HEALTHCARE ORGANIZATIONS THAT strive for excellence in patient care work in such an arrangement that all the systems, functions, processes, departments, units and people in the organization work together, in sync with the organization's mission, vision, values and strategic direction, to cater to the requirements of the customer, i.e. the patient. The customers are the centre of all service delivery. While the top management is responsible for a strong culture of patient safety, the Quality Department is equally accountable for supporting leadership in developing processes that improve outcomes and reduce and mitigate errors. Although the leaders in such organizations express their support for the quality strategy, the quality champions make a personal effort to walk the path of quality.

The leaders express their commitment to driving and implementing the quality department's annual operating plan, and support in delivering best practices to achieve the best clinical outcomes for their patients. They work directly with the quality team, integrating all operational quality improvement initiatives with overall quality Annual Operating Plan (AOP). They provide constant support to the quality team, with the required budget and resources to carry out quality improvement initiatives within the organization. They also plan for a strategy to achieve the system-level quality goals, and oversee the execution by reviewing the compliance status of quality activities and attending all clinical governance committee meetings. Further, they report the performance of the quality matrix periodically and seek their inputs to enhance the quality performance in their organization. The leaders thus drive the culture of quality and patient safety across all levels of the organization.

Team Competencies/Capabilities

A competency framework of organizations is a model that broadly describes employees' combination of skills, knowledge, attributes and behaviours that enable them to perform a task or an activity successfully within a given job. Competencies are measurable behaviours essential in defining job requirements and recruiting, retaining and developing staff. It comprises a competency matrix—a tool to map required and desired skills.

The competency matrix defines the competencies that your team should possess in order to reach these goals. The main components of the competency matrix include core and functional competencies. Core values are ideologies that stimulate people's actions and the choices they make. Core competencies provide the basis of the matrix, describing the behaviours of staff members. Functional competencies on the expected duties and responsibilities are assigned to the staff members for a given job.

Competencies empower the staff of an organization to have a clear understanding of the behaviours and the levels of performance anticipated to achieve organizational goal, as a hint of the behaviours and actions that will be valued, recognized and rewarded. Therefore, a well-structured and well-defined competency framework plays a pivotal role in achieving an organization's goals in line with its mission and vision.

Competency Framework for Healthcare Quality Professionals

Accountability

Accountability is nothing but ownership. It involves accepting responsibilities for one's actions, owning mistakes and correcting them—thus achieving measurable high-quality, timely, and cost-effective results. Accountability is about being committed to working in an effective, efficient and ethical manner by determining objectives, setting priorities and delegating work.

Analytical Thinking

Applies to the person's ability to identify problems through data analytics, to recommend meaningful solutions for process improvement. It applies to the person's ability to derive logical and accurate outcomes from the available information and analysis. This requires critically identifying key issues, opportunities, risks and challenges of a process through data patterns, trends and root causes to anticipate potential challenges and recommend solutions and mitigation plans to prevent them.

Teamwork

This competency demonstrates an ability to work in a group cooperatively and effectively, without hassles or discord, towards a common goal and objective. It involves the development of group identity based on trust, commitment and mutual respect for diverse personalities, and meets ambiguity with resilience. This skill enhances loyalty in the organization through transparency as a means of building team spirit and harmony among employees of the organization.

Problem Solving/Technical Credibility

This skill demonstrates the person's ability to identify and analyse problems, guide colleagues and team members by generating and evaluating available alternatives, and make recommendations on methods of implementation of the processes and approaches. It also helps the person understand and appropriately apply principles, procedures, requirements, regulations and policies. The person should be aware of the latest developments in the field of expertise to provide authoritative advice to senior management when in need. This competency thus translates to increased productivity and growth among employees.

Decision-making

This skill enables a person to take responsibility for and demonstrate a commitment to right, well-informed and effective decision-making. It may also require the person to consult with and seek advice at a senior level when making complex decisions; facilitate discussion and development of best practices to support decision-making; comply with policies, rules and directives; and solve emerging problems.

Persuasion and Influence

This skill demonstrates the person's ability to develop agreement on ideas and recommendations affecting or transforming the team's opinion by facilitating discussions in the interests of team members. Such a skill helps create broad consensus around everyone's approaches and plans, by finding common ground and adopting a mutual approach to accomplishing goals.

Resilience

This skill demonstrates the person's ability to be calm and tolerant, even in difficult or adverse circumstances, by continuing to perform when faced with time pressures, adversity, disappointment or opposition. A person with such skills is prepared to make difficult decisions by remaining focused, composed and optimistic in difficult situations, and thus overpowering failures.

Good Communication Skills

This skill demonstrates a person's ability to express thoughts and ideas effectively by using oral and written communication skills. By being an active listener, one can learn to be a good communicator, which involves paying attention to what the other person is saying. This skill enables a person to pass on brief, concise information to create an impact. Moreover, body language, eye contact and tone of voice ensure effective communication. A good communicator should also give and receive feedback suitably with an open mind.

Innovative

This competency demonstrates the person's ability to share knowledge and ideas to improve current processes and foster positive outcomes. By pioneering innovation, one can envision situations from multiple perspectives and think critically about the best methodology to address a problem. The person performing this job is expected to demonstrate acceptance of new ideas and be willing to make modifications as needed. He identifies glitches, solves them and goes beyond the call of duty to resolve a problem. He recommends different approaches and methods to achieve the best results; responds to fruitful feedback from others by making alterations as appropriate; identifies and addresses concerns if any; and advocates changes that result in improvement.

Commitment to Continuous Quality Improvement

This competency demonstrates the person's ability to assess the effectiveness of current practices as per the required quality management standards; redesign standards and processes; and develop innovative methods for the implementation of set processes to minimize nonconformity. The person with this skill develops an understanding of quality management standards, ensures the formulation and implementation of the standards, and regularly evaluates processes and systems with teams to identify required enhancements and apply them to practice. Such a person is also capable of evaluating the results to identify training needs and, subsequently, develop, monitor and sustain the implementation of new standards and processes.

Mentorship and Competency Development

Mentoring helps encourage and support staff to enhance their skills and potential, improve their performance, develop their knowledge and become the person they aspire to be. Mentorship introduces them to new ways of thinking, fresh ideas and innovative ways of problem-solving.

Mentoring is a demonstration of leadership by acting as a role model, inspiring others and providing clear direction for achieving the organization's goals. Moreover, mentorship may lead to motivation and empowerment of staff, and recognition of individual and team contributions to the organization's success. Finally, it can help the organization achieve the highest standards of quality and efficiency. The leader supports the team and enables a favourable environment for others to reach their full potential. They promote elasticity and approachability to emerging strategic issues and opportunities, and see bottlenecks or uncertainty as a chance to improve processes and services. The leader also listens carefully, encourages team members, handholds them, builds trust, and nurtures their talent for better performance.

The organization should institutionalize coaching as part of the departmental functioning training programme to create a learning atmosphere and opportunity for the staff's growth and development. Promoting a platform for knowledge-sharing for effective learning will also enhance the department's and organization's performance. Mentoring and competency development improves the team's ability to make sound judgements and collaborate as one team to achieve organizational goals. It encourages the team to think creatively and seek new and innovative approaches to solve issues. Such opportunity for staff to take independent decisions also enables them to take complete ownership of the decisions taken for any changing situations.

Mentoring and competency development lead to continuous quality improvement initiatives across each department, by teaching the team the requirement of established quality standards and providing training on quality improvement tools to check on the existing process. This fosters a culture that promotes quality and process efficiency through advocacy and use of advanced quality tools, techniques, technology, practices, policy, procedures and training.

Some of the functional competencies of a mentor are analytical thinking, supervising, change management, knowledge-sharing and learning, decision-making, developing communication skills, resilience, and commitment to continuous quality improvement.

Therefore, mentoring brings in many benefits at all levels of the organization—from personal development and mental health to employee retention.

Roles and Functions of Other Stakeholders in Quality Assurance

It's essential to involve doctors, nurses and other team members in driving the organization's mission and vision. This ensures increased accountability and efficiency, and improved quality of healthcare delivery, helping stakeholders take collective strategic decisions as a multidisciplinary team.

Doctors

Doctors play a very crucial role in patient care. They constantly engage with patient needs, identify patient's clinical diagnosis, provide appropriate treatment, address risks involved and explore alternatives to the treatment. They provide patients with all the information required for them to make informed decisions about the treatment and care offered.

They constantly engage with the patients during the treatment process, update them with the change in their medication conditions by appropriately assessing and reassessing their clinical progress, and develop care plans to order required medication and investigations. Doctors identify their discharge needs at the time of admission.

Finally, doctors keep a close tab on the treatment journey of each of their patients. They use clinical pathways to review the patient progress, by reviewing data and trends of the defined clinical protocols. They work closely with the quality team in clinical quality improvement projects to streamline the process. Clinicians are also a part of various clinical governance committees involved in making strategic clinical decisions in collaboration with the management.

Therefore, incorporating physical engagement strategies in quality of care, transparency and effective communication between physicians and system administrators will go a long way in establishing a culture of teamwork and respect.

Nurses

Clinical skills and commitment to patient support are essential qualifications for risk management roles. Nurses play an active role in quality assurance, to prevent patient safety errors on floors that cause serious harm to patients.

- Multiple instances occur when patients are misidentified and miscommunicated with during their treatment journey.
- Surgeons accidentally leave foreign objects inside patients' bodies.
- Wrong medications are given to patients.
- Patients acquire infections while in the hospital.

After analysing the problem, nurses can recommend steps to improve the procedures and avoid the likelihood of recurrence. Good quality hospitals view nurses as the quality champions in preventing errors. Quality and safety initiatives and improvement projects cannot function optimally without nurse involvement. Nurses vigilant teams on floors support physicians and the rest of the care team in these efforts.

1. **Prevent medication mistakes from reaching the patients:** Patients are transferred from floor to floor before they get discharged. The nurse's role in medication management becomes equally pivotal in most inpatient areas; assigned medication nurses cross-verify all the prescribed medications

that need to be administrated by the nurses as per the doctor's orders. In the outpatient setting, nurses are often part of the medication reconciliation process. They check for drug interactions and therapeutic class duplications and inform the doctors of impending errors due to wrong medication prescriptions. To reduce patient falls in the inpatient setting, trained nurses follow several precautions that reduce the risk of falls while ambulating patients. They are on constant vigil for vulnerable, post-surgical patients, patients who need assonance while mobilization, tripping hazards, and managing the turning and toileting needs of patients too ill or weak to care for themselves. The call bells at the bedside and washrooms help the patients constantly reach out to their nurses when they need support.

2. **Monitor patients for decline in their clinical conditions:** Physicians are not always available at a patient's bedside to check on their clinical condition. They, therefore, depend a lot on their nurses, being a critical part of the clinical care team to constantly monitor patients for signs of worsening clinical conditions—in both inpatient and outpatient locations. Nurses help monitor unplanned post-op re-exploration, a wound that is not getting cured, lack of improvement in the situation of an elderly patient for palliative care, and the child whose mild condition has worsened. They are often unrecognized heroes in providing quality clinical care and patient safety.

Paramedics

Another feature of patient satisfaction and expectations is directly related to the attitude and responsiveness of the paramedical staff. Healthcare professionals (physicians, doctors and surgeons) intermittently visit the patient care areas for their daily rounds or during on-call emergency duties. The paramedical team comprises:

- technicians,
- physiotherapists,
- pharmacists,
- dieticians, etc.

They are available in-patient care areas catering to the requirements of patients. They help them collect patient samples for laboratory testing, assist patients with their medicines at regular intervals as per the doctor's orders, assist the patients with timely food by the nutritionists, and manage housekeeping employees looking after their comforts in the healthcare facility, etc. If paramedics do not treat patients with empathy and respect, patient recovery may be adversely affected. Some patients admitted to the hospital are so anxious about their clinical condition and care progression that they, or their family members, may ask numerous, sometimes unrelated, questions to the staff. In such situations, the staff should not express annoyance and continue to behave politely, to give them the utmost comfort and make them feel at ease. Hence, training should be provided periodically to the paramedical staff on interpersonal skills in handling difficult patients, while keeping in mind that 'empathy is the key'.

Operations Managers

A hospital is a highly challenging and stressful workplace, with everyone working in a volatile environment. There could be bottlenecks that may worsen the efficiency and services being delivered to patients, as all the processes are interlinked, and any error in the process may adversely impact the entire patient care workflow. Therefore, brand reputation depends on how quickly operations managers resolve the problems raised, without compromising on quality and patient satisfaction. Spontaneity in addressing any situation is possible only with a strong operations management team. The team is accountable for handling all operational processes of clinical and non-clinical departments to enable a seamless working environment.

Healthcare operations include all administrative, financial, legal and quality improvement activities necessary to run its business and to sustain the fundamental functions of treatment and payment. All administrative aspects affect the outpatient department, inpatient department, emergency services, operation theatre (OT), diagnostics and other medical services provided by the hospital (day surgery, homecare, etc.): for example, appointment scheduling, patient registration, queue management, billing and payment, investigations, inpatient admissions and discharge, managing beds, OT availability and scheduling, and diagnostics reports delivery.

An operations manager ensures seamless workflow so that patients get the best service. Healthcare operations include case management, care coordination, business administration and general administrative activities. They must also handle and resolve patient queries and complaints, and manage the staff performing all the operational activities. Additionally, they have to work with clinical and other teams to speed up turnaround times—quick completion of discharge documentation to speed up the discharge process, optimum utilization of the OT, and so on.

Operations managers also work with nurses and the housekeeping department to ensure beds are ready for the next patient in a shorter time. They make sure food is served on time to the patients, as per their diet requirements.

Finally, operations managers must look up innovative ways to improve the process of patient care delivery. For example, they may need to work with the IT Department to build a better system for managing a doctor's appointment or systematize billing and payment. They would also have to consistently improve processes and facilities to enhance the overall patient experience. Their work also involves managing the operations of the entire hospital facility, including laundry, housekeeping, maintenance and kitchen.

Facility Managers

Hospitals are striving to reach long-term goals. While codes and regulations ensure safety compliance, hospitals are putting extra effort to ensure a safe environment. Factors such as seamless access to inpatient rooms after admission through simplified workflow augment patient satisfaction, by preventing stress, tiredness, disturbances and breaks in communications and process flow among healthcare staff duties. This ensures patient safety.

In addition, systems are deployed in the hospital to prevent cross-contamination and infection prevention, such as room-pressure indicators and alarms for monitoring the direction of airflow in or out of a room. Hospitals also have positive and negative pressure indicators in isolation rooms, which offer visual cues (red or green ping-pong-sized balls), indicating proper or improper airflow direction.

To ensure safe facilities for patients, hospitals are adopting technologies such as:

- ultraviolet technology;
- fogging and misting using ozone mists;
- vaporized hydrogen peroxide; and
- adenosine triphosphate monitoring systems to measure organic matter on surfaces.

Due to the pandemic, in every hospital, alcohol-based hand disinfectants have become an essential germ killer. Thus, facility managers continue to look out for new solutions to resolve old and emerging patient safety issues in the hospital.

Should Patients Have a Role in Patient's Safety?

In the modern system, many hospitals seek patients' opinions in improving the quality of care and enhancing patient experience by seeking active feedback on the services they avail in the hospital. Since the patients know more about the development of their symptoms and their treatment, they can actively participate in the safety of their care processes by checking on themselves whenever needed. If a sign or symptom changes, the patient will be the first to relate to the change and will have the opportunity to communicate this change to the staff in the nursing station through the call bell. Hospitals are now actively putting in a lot of effort to engage patients in redesigning and executing patient safety protocols. Thus, patient involvement is required so that patients and professionals collaborate as partners in the care delivery process. This will help patients build trust in the hospital, promote transparency, prevent barriers to communication and ensure timely delivery of care to the patients as per their expressed needs. Patients may also be involved in the decision-making process of therapeutic intervention, but that may require the discretion of the treating doctor as to what extent such involvements may be permitted.

Ultimately, we need to modify our outlook if we want patients to participate in the patient safety process in the hospital.

References:

1. *Infographic: The Future of Nursing* (Washington DC: The National Academies Press, 2011), https://nap.nationalacademies.org/visualizations/future-of-nursing/
2. Centres for Disease Control and Prevention (CDC), https://www.cdc.gov/media/releases/2016/p0922-older-adult-falls.html.
3. Vasilis Bouronikos, 'Importance of Technology in Healthcare', Institute of Entrepreneurship Development (iED), 17 November 2020, https://ied.eu/blog/importance-of-technology-in-healthcare/
4. Yasser K. Alotaibi and Frank Federico, 'The impact of health information technology on patient safety', *Saudi Medical Journal* (December 2017), Vol. 38, No. 12, DOI: https://doi.org/10.15537/smj.2017.12.20631
5. 'The Importance of the Front Desk in a Medical Office', Study.com, video, 3.23, http://study.com/academy/lesson/the-importance-of-the-front-desk-in-a-medical-office.html.
6. 'Front office Associate Job duties and skills', Jobawareness.com, http://www.jobawareness.com/front-office-associatejob.asp
7. K. J. Henderson, 'Duties of a Front Desk Receptionist', Smallbusiness.chron.com, 8 March 2019, http://smallbusiness.chron.com/duties-front-desk-receptionist-1336.html.
8. 'Front Office Executive at Apollo Hospitals', Naukri Apollo: Recruiter Box, https://naukriapollo.recruiterbox.com/jobs/fk0rmn.
9. Mohana Pillai, Oviya Senthilraj and S. Swaminathan, 'Role of Human Resources Management in Healthcare Organizations: A Review', *International Journal of Health Sciences and Research* (January 2019) Vol. 9, Issue 1, https://www.ijhsr.org/IJHSR_Vol.9_Issue.1_Jan2019/34.pdf.

2

Hospital Accreditation: Our Journey

Accreditation is viewed as a reputable tool to evaluate and enhance the quality of the healthcare system. It aims to systematically review the impact of healthcare quality indicators on hospitals.

Accreditation can simply be defined as an 'external assessment', wherein the organization undergoes a structured and detailed peer review by respective experts, in which it is assessed how well the organization has implemented the standards on ground.

There are reasonable evidences to support the notion that compliance with accreditation standards has multiple plausible benefits in improving the performance in the hospital setting.

'Quality means doing it right when no one is looking.'

—Henry Ford

FUNDAMENTALLY, HOSPITAL ACCREDITATION aims to enhance the delivery of healthcare in a more structured manner. Hospitals have been functioning for the last so many decades, but healthcare standards have received a spotlight only recently. Though all parameters, as demanded by various accreditation standards now, already existed, a systematic and structured approach was lacking in healthcare delivery. Moreover, the idea of evaluation by an external peer review was never imagined. The majority of the audits per say were only restricted to morbidity and mortality audits, complaints by patients or external agencies, and cases or inspections by government agencies.

With the advent of the National Accreditation Board for Hospitals and Healthcare Providers (NABH), under the aegis of the Quality Council of India, the Indian healthcare industry is now setting global standards, leading to a sea change in the manner in which healthcare delivery is provided to patients.

Accreditation can simply be defined as an 'external assessment', wherein the organization undergoes a structured and detailed peer review by respective experts, in which it is assessed how well the organization has implemented the standards on ground.

NABH has defined accreditation as 'a self-assessment and external peer assessment process used by healthcare organizations to accurately assess their level of performance in relation to established standards and to implement ways to continuously improve'. Accreditation is a quintessential component in patient safety and one of the many paths leading to (and sustaining) patient safety.

Accreditation standards are not just about drafting standards for the healthcare industry. It involves a lot of brainstorming among the experts, critical and analytical deliberations; reviews by industry experts; and 360-degree feedback from all stakeholders, including healthcare providers and patients. It also takes into consideration global best practices, evidence-based medicine, and recommendations by expert groups and organizations (e.g., CDC, ASHARE, NBC, government advisory, NOTTO, specific statutory and regulatory rules and regulations).

A healthcare facility is governed by statutory and regulatory compliances, which denotes minimum quality and safety parameters, whereas accreditation encompasses holistic pathways to quality and patient safety. An accredited organization gives a sense of confidence to patients and other stakeholders such as insurance, and external agencies, that the hospital systems and processes are good enough to provide good clinical outcomes in a safe manner. Under the quality framework, all departmental systems and processes have a monitoring system to ensure continuous quality improvement. Thus, an accredited hospital will provide good clinical outcomes, credentialled staff, quality of care, innovations and improvements in system and processes, which surely provides a competitive advantage to the organization by fostering community confidence.

Presently, the accreditation process is voluntary, which means that if a healthcare provider really wants to improve its systems and processes, it will apply for the accreditation. The accreditation is a self-assessment as well as an external peer review system. The organization evaluates itself against the standards requirements, which is then followed by another evaluation by a team of external assessors.

In this global economy era, more and more human beings are choosing to access healthcare. Medical tourism, too, has taken a significant leap. Every healthcare provider, especially in India and some Southeast Asian countries, is catering to international patients. Now, the accreditation agencies such as JCI are also promoting internationally accredited organizations and advocating that patients and fellow citizens opt for accredited hospitals. Thus, Global Healthcare is a primary in international healthcare accreditation and cannot be ignored at any cost.

Here's why patients seek medical tourism options:

(a) high cost of healthcare
(b) long waiting lists
(c) non-availability of certain high-end treatment modalities in some countries

All healthcare facilities must strive to offer a safe environment for patients, staff and stakeholders. At hospitals and healthcare services, quality and patient safety have become the major factors of consideration by stakeholders, e.g., government bodies, NGOs, insurance agencies, professional organizations representing healthcare workers and patients. The focus of all accreditation standards is to build high standards of quality and safety in an objective manner with respect to the various requirements of accreditation. The rule of thumb is to encourage all healthcare organizations to pursue continual excellence.

In comparison to the old practice of medicine, healthcare delivery has now become a complex system; hence, there are high chances of variations in patient care, which can lead to complications in clinical outcomes as well as patient harm in hospitals. A systematic approach through healthcare accreditation is one of the best approaches for improving the quality of hospitals.

Benefits of Accreditation

For Patients

- Patients are the supreme beneficiaries.
- Accreditation leads to better care and patient safety.
- The patients are serviced by credentialled medical staff and their rights are respected and protected. Their satisfaction levels are prioritized and regularly measured.

For Staff

- The staff feels satisfied as they get continuous learnings, excellent leadership and working environment.
- Accredited hospitals focus on improving efficiencies and competencies of staff.
- Overall professional development, knowledge and competencies are improved in systematic ways.
- Defined ownership and accountability of all the staff including medical and para medical staff.

For Organizations (Hospitals, Regulatory Bodies, etc.)

- It incentivizes continuous improvement.
- It enables the organization to demonstrate its commitment to providing quality care, patient safety, and consequently, world-class clinical outcomes.
- It raises community confidence in the services provided by the healthcare organization as the patients are serviced by credentialled medical staff.
- It provides an opportunity to healthcare units to benchmark with the best.
- An accreditation status also provides marketing advantage in a competitive healthcare industry.
- It provides an objective system of empanelment by insurance and other third parties.
- Accreditation provides access to reliable and certified information on facilities, infrastructure and level of care.

Assurance by an Accredited Hospital for its Patients

Getting an accreditation fully endorses the fact that the quality of patient care at the hospital is ethical, safe and at par with national/ international standards; that the patient's interests are kept foremost, and patient and family's rights are respected. A culture of continuous improvement exists, and objective criteria are in place to explicitly provide evidence of the high quality of care.

- The accreditation standards measure the complete journey of the patient in a hospital. It emphasizes all aspects of patient care, right from access to the facility, patient rights, medication and facility safety, infection control and clinical outcomes. Since quality has three primary building blocks, i.e., structure, process and outcomes, the total concept of 'patient centricity' should revolve around these three. This includes a safe facility and meeting building norms that are best suited for patient care and safety, staff training and skills, environment, technology, and systems and protocols. Key monitoring indicators provide objective evidence of the highest quality of care, such as infection rates, mortality rates and morbidity rates, which are checked during the assessment process.
- The standards begin with asking the hospital to ensure that patients and their attendants know about the services that the hospital provides, and that these are easily accessible through displays and brochures. The staff is trained to guide the patients about the services.
- There is an emphasis on respecting patient rights. This means that patients have a right to know about their illness, the treatment options, medications, procedures, surgeries, costs involved, and have a right to decide what choices to make. Tariffs are available to the patient along with related billing information in a totally transparent and ethical manner. Consent for treatment has to be explicit and informed. The hospital is bound to protect the confidentiality, privacy and safety of the patients while they are undergoing care.
- Understanding and reaching out to the patient and the family is integral to the treatment process, be it respecting

their wishes for spiritual or psychological needs, organ donation, or choosing a particular treatment over others, where options exist.

- Extra safety precautions are provided for vulnerable patients such as senior citizens, children and the disabled. Transporting patients while they are on a wheelchair or trolley, through lifts and corridors, is done with utmost care, using safety belts, appropriate staff and medical equipment accompanying them wherever necessary.
- Knowing that the hospital environment gets contaminated due to infectious patients, stringent norms are followed by all staff dealing with patients so as to ensure that infections are not spread to other patients or staff. This includes washing hands frequently between patient care, wearing gloves, masks and gowns where appropriate, and ensuring all biomedical waste is disposed of properly. The engineering and air-conditioning systems have to meet stringent quality control criteria for maintaining proper temperature, humidity and filtered air so as to ensure the cleanliness levels required.
- Care is provided in a uniform manner, with emphasis on systems, processes and protocols. All staff in the clinical areas is trained to follow latest evidence-based care protocols, be it in the operation theatre, ICU or wards. Admitting and treatment criteria for various clinical areas are developed with the patient's best interest and likely benefit in mind, including cost, efficiency and appropriateness. This is especially so for critical care areas. Throughout a patient's hospital stay, the progress of their condition is continuously monitored and treatment modified as per progress. Patients are transferred to other wards or discharged on the basis of

objective criteria, so that they receive care in a setting that is most appropriate.

- There are standards for safe medication practices—with stringent controls to double check the identity of patients, the dosage, type and route of medications—to ensure that the right medication reaches the right patient.
- An antibiotic stewardship programme is in place, and appropriateness of medication and rational use of antibiotics is ensured.
- Patients and their families are encouraged to understand and participate in their treatment process. Wherever a patient needs to manage their own illness, such as through self-medication of insulin after discharge or by changing lifestyle to control risk factors and slow the progress of disease, they are especially educated on the same. Thus, patients benefit from the hospitalization and also gain information about aftercare, prevention of disease, immunizations, rehabilitation and pain management.
- Feedback is welcomed from patients, and internal quality audits are carried out routinely to ensure that all aspects of the standards are continuously met. Patient satisfaction levels are measured, and suggestions are incorporated to further improve the system. In case a patient is not satisfied with the care, he/she has a right to have the grievance heard and addressed.

Preparation for Accreditation

Every journey starts with the first step. For accreditation, this first step is the management's vision and support. The management needs to steer this journey from the very beginning and inculcate in all employees the idea that quality and patient safety is centric to patient care. The accreditation is an automatic by-product of the sincere efforts in patient care. Of course, the resources, workforce, budget allocation, etc., also need to be provided by the management to start this journey. We begin the entire implementation process by preparing the organizational strategy with top management; once consensus achieved, we identify core quality team members and the senior management is involved from the beginning. Based on the hospital's scope of services and its bed strength,[1] we need to carefully select the type of accreditation, e.g., Full HCO or SHCO. In case the organization is not confident at this stage, it may choose to go for pre-entry standards.

1. Leadership decision: whether to go for national or international accreditation, or not
2. Depends on:
    - Quality vision and commitment
    - Market
    - Cost
    - Benefits
    - Existing infrastructure

Fulfilling the Statutory, Regulatory and Legal Compliances

The organization needs to be fully aware of all the applicable compliances required for the organization. A tracker with a

1 Please note that the sanctioned bed strength is taken into consideration in the NABH application.

responsibility matrix must be in place, so that all requirements can be adhered to for the smooth functioning of the hospital. As per the current practice, the organization needs to upload all the applicable licences and other documents at the time of filling the accreditation application. Hence, it is mandatory to have all approved licences in place.

Conducting a Baseline Assessment

The self-assessment sheet consisting of all standards and objective elements is filled up and compliance in terms of structure, process and outcome—including SOPs/protocols/policies/forms and formats—are mapped. For each objective element, evidence remarks are filled for compliance. This exercise provides a complete gap analysis for non-compliances in the system with respect to the accreditation standards.

- To identify whether the hospital is within the scope of accreditation norms, the following need to be considered:
    - Bed space, infrastructure, manpower, etc.
    - SOPs, policies, procedures, documentation, signages, forms and formats
    - Quality programmes already in place
    - Costs

Figure 1. Gap Analysis: Compliance to Standards Requirements

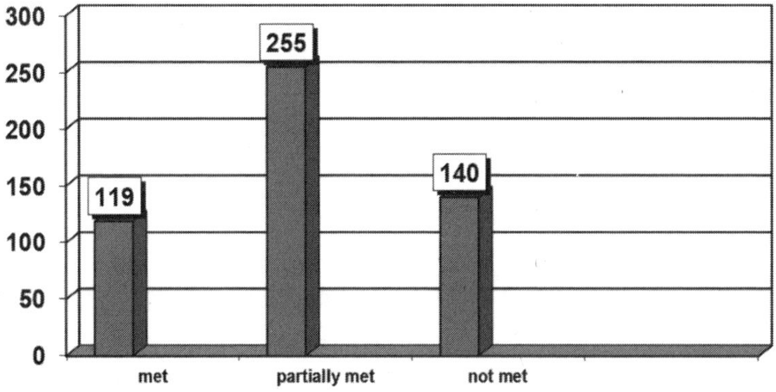

Courtesy: Apollo Hospitals

No. of objective elements of standards met/partially met/not met out of total standards/MEs

Figure 2. Gap Analysis: Compliance to Accreditation Standards Requirements

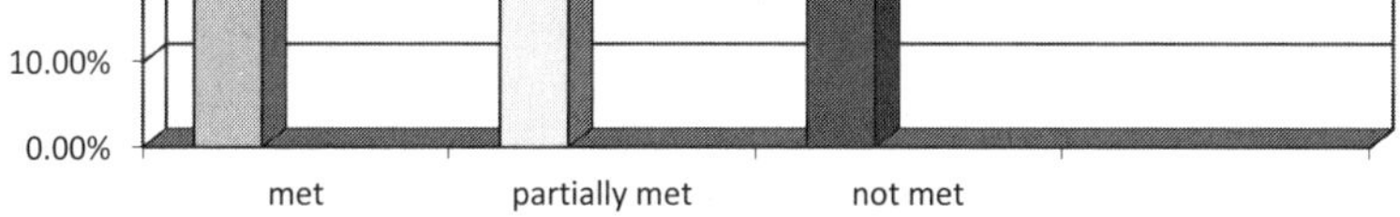

Courtesy: Apollo Hospitals

% Compliance: Objective elements of standards met/partially met/not met out of total standards/MEs

Setting Time Frames

Setting time constraints for timely completion of tasks promotes better focus and efficiency levels. Making small extra efforts towards time management can also help you recognize potential problems before they arise. Hence, you can prepare action plans for tackling them.

Figure 3. Accreditation Plan

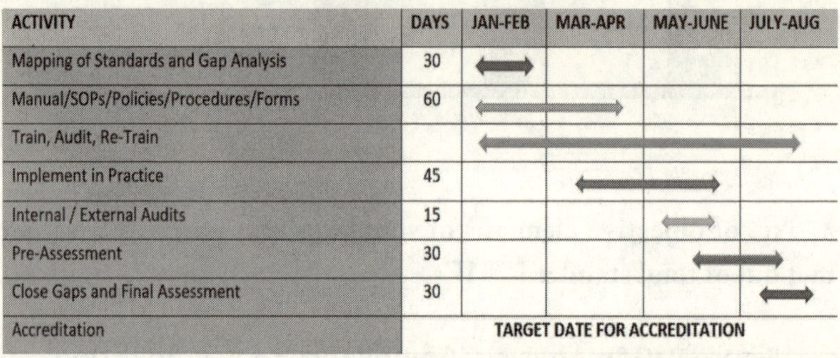

Courtesy: Apollo Hospitals

Identifying Core Team

Core teams are small and cross-functional, and take on the responsibility and authority for a whole department. The core team approach goes well beyond a gathering of functional liaisons. The team members represent every area of a department contributing to innovation and are jointly accountable for market success. These teams effectively break down functional silos with their decision-making and accountability towards a project-centric model where development happens concurrently across functions and market success is the primary measurement of team-member success. In addition to the core quality team, we have introduced the concept of

'Chapter Champion', based on NABH's 10 Chapters, e.g., the Care of Patient (COP) Chapter given to the Nursing Superintendent. We select ten Chapter Champions, who are given the responsibility to implement standards requirement in the hospital. The Chapter Champions are required to give updates during the management reviews.

Trained employees are nominated as Internal Quality Auditors and different teams are constituted to undertake internal audits across the unit. The composition of a team is Doctor–Nurse–Administrator, so that all aspects of the standards can be audited.

Training the Core Team

To initiate your journey towards accreditation, it is very important to create a pool of talented and trained personnel. The initial first steps are:

1. Familiarization with NABH Standards
2. Review of NABH requirements through their website
3. Exploring the training opportunities on NABH standards

The aim of the sensitization workshop is to improve the knowledge and skills of the core team that will further educate and develop their department. After the selection of the type of accreditation, the journey begins with acquiring relevant NABH Standards and getting acquainted with the same. It is always better to undergo a structured training programme on NABH standards. Nowadays, NABH and a few other organizations provide structured three-day programmes to train the employees on NABH standards.

Implementing the PDCA Cycle

The PDCA model set up by the core team for standards requirement is shown in the figure below.

Figure 4. PDCA model

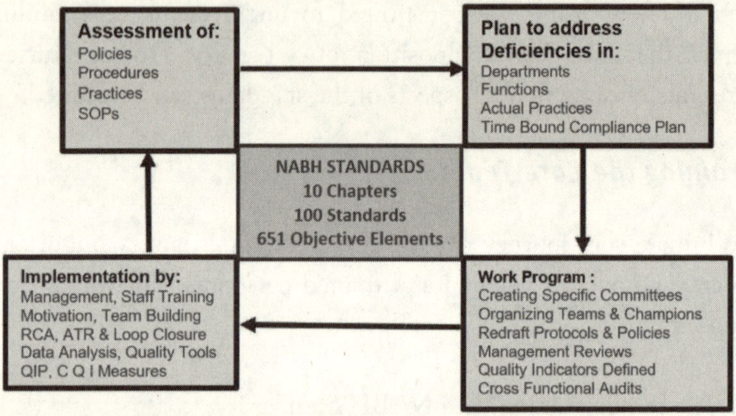

Courtesy: Apollo Hospitals

This involves categorizing each element, chapter or standard of an accreditation requirement to a particular department, and identifying if any gap exists between the already laid down structure and the new requirements. Categorization helps easily distribute the workload and give responsibilities to the team members who are going to get the work done. At the heart of our model, we put the NABH standards with all application standards and objective elements. The core team starts the assessment of current SOPs, policies, procedures and practices with respect to the NABH standards. This assessment identifies gaps in compliance, and a plan is made to address the deficiencies in all departments for structure/

process/outcome measures and actual practices. A time-bound compliance plan is made, with responsibility and timelines.

Creating a Governance Structure

To achieve the accreditation in a systematic way, a governance structure is created by constituting various committees that can work on behalf of management and address specific issues for standards' compliance.

Root Cause Analysis, Action Taken Report and Loop Closure Meetings, CAPA

These techniques help in problem-solving aimed at a particular problem or a particular area along with collecting information, analysing information, identifying and investigating the issues, and taking corrective measures to prevent a recurrence.

Implementing the Accreditation Process

Creating Quality Structure

- Accreditation's chapter/standard champion needs to be identified.
- Each department should be assigned its own quality coordinator.
- Committees should be created and given authority so that they can carry out and adhere to the accreditation standards.
- The accreditation committees should regularly give updates on their progress and achievements in meetings.
- The decisions taken and changes implemented by the committee should be well documented, which should contain

the details of the role in change, the timeline associated with the decision, and an action taken report.

Policies, Documents, Procedures

Each standard or objective element that must be achieved should be read and understood properly. The importance of the standards and the process of implementation for each standard should be noted.

With these, we can identify a list of:

Manuals – Apex, Quality, Safety, Infection Control

- SOPs, policies and procedures (hospital/departmental)
- Clinical guidelines
- New forms and formats
- Other document needs, for e.g., patient rights and responsibilities, consent forms, pain management

Examples of new procedures or policies that can be implemented:

- CPR form, early warning signs
- Sentinel event reporting
- ADR, medication error
- Drug requisition
- Pain score and questionnaire
- Clinical, medical audit
- Nutritional assessment
- Anaesthesia, sedation monitoring sheet
- Incident reporting
- In-house transfer form

New System Requirements

- Identification of new processes should be carried out.
- Patient satisfaction surveys should be carried out to check the implementation of the new standards and their impact on patient satisfaction.
- Measurements/indicators: Clinical and non-clinical
- Clinical credentialling/privileging
- Employee satisfaction surveys
- Clinical audits/mortality and morbidity review/MRD audits
- Antibiotic stewardship programme

The responsibility of implementation should be allocated to the chapter champions or the department heads with proper resource allocation.

Training

- Training needs should be identified and carried out according to the requirements of different standards.
- Faculty with expertise in different domains or in general should be identified.
- Planning of the training should be done with the help of a planning calendar, and the training should be rolled out. Pre- and post-training measurement should be done to enable tracking.
- Feedback and evaluation should be a major part of the training activities as they will help in identifying faults and gaps in our training plans and hence, in improving them.
- Audits, which include both external and internal audits, should be established.

Implementation

- After trainings and modifications, implementation of the standards should be done in day-to-day practice, to merge with operations rather than be seen as separate 'extra' work by employees.
- Creation of Quality Circle teams in departments should be done to discuss bottlenecks and define measures for optimum operational efficiency.
- Changes should be rolled out in a phased manner.

Continuous Measurements

- Measurable indicators should be defined for various departments.
- Tracking sheet for each of these quality indicators should be put in place.
- Review meetings should be done for improvement trends.

Internal Audits

- Cross-functional internal audits should be implemented.
- Gap analysis should be done for each department.
- Using reports from this analysis, gaps should be closed using timeline and action taken report.

Challenges: Quality Management in the Hospital

Quality management is a profound change in the hospital that leads to transformation of its organization. This transformation concerns every actor within the organization. It implies a change in culture, habits and behaviour, and disrupts sociological hierarchy and power systems.

Quality Management in the Hospital

- The hospital environment is not a particularly favourable terrain for changes.
- Quality management is the exact opposite of bureaucratic management.
- Professional motivation, confidence and responsibility are mandatory prerequisites.
- Quality management can lead the hospital to change through participative and delegated management.

Involving Clinicians and Getting their Support

Clinicians participate if:

- Their HODs and peers are 'for it'.
- Their professional body endorses it.
- They are given a sense of ownership.
- They are convinced about it scientifically.

Challenges that need to be addressed

- Knowledge about quality as a subject; capability very limited and not known to all
- Building competent and frontline quality champions
- The difference between policy and procedure

- How a policy is to be made
- Focus on documentation *and* practice
- Getting top team commitment
- Reaching out to all clinical and other HODs through sensitization
- Training (e.g., daily training nurses)
- Separate trainings for doctors (extracting 55-odd elements that are directly relevant to them)

Key to Successful Preparation

The success of accreditation preparation is majorly determined by whether the HCO gets accredited. Some key points that help in making the preparatory activities a success are given below.

Dedicated and motivated core team: Core team is the key to success as it plays a pivotal role in accreditation preparation. Motivation is a requisite, and working towards attaining a tangible result in itself is a motivation and recognition of the work lot.

Involvement of staff: Implementation of accreditation requirements is the ultimate check, which cannot happen without sufficient involvement of most of the staff. Closer connect with staff on the job and with their in-charges and supervisor is essential.

Continuity of effort: Mostly, HCO initiates with full force but the level of effort and dedication reduces with time. Consistently making the efforts till the end is what brings astonishing results.

Expertise: Correct understanding of accreditation requirements and how to address them is crucial to successful preparation. Thus, having a subject expert in the core team or as an advisor can be a huge advantage.

Management support: Keeping accreditation as a priority and fostering the necessary cooperation from management is essential.

Conclusion

Adoption of accreditation standards means ensuring that the quality of patient care at the hospital is ethical, safe and at par with national and/or international standards. Healthcare Accreditation Standards have emerged as an initiative for improvement in the quality of patient care. A structured and well-defined methodology needs to be adopted by the hospitals to improve the current system and processes, in compliance with the accreditation standards. The first step should be gap analysis to identify where the hospital stands in terms of requirements for accreditation. This needs to be followed by a review of policies, procedures, formats, manuals and documentation issues. The third step is to identify new quality initiatives needed, and the fourth to narrow down on the training needs. Internal audits and steering committees are all part of the process. A timeframe of six to nine months is essential for the entire process. Challenges in the process include ensuring commitment from the top management, sensitization of clinical staff and HODs, training, and separate training for clinical staff (especially doctors).

References:

1. National Accreditation Board for Hospitals and Healthcare Providers, https://www.nabh.co/
2. Joint Commission International, https://jointcommissioninternational.org/
3. 'Tools and Strategies for Quality Improvement and Patient Safety', in R. Hughes eds, *Patient Safety and Quality: An Evidence-Based Handbook for Nurses* (Rockville, MD: Agency for Healthcare Research and Quality, 2008), https://www.ncbi.nlm.nih.gov/books/NBK2682/
4. S. Hanney, M. Gonzalez-Block, M. Buxton and M. Kogan, 'The utilisation of health research in policy-making: concepts, examples and methods of assessment', *Health Research and Policy System* (2003), Vol. 1, No. 2, https://doi.org/10.1186/1478-4505-1-2
5. 'Quality Improvement Essentials Toolkit', Institute for Healthcare Improvement, https://www.ihi.org/resources/Pages/Tools/Quality-Improvement-Essentials-Toolkit.aspx
6. Leslie Falk and Ann Tinker, 'The Top Five Essentials for Quality Improvement in Healthcare', Health Catalyst, 2017, https://www.healthcatalyst.com/wp-content/uploads/2016/06/Top-Five-Essentials-for-Quality-Improvement.pdf
7. B. Jones, E. Vaux and A. Olsson-Brown, 'How to get started in quality improvement', *BMJ* (January, 2019).
8. Pamela H. Mitchell, 'Defining Patient Safety and Quality Care', in R. Hughes eds, *Patient Safety and Quality: An Evidence-Based Handbook for Nurses* (Rockville, MD: Agency for Healthcare Research and Quality, 2008), https://www.ncbi.nlm.nih.gov/books/NBK2681/

9. World Health Organization, 'Patient Safety', https://www.who.int/news-room/fact-sheets/detail/patient-safety
10. Cleveland Clinic, https://my.clevelandclinic.org/departments/patient-experience/depts/quality-patient-safety
11. American Hospital Association, 'Quality & Patient Safety', https://www.aha.org/advocacy/quality-and-patient-safety
12. 'The patient comes first', ISO.org, 7 March 2016, https://www.iso.org/news/2016/03/Ref2055.html
13. Michael G. Crago, 'Patient Safety, Six Sigma & ISO 9000 Quality Management', Quality Digest, https://www.qualitydigest.com/nov00/html/patient.html
14. National Patient Safety Implementation Framework (2018–2025), Ministry of Health and Family Welfare, Government of India, https://main.mohfw.gov.in/sites/default/files/national%20patient%20safety%20implimentation_for%20web.pdf
15. Anupam Sibal, R. S. Uberoi, Arpita Malani, 'An approach to improve patient safety and quality beyond accreditation', *World Hospitals and Health Services* (2016), Vol. 52, No. 2, https://pubmed.ncbi.nlm.nih.gov/30716235/

3

Quality Improvement Essentials: First Step of Improvement

Quality Improvement is one of the challenging and complex aspects for the healthcare industry that focuses on improving patient experience since they need to align industry changes with the different levels and processes of their organization.

In this chapter, healthcare professionals, researchers and students will understand the best ways to deal with challenges by leveraging the established Quality Improvement approaches with improved technologies, making policies of effective assistance, offering training, implementing SOPs and making patient and employee-centric decisions.

'Improvement usually means doing something that we have never done before.'

—Shigeo Shingo

AN ORGANIZATION'S SERVICE delivery system is directly linked to the kind of quality the hospital plans on providing to the patients. Quality plays a very major role in the way the patients perceive our system. From patients' point of view, even minute details such as technical performance or cost-effectiveness calculations matter a lot.

Quality Improvement (QI) consists of various systematic and continuous actions that eventually lead to measurable improvement in the quality of care provided to patients. The QI in any organization rests on a base of certain fundamental concepts. In healthcare, the following six dimensions are the simple rules for redesigning healthcare:

- Safe: Patients look for a safer environment when interacting in a medical surrounding.
- Timely: Less waiting time is the key for better patient experience.
- Effective: No matter how easy or complex the procedure is, the best standard of care should be provided to the patient.

- Efficient: Cost-effective care and treatment should be provided to every patient.
- Equitable: No matter what the socio-economic class of a patient might be, treatment and care should be given without any partiality.
- Patient-centered: All the system of care should revolve around the patient and his/her care.

For any organization or a process to function well, we need to ensure that guidelines are set in order. These should be in a documented format and should guide the teams to execute in the manner they are expected to be. These guidelines include policies, procedures (standard operating procedures), manuals and checklists to name a few.

Imagine a new nurse who joined your hospital two weeks back and is faced with a concern that she doesn't know how to deal with. A patient asked her if he can get his family doctor to visit him late in the evening. If guidelines are in place, the nurse can simply browse through the process of 'visiting rights/second opinion' policy and communicate accordingly. This is where the true value of these protocols is reflected right.

Understanding 'Guidelines'

Policies

Policies, in general, are kind of a standard answer for recurring questions. It is what guides the decision-making to achieve the long-term goals. One of the key reasons for the formulation of the policies is to direct and exert influence on all the major decisions made within the organization, and to keep all the business activities within a set of boundaries that have been established.

For effective assistance, it is advisable that the organization ensures that the developed policies are made easily available to every employee of the organization.

Processes

In simpler words, a systematic way for execution of tasks is 'process'. It is an ongoing presentation of all the activities, and not just a one-time step. This helps foster growth in a much more productive way.

An essential aspect of processes is the achievement of the pre-defined objectives.

Procedure

To achieve a result, the series of steps that are taken together is defined as a procedure. It could be a particular way of achieving or accomplishing an end result. A procedure does not typically change and is performed in the same way each time, to make sure that consistent and standardized results are obtained.

Standard Operating Procedures

The more the number of processes, the more complicated the procedure becomes. To standardize the procedures, departmental Standard Operating Procedures (SOPs) are being made. An SOP includes the set of procedures required at different levels. It helps in reflecting the difference in opportunities, capacities and vulnerabilities of the staff at different levels of the organizational system. These are the specific sets of practices that are required, initiated and followed as the circumstances arise.

The main purpose of SOPs is to provide a clear and detailed description of every step-by-step routine action of the service providers in particular facilities. With respect to healthcare, SOPs are developed for the healthcare facilities based on the healthcare standards, which are primarily involved in the health services.

SOPs help ensure that the important elements of processes are performed consistently in the best-known way. SOPs help to describe what should be done for an expected outcome, and relevant information is incorporated—for example, who should do what and when, where and how it should be done. Changes in SOPs are made whenever there is a modification in the existing process/procedure. Any revision in the existing process should be updated in the SOP with the revision date, revision number and summary of the revised update.

Standardization of processes through SOPs can:

- increase reliability;
- reduce costs;
- improve employee performance;
- increase safety;
- keep processes in control;
- ensure continuous improvement; and
- enable quick change in a framework, which can then be easily communicated to all employees, allowing for rapid response to changing organization, staff and customer needs.

SOPs will help us evaluate more than what we're actually looking for, and they also help us consider the bigger picture while moving forward. Thus, it is a useful business tool for ensuring that we have a very structured quality system and process in place, while also contributing to creating a motivating workplace. This can indeed help eliminate disorganization and improve operations to a greater extent.

Figure 1. Purpose of SOPs

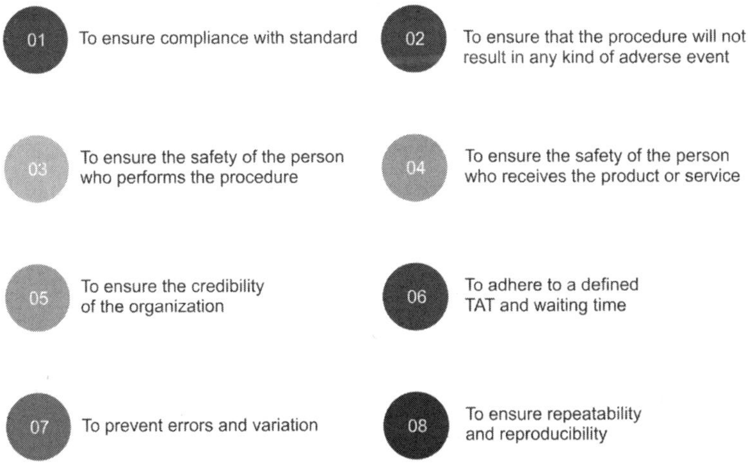

Steps to Create an SOP

Beginning and Defining

Begin with defining what the end goal is, and what we want to convey through the SOP. Before this, make sure that the need and actual requirement of this SOP is clear. Once we have defined the same, we can work towards accomplishing the identity of the particular SOP.

All organizations have certain processes or procedures that are repeated daily, weekly and monthly. The management of the organizations should make sure before proceeding with the making of the SOP if there is a specific goal for including a particular goal in the set SOP. Once known, it is simpler to make an outline and design for the SOP.

Choosing a Proper Format

There are different kinds of formats that could be implemented during the making of the SOP, depending on the need and requirement of the organization.

For example, a simple step format could be used for routine procedures that are short and easy to follow, simply numbered or bulleted with very short, crisp and clear sentences/statements that are clear and easy to read. A hierarchical format could be used if numerous steps are involved in a certain kind of decision-making, which includes the use of bulleted and numbered lists with specific subsections. In case the results are unpredictable, a flow chart could be used to map out and plan the procedures that may include the possible outcomes.

Other factors to be implemented are as follows:

- Name and logo of the organization
- The title and document number
- Issue and revision date number
- Names, signatures, roles and responsibilities of all those involved in the document
- Content table
- A description on the SOP, i.e., scope, purpose and limitations
- Department reporting structure
- Simple language for the reader and clarification of the terminology, if any used
- Detailed explanation of all the points explained in the content table, along with all the forms and records related to the particular SOP

- Any reference used
- It is also a good idea to add a summary page with clear expectations, if the policy/procedure runs into several pages.

Asking for Input

The SOP should be a full team effort. The whole team should be invited to give their inputs and to make any additional suggestions. Evaluation of the best practices that could be incorporated in the SOP should be considered.

Reviewing, Testing, Editing and Repeating

Like the above-mentioned point, ask for an input by sending in a draft to the team members for their review and valuable feedback. The data and suggestions could be incorporated to improve the document further.

Repeat the steps of reviewing, testing and editing the SOP, until the document is approved by all stakeholders. Once the approval is confirmed, implement the SOP and make it easily accessible to all the relevant people.

Implementation

To make sure that the SOPs are implemented and actually effective, they must be readily accessible to all the stakeholders. For the staff who are newly recruited, it is advisable that the SOPs are not only made easy to access but also explained during the induction/orientation process. A well-designed SOP should answer as many questions as possible for a new employee. For already experienced staff, SOPs should be explained during refresher training.

Training

Once the SOPs are fully documented and completed, there should be a process of training the staff on the newly defined process, as effective SOP implementation is very critical for preventing even minute mistakes that could cost a fortune to the organization.

The purpose of training is to ensure that all process users perform procedures in the same way and results are repeatable and reproducible.

- While training, the focus should be on the most critical aspects of the SOP.
- The reason for any and all changes made in the process should be explained to the staff, to seek their support for effective implementation.
- Since no staff can learn everything at once, there should be repeated sessions conducted for effective learning.

Once completely implemented, regular audits and check-ins with the team are required to make sure that the team is following the SOPs.

Access and Availability

One common mistake observed in many units' departments is that these documents are often available in a single room. We should remember that these SOPs are made for employees, who have day-to-day functions and associated challenges. Thus, they should have easy access to these documents, whether manual or electronic, such that they are quickly available when needed.

Monitoring

To ensure long-term sustenance of an implemented process, it is important to seek the management's support in monitoring key measures, reviewing work methods and procedures, and taking appropriate action when a problem occurs.

An SOP should be reviewed at pre-defined intervals or as necessary, to identify areas where it can be improved and to reflect any new changes that have been made to current procedures. It is a good idea to review and revise all SOPs once in a year, and no longer than once in three years. However, in the case of accidents, technology changes, process changes, or goalpost changes, policies/procedures must be revised and SOPs reviewed immediately.

1. **Policy:** The guidelines for decision-making.
2. **Procedure:** Documents instructing the execution of work activities of a business process, as well as the sequence and specifics of each step.
3. **Mission Statement:** The purpose of the existence of the organization.
4. **Vision Statement:** The direction that the organization wants to chart.

Policy development is a dynamic and cyclical process, which requires planning and collaboration to a very great extent. An organization needs to constantly assess the activities and responsibilities to identify the sheer need of any kind of policy or procedure.

References:

1. '7 Reasons Why Your Business Needs Standard Operating Procedures', Solvo Global, https://solvoglobal.com/2020/04/08/standard-operating-procedures-2
2. Express Healthcare Management. Tracer survey method – A great tool for achieving operational excellence in hospital, The Healthcare Manager, 4 May 2018, https://expresshealthcaremanagement.blogspot.com/2018/05/tracer-survey-methodology-hospital-JCI.html
3. 'Top 5 Most Important Standard Operating Procedures in Healthcare (How to Develop Them), Digitalis Medical, https://digitalismedical.com/blog/standard-operating-procedures-in-healthcare/
4. 'Healthcare Standard Operating Procedures', Fhyzics, http://fhyzics.com/healthcare-standard-operating-procedure.html
5. Bryan Jones, Esther Kwong and Will Warburton, 'Quality improvement made simple: What everyone should know about healthcare quality improvement', The Health Foundation, https://www.health.org.uk/sites/default/files/QualityImprovementMadeSimple.pdf
6. R. Hughes, 'Tools and Strategies for Quality Improvement and Patient Safety', NCBI, https://www.ncbi.nlm.nih.gov/books/NBK2682/
7. 'Quality Improvement Processes: Basics and Beyond', Smartsheet, https://www.smartsheet.com/quality-improvement-process
8. J. Grimshaw, 'Systematic reviews of the effectiveness of quality improvement strategies and programmes'.

9. S. Hanney, M. Gonzalez-Block, et al., 'The utilisation of health research in policy-making: concepts, examples and methods of assessment'.
10. H. Greenwood, 'Healthcare Policy: What Is It and Why Is It Important?' University of St. Augustine for Health Sciences, October 2021, https://www.usa.edu/blog/healthcare-policy/
11. 'Quality Improvement Essentials Toolkit', Institute for Healthcare Improvement (IHI), https://www.ihi.org/resources/Pages/Tools/Quality-Improvement-Essentials-Toolkit.aspx
12. Leslie Falk and Ann Tinker, 'The top five essentials for quality improvement in healthcare'. https://www.healthcatalyst.com/wp-content/uploads/2016/06/Top-Five-Essentials-for-Quality-Improvement.pdf
13. B. Jones, E. Vaux, and A. Olsson-Brown, 'How to get started in quality improvement.'
14. R. Kronick, 'AHRQ's Role in Improving Quality, Safety and Health System Performance.'

4

The Right Plan Is the Base for the Right Execution

This chapter examines the association between the scope of quality improvement (QI) implementation in hospitals and hospital performance on selected indicators of clinical quality.

To evaluate improvements and goals, the QI Plan should be reviewed on a regular timeframe for each key process. The Quality Improvement (QI) Plan aims to offer a formal ongoing process that can be utilized by organization and its stakeholders to monitor and evaluate the quality of services, both clinical and operational, given to the patients. It defines and facilitates a seamless approach to finding and pursuing opportunities to constantly enhance services and get solutions for the already identified problems.

'I have not failed. I've just found 10,000 ways that won't work.'

—Thomas Edison

'FORM FOLLOWS FUNCTION', a concept founded in the field of architecture, describes the importance of understanding what you want to do before you determine how you are going to do it. The thought behind the principle also applies when an organization is deciding what quality improvement plan to adopt.

What Is a Quality Improvement Plan?

A Quality Improvement (QI) Plan is a formal, documented set of commitments that a healthcare organization makes to its patients/clients/residents, staff and community to improve the quality of service through focused targets and actions.

The QI Plan is a detailed organizational work plan for the organization's clinical and service quality improvement activities. The QI Plan is generally developed by hospital leadership, along with various heads of the departments and quality team, and is approved by the organization's governing body (i.e., the Board of Directors).

It serves as a blueprint for all quality activities, including both operational and clinical. All QI projects are within the purview of the QI Plan and for the current/subsequent year, the plan usually highlights the specific focus areas (clinical as well as non-clinical).

Often, the QI Plan is developed as a projection of the evaluation of the previous year's QI activities, organizational priorities and organizational programme requirements.

A QI Plan should have the following characteristics:

Figure 1. Characteristics of a QI Plan

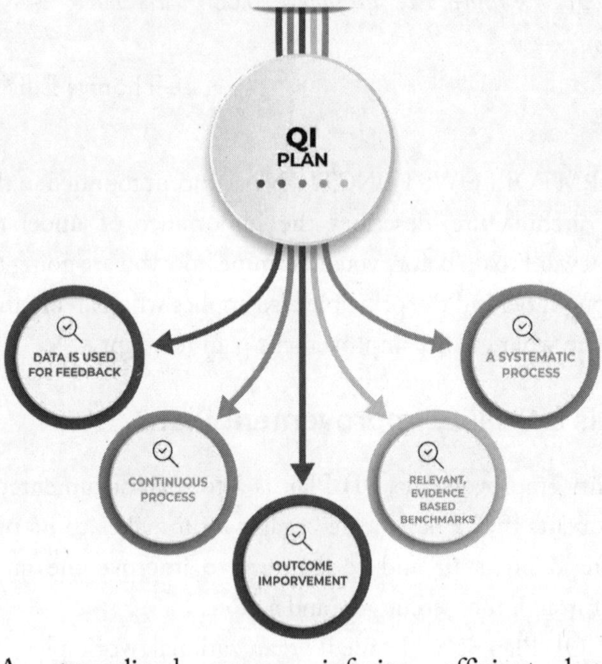

- A streamlined process infusing efficient leadership, accountability and dedicated resources.
- Leveraging data and measurable outcomes to monitor progress toward practical, evidence-based milestones.
- Lay emphasis on linkages, efficiencies and expectations of patients in addressing outcome enhancement.
- Continuous process that can be easily adapted to change and sets within the pre-set framework of other programmatic quality assurance and quality improvement (QI) activities

(i.e. JCIA, NABH, and other national and international accreditation and benchmarking programmes);
- Gathered data is used to analyse feedback into the process and assure that targets are achieved and are concurrent with improved outcomes.

The Purpose of a QI Plan

A QI Plan has the following purposes:

- To provide a framework for a systematic and organization-wide approach to improving organizational performance.
- To provide an integrated and comprehensive Quality Management (QM) Programme, which monitors, assesses and improves the quality of patient care services delivered.
- To guide all components of the organization towards obtaining patient outcomes of the highest quality and providing services that meet or exceed the expectations of our customers.

The Quality Improvement (QI) Plan aims to offer a formal ongoing process that can be utilized by organization and its stakeholders to monitor and evaluate the quality of services, both clinical and operational, given to the patients. It defines and facilitates a seamless approach to finding and pursuing opportunities to constantly enhance services and get solutions for the already identified problems.

A pivotal role is played by leadership and the organizational structure to develop and implement a QI Plan. Leadership coordinates directly to improve quality by setting priorities, focusing on core values and supportive policies, promoting a learning atmosphere, considering recommendations, and allocating resources for improvement.

A clear delineation of oversight roles and responsibilities and accountability are required to successfully implement a QI Plan.

Developing a QI Plan

A QI Plan serves as the pathway for the quality management effort of the healthcare organization. The following steps are key in the development process:

- Define organizational priorities
- Define organizational mission, vision, and scope of service
- Define goals and objectives—both clinical and operational
- Include S.T.E.E.P. analysis, i.e., safety, timeliness, effectiveness, efficiency, equitability, and patient centeredness
- Data collection and analysis planning—to decide frequency and assign responsibility
- Identification of opportunities for improvement

While developing the plan, we need to ensure that:

1. We have clarity in expectations by the board, community, patients, families, staff and the unit leadership.
2. Data, if available, should be analysed to identify what worked well/has been working well and what is not.
3. Priorities are identified for the year (should not be more than four or five).
4. Execution map for every identified priority for the year is detailed out.
5. While designing execution maps, the following are covered:
    - Baseline state and future expected state

- Initiatives to consider reaching the desired state
- Resources required
- Engagement and training of stakeholders
- Pilot/implementation
- Monitoring
- Sustenance
- Governance

Figure 2. Developing a Quality Plan

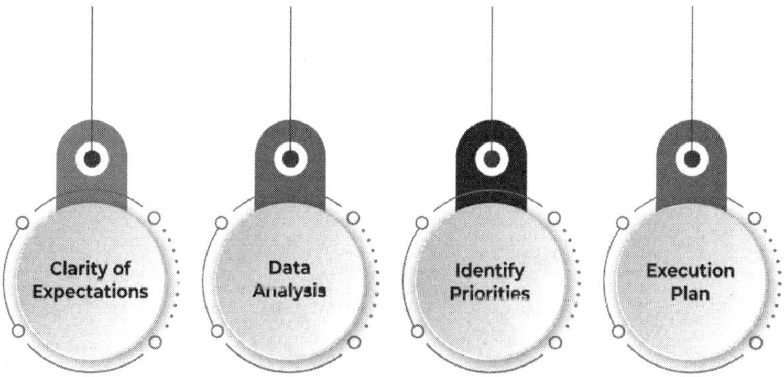

Following are some of the systems and processes that guide quality improvement plans today. These quality improvement approaches, or themes, are derivatives and models of the ideas and theories developed by the thought leaders.

- PDCA/PDSA (Plan–Do–Check/Study–Act)
- Lean Thinking
- Six Sigma

The annual quality plans can be based on any of the three themes, depending on the maturity of the organization or the priorities set for the year.

PDCA or PDSA Cycle

In the 1920s, Walter Shewhart developed the PDCA cycle, used as the basis for planning and directing performance improvement efforts. The PDCA cycle is a way of continuously checking progress in each step of the process.

Figure 3. PDCA Cycle

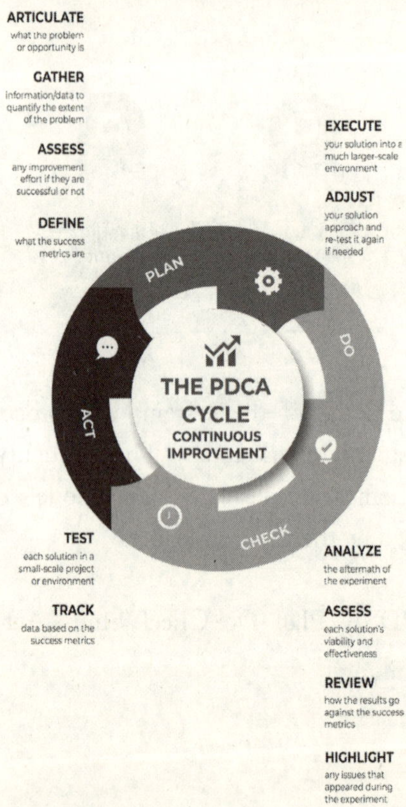

Plan

- Objective: What are you trying to accomplish? What is the goal?
- Questions and predictions: What do you think will happen?
- Plan to carry out the cycle: Who? What? When? Where?

Do

- Educate and train staff.
- Carry out the plan (e.g., try out the change on a small scale).
- Document the problems and unexpected observations.
- Begin analysis of the data.

Study/Check

- Assess the effect of the change and determine the level of success as compared to the goal/objective.
- Compare results to predictions.
- Summarize the lessons learned.
- Determine what changes need to be made and what actions will be taken next.

Act

- Act on what you have learnt.
- Determine whether the plan should be repeated with modification or a new plan should be created.
- Perform necessary changes.
- Identify remaining gaps in process or performance.

- Carry out additional PDCA/PDSA cycles until the agreed-upon goal/objective is met.

Figure 4. Example of a PDCA model

Quality Improvement Priority – Operation Theater
Improvement in Surgeries done Vs Booked Schedule

It was identified from the OT committee meeting discussions and from the feedbacks from Operation Theater staff that surgeries done as per booked schedule is less and there is an area of improvement to increase compliance. Hence, this QI project was identified as one of our Quality Improvement Priorities.

Plan	1. Discussed and deliberated with Surgeons and OT staff to understand common measures and plan to improve this process of actual surgery done VS surgery booked schedule. 2. Baseline of 70% was identified and a target of 88% was decided as internal benchmark. 3. Consultants and staff were sensitized by re-training and motivated them to participate in this type of Quality Improvement Priority. 4. Templates for data collection and staff were trained to populate data collection sheets.
Do	1. Inputs from Surgeons, and OT staff were converted into executable actions and implemented. 2. It was decided to follow minimum booking details of patient to prevent additional booking and control booking cancellations. 3. Communication regarding stringent booking process was forwarded from Medical Head office to all Surgeons. 4. Staff of OT booking and OT were empowered to achieve compliance towards our booking policy.
Check	1. On ground implementation of Action plan were checked and confirmed. 2. Trend for surgery done VS surgery booked schedule were checked as a part of our OT Committee agenda. 3. Deviation or non-compliance was escalated and corrective actions were taken.
Act	1. As the trend showed the continuous improvement in Surgery done VS booking, we continued to follow the same action plans.

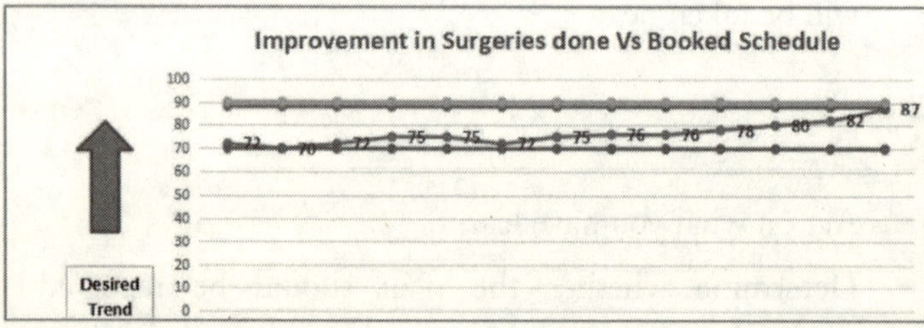

Courtesy: Apollo Hospitals

Lean Thinking

It can be seen as a conceptual framework aimed at offering an innovative way to think and organize human activities to deliver more benefits to society and value to individuals while eliminating waste. Lean Thinking focuses on the removal of waste (*muda*), which is defined as a non-value-adding component that is unnecessary for producing the product or service.

The focus of this methodology is a 'back to basics' approach that places the needs of the customer first, through the following five steps:

1. Defining value as determined by the customer and identified by the provider's ability to deliver the right product or service at an appropriate price
2. Identifying the value stream, i.e., the set of specific actions required to bring a specific product or service from concept to completion
3. Making value-added steps flow from beginning to end
4. Letting the customer pull the product from the supplier, rather than pushing the products
5. Pursuing perfection of the process.

Although Lean Thinking focuses on removing waste and improving flow, it also has some secondary effects. Quality is enhanced. The product spends much lesser time in the process, diminishing the percentage of damage. Streamlining of processes results in less variation, more uniform output and less inventory (Heim 1999).

Six Sigma

Six Sigma (3.4 defects per million) is a system for improvement developed over time by Hewlett-Packard, Motorola, General Electric, and others in the 1980s and 1990s. What makes Six Sigma appear new is the rigor of tying improvement projects to key business processes and clear roles and responsibilities for Executives, Champions, Master Black Belts, Black Belts, and Green Belts.

The aim of Six Sigma is to reduce variations and eliminate defects in key business processes. By leveraging a set of statistical tools to know better about the fluctuation of a process, leadership can predict the expected outcome. If the outcome is unsatisfactory, leadership can bring associated tools to use and further know the elements influencing a particular process.

Six Sigma includes five steps—define, measure, analyse, improve, control—commonly known as DMAIC.

- Define: Identify the customers and their problems. Determine the key characteristics important to the customer, along with the processes that support those key characteristics. Identify existing output conditions along with process elements.
- Measure: Categorize key characteristics, verify measurement systems, and collect data.
- Analyse: Convert raw data into information that provides insights into the process. These insights include identifying the fundamental and most important causes of the defects or problems.
- Improve: Develop solutions to the problem and make changes to the process. Measure process changes and judge whether they are beneficial or another set of changes is necessary.

- Control: If the process is performing at a desired and predictable level, monitor it to ensure that no unexpected changes occur.

The primary theory of Six Sigma is that focus on variation reduction will lead to more uniform process output. Secondary effects include less waste, less throughput time, and less inventory (Heim, 1999).

Six Sigma Project Example: Reduction of Material Cost and Consumption

Defining CTQ

Business Case:

1. Increased costs
2. Adverse effect on the financial performance of company
3. More material consumed than required
4. Reduction of the operational efficiency

Big Y/CTQ:

1. Control—High (Proper analysis, evaluation, training and monitoring can appropriately address issues related to material consumption)
2. Impact—Very high
3. (CTQ)—Optimized material consumption
4. Quantitative Business Specification (CTQ)—Decreasing the material consumption, up to the optimization reached

Problem Statement

Consumption of all materials consumables and non-consumables, which are being issued to various areas from central materials for various surgeries and procedures.

Operational Definition

Metrics: Material consumption

Goal: 2 per cent reduction

Goal Statement: Reduce the material consumption by 2 per cent over a period of six months. Projected business benefits are defined, scope is defined, and project timelines are decided for each step. Project team members are identified and supported by leadership. Process mapping is done. Definitions for each parameter are defined and discussed with team. Data collection approach is decided. Analysis is done after data collection at defined intervals.

Figure 5. Process Mapping

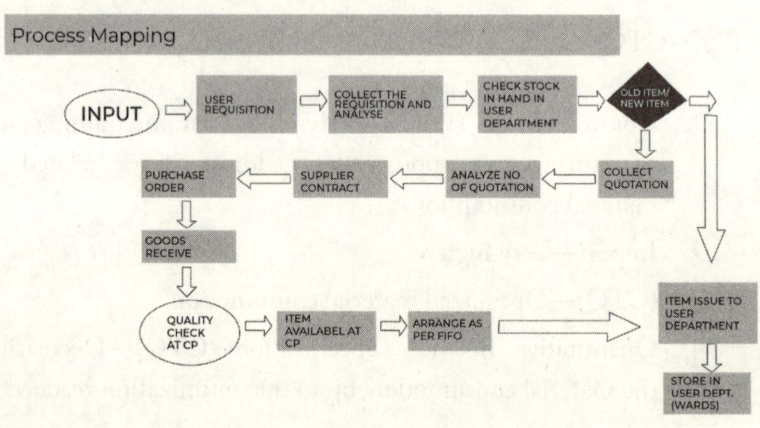

Figure 6. Fishbone Analysis

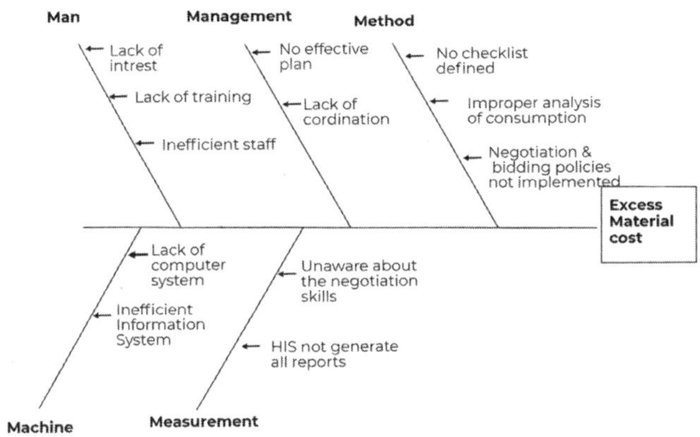

Interventions are implemented. Trends are analysed and briefed to the management at regular intervals and inputs are incorporated. The impact of project is verified and validated.

Quality Tools

One of the difficult things about quality is explaining how a tool is different from a process or a system. We can see people using various tools and methods for improvement.

There are many established quality tools and techniques available, which are designed to support quality systems and improvement. The American Society for Quality (2007) has described six categories of quality tools as under:

1. Cause analysis
2. Evaluation and decision-making
3. Process analysis
4. Data collection and analysis

5. Idea creation
6. Project planning and implementation

The tools can further be organized in three categories:

1. Basic quality tools, such as Control Chart, Histogram, Cause-and-Effect/Fishbone Diagram, and Pareto Chart
2. Management and planning tools, such as Affinity Diagram, Matrix Diagram, Priorities Matrix
3. Other quality tools, such as Benchmarking, Failure Mode and Effects Analysis, 5S

Implementing a QI Plan

For the successful and systematic implementation of the QI Plan in an organization, we need to first identify the organizational problems and solve them in a structured manner. Ongoing education and training for the entire staff is required within the organization and emphasis should be laid on the principles, tools, and techniques of continuous improvement. Furthermore, it is very essential that the mission and vision of the organization are clearly understood by all the staff and that they are fully committed to quality improvement as part of their daily routine activities.

Transfer of Knowledge

The ability to learn the lessons, transfer that knowledge and replicate the success in other areas of the organization are the key components of any quality improvement plan. However, this cannot be achieved without challenges and roadblocks. The common issues that are faced are organizational culture, miscommunication, lack of leadership support, etc. Organizations usually end up with unnecessary waste, inconsistency in organizational performance, and missed opportunities in achieving benchmark levels of operational performance, in case if they fail to transfer the knowledge effectively.

Staff Buy-in for Improvement

An important element of the success of any QI Plan is staff buy-in. They need to believe that the change will improve their performance. Institute for Healthcare Improvement (IHI) developed a rapid cycle testing, wherein many small sample sizes were used with multiple PDSA cycles. The resultant lessons learnt in this short period helped significantly in gaining buy-in from staff involved in those changes. At the same time, such testing also helps the organization to significantly decrease the cycle time of new process implementation. It certainly prevents unnecessary delays and fastens the actual implementation.

Quality Circles

Kaoru Ishikawa pioneered the concept of quality circles. A quality circle or quality control circle is a group of workers/employees who do same or similar work, who meet regularly with support of management to identify, analyse and solve work-related problems. Such staff, who are involved in quality circles, generally develop ideas for improvement and also approach management to propose solutions for betterment and quality improvement. They suggest and recommend the best practices for further adoption. The primary objectives of the quality circle activities are to:

- contribute to the quality improvement and overall development of the organization;

- review human interactions and build a culture around productivity and job satisfaction; and
- deploy human capabilities fully within the given resources and draw out maximum results out of it.

Highlighted below are a few organizational processes to assist in the successful implementation of a QI Plan.

Looking Back and Evaluating

The QI evaluation is often an annual evaluation of the prior year's quality improvement activities, which also includes recommendations for the next year. During this process of evaluation, the QI Plan is updated and put up to leadership and the Board of Directors for approval. The QI Plan is a detailed, on-year work plan and schedule of the organization's clinical and service quality improvement activities for the current year. The QI Plan specifies the actions and timeframes for each individual quality improvement project.

Continuous Monitoring

The process for developing and implementing a quality improvement plan incorporates the following:

1. A problem is identified through a variety of sources (e.g., member complaints, providers, over or under-utilization, clinical quality or safety, or administrative quality indicators).
2. The issues with the greatest impact on the enrolled population are identified based on demographics, utilization and the cost of care. Quality indicators are then selected (i.e., what will be measured and how it will be measured). Through this step, it is determined what data is appropriate for measurement.

3. Data is collected and reviewed for performance and/or outcomes.
4. Targets for improvement are set.
5. A specific work plan is developed to lead to improvement in performance and/or outcomes.
6. The plan is approved or modified as necessary and implemented.
7. After an appropriate time period, new data may be gathered to assess the success of the plan for improvement or data may be gathered at regular intervals on an ongoing basis for continuous assessment of performance.
8. Through the analysis of the data, barriers to improvement are identified.
9. Based on the analysis, a decision is made regarding the next step:
    a. Continue the process as is, with the same indicators/ data monitoring
    b. Continue the process with modifications (i.e., implement additional interventions to developing and implementing a QI Plan and remove identified barriers)
    c. Add new monitors/quality indicators
    d. Stop monitoring.
10. New thresholds are developed, or current targets are maintained.
11. A new work plan is developed.

To evaluate improvements and goals, the QI Plan should be reviewed on a regular time frame for each key process. Objective feedback measures may include a display of improvement data (how much cycle times have been reduced, how many complaints have been received, and so on). This enables an organization to take action on less than satisfactory performance. Organizations meeting the thresholds can also determine priority areas that may require improvement outside of identified measures.

Conclusion

The continued success of an organization depends on the strength of the foundation on which it was built and the systems, processes, tools, and methods it uses to sustain benchmark levels of performance. Healthcare will continue to build on these principles as it strives to maintain benchmark levels of performance by working to provide the right care for every patient at the right time—every time.

References:

1. Armand V. Feigenbaum, The Feigenbaum Foundation, https://www.feigenbaumfoundation.org/about/dr-armand-v-feigenbaum/
2. Julius Sydney Floyd, *Certified Quality Manager Handbook* (Milwaukee, WI: ASQ Quality Press, 2005).
3. D.A. Berwick and L.L. Leape, 'Five Years After to Err Is Human: What Have We Learned?', https://www.ihi.org/resources/Pages/Publications/FiveYearsAfterToErrIsHumanWhatHaveWeLearned.aspx
4. ASQ Books & Standards, https://asq.org/quality-press.
5. W. Edwards Deming, *The New Economics for Industry, Government, Education*, Second Edition,(Cambridge, MA: MIT Press, 2000), https://mitpress.mit.edu/books/new-economics-industry-government-education-second-edition; https://www.amazon.com/New-Economics-Industry-Government-Education/dp/0262541165
6. L. Rad Dillion, 'Health Care and ISO 9000: An Interview with Dr. Michael Crago', Quality Management (July–August 2002), https://kipdf.com/this-time-we-are-going-to-do-something-different_5ac794f21723dd2cda2641ee.html; 'The Feigenbaum Constant (4.669) - Numberphile', Numberphile, Youtube video, 18.54, https://www.youtube.com/watch?v=ETrYE4MdoLQ
7. A. V. Feigenbaum, *Total Quality Control* (New York: McGraw-Hill, 1983), https://archive.org/details/totalqualitycont00feig_0
8. American Society for Reproductive Medicine, https://www.asrm.org/events/upcoming-meetings/events/2022-10-22
9. 'Developing and Implementing a QI Plan', Health Resources and Services Administration, US Department of Health and Human Services, April 2011, https://www.hrsa.gov/sites/default/files/quality/toolbox/508pdfs/developingqiplan.pdf

5

Team Engagement: A Silent Driver of Quality Patient Care and Safety

Health service administrators continually investigate new and better ways to improve the safety and quality of health services. A positive and powerful relationship between employee engagement and patient safety is pivotal and steps can be taken by the healthcare organizations to enhance engagement to improve the safety of health service. While keeping up with the advancements in technology, developing partnerships within the care continuum, and building high-reliability organizations towards the transformation of service delivery, administrators should always keep in mind that, ultimately, patient care is delivered by their employees.

'Teamwork is the ability to work together toward a common vision. The ability to direct individual accomplishments toward organizational objectives. It is the fuel that allows common people to attain uncommon results.'

—Andrew Carnegie

THE SAFETY OF patients within a healthcare setup is one of the most important aspects of quality patient care delivery. Each year, numerous lives are lost due to safety issues in hospitals—surpassing the death rate of infectious diseases or non-infectious lifestyle conditions. This trend is common not only in poor and developing nations, but also in developed nations that have a sturdy healthcare system.

Thus, every responsible healthcare organization makes safe and quality patient care its top priority. Even with all the technological advancements, the current healthcare delivery is very much dependent on the human aspects, and all the behaviours and emotions related to that cannot be eliminated. The interactions that happen between the hospital staff and the patients have a very important role in patient satisfaction levels, which organizations continually strive to improve.

To this end, keeping the hospital staff engaged and happy is one of the most significant steps, which, in turn, leads to better patient and employee safety as well. Engaged employees help organizations perform better in any industry. Moreover, in the healthcare industry, this has been proven to directly impact the hospitals' safety measures and patient outcomes.

What Is Employee Engagement?

Employee engagement may be defined as the connection between an employee and their workplace, which includes their team/department/area, the kind of work that they do, the organization's culture, and the organization itself. There is an obvious relationship between employee engagement and the efficiency, effectiveness and well-being of an employee.

Engaged employees display enthusiasm and dedication towards their work, and are more likely to go beyond their call of duty to help their team members and the organization in succeeding. Such employees are satisfied with their jobs and stay loyal to the organization, without feeling the need to seek opportunities elsewhere. They are also more likely to endorse their employer to their family and friends as a great place to work.

Employees who lack engagement would show poor morale and often spread negativity among the team members. They also fare poorly in performing their tasks due to increased absenteeism and decreased productivity. These employees are also more likely to make easily avoidable errors in their jobs.

Employee Engagement and Hospital–Patient Experiences

Every healthcare organization sets for itself the goal of delivering the best patient care and outcomes. And in this aspect, there is a very strong positive correlation between employee engagement and the quality of the healthcare services received by the patients, which is also backed up by a lot of research and literature.

According to research by Press Ganey, employee turnover as a result of disengaged employees comes at a high cost in the healthcare industry compared to other sectors. In addition to the cost of recruitment, the high staff turnover impacts the patients in the form of decreased access and compromise in the safety and quality of care received. Additionally, the employees who are disengaged but do not quit contribute to poor patient outcomes due to stress, burnout and increased workloads.

Research done by Workhuman and IBM has indicated that employee engagement levels are directly proportional to patient satisfaction levels in a healthcare setting. Relationships have also been established between healthcare professionals' engagement or disengagement and healthcare organization's performance with respect to service efficiency, patient satisfaction, patient revisits, and the instances of the healthcare services being recommended by the patients to others.

According to an HR solutions case study, a genuinely caring attitude towards the patients was displayed by as many as 85 per cent of the employees who were engaged. This number was as low as 38 per cent among disengaged employees. Researchers have also found that the nurses' level of engagement was the biggest correlating variable to mortality. A recent Johns Hopkins study found that more than a quarter million hospital deaths each year occur due to medical errors, locking in as the third-leading cause of death in the United States.

Team engagement results in better experiences for all the stakeholders in a healthcare setup, driving quality care with patient safety, lower mortalities and improved reporting of errors—while also boosting the organization's revenue performance. Improvement in patient experience or team engagement shows an evident change in how patients rate the care provided, and a hospital that strives to improve both gets the double benefit. Hence, improving team engagement levels is much more impactful than limited interventions addressing a specific safety risk. This is particularly so given the complicated, interdisciplinary and collaborative nature of healthcare.

A lack of employee engagement in healthcare can be extremely grievous, while improved team engagement can result in various positive impacts on the workforce.

Figure 1. Team Engagement

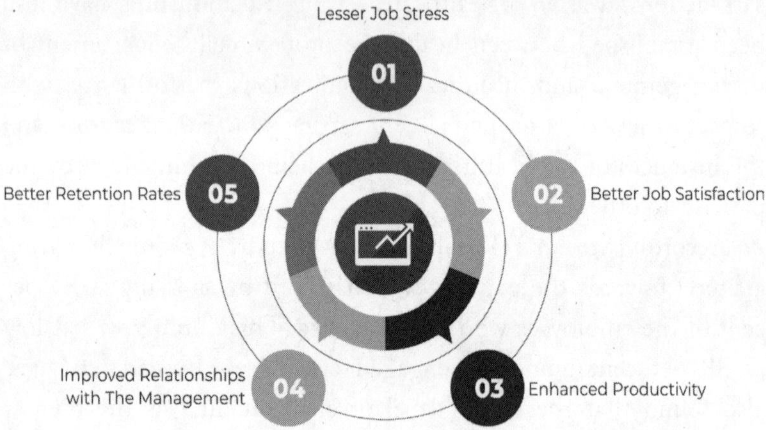
Lesser Job Stress
01
02
Better Job Satisfaction
03
Enhanced Productivity
04
Improved Relationships with The Management
05
Better Retention Rates

Unfortunately, hospital top management teams usually mix up employee engagement with staff appreciation or employee satisfaction, setting the bar too low for achieving the required goal. A satisfied person may show up to work punctually and do the tasks assigned to them. However, true employee engagement is much deeper than this.

A truly engaged employee is committed emotionally to the organization and its goals. A sense of pride and ownership towards their performance and their team is reflected in their conduct and performance. Employees who are engaged provide discretionary effort and go the extra mile for their patients.

Following are some of the indicators of an engaged team:

- Employees make eye contact with patients, with a sincere smile, and are welcoming.
- Rather than just giving the right directions, the team member escorts the patients to their destination or helps family members find their loved ones.
- Instead of only hearing out the patients, clinicians listen to a patient in an unrushed manner and try to answer their queries regarding medications and discharge instructions.
- A medical officer checks in on the patients one last time before completing their shift and leaving.
- Engaged staff does not forget to follow infection control practices, such as washing hands at every opportunity.
- Engaged teams are proactive in reporting errors and trying to learn and improve from the incidents. This eventually leads to fewer mistakes.
- Patient care and safety is prioritized above anything else.

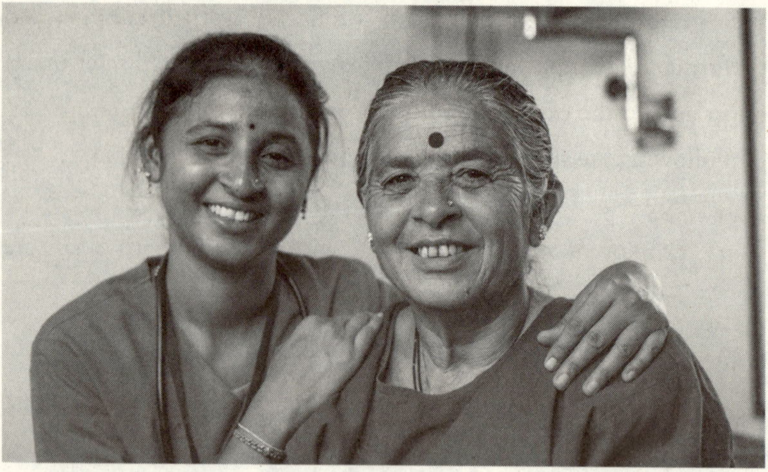

Courtsey: iStock by Getty Images

Happier Workplace to Improve Patient Loyalty

The habits and behaviour of engaged employees help create a better, happier and safer atmosphere at the workplace. A happier and invested healthcare worker will show genuine care towards their patients, which, in turn, can be sensed and experienced by the patients.

Overall, better team engagement results in:

- Better quality of care
- Improved patient loyalty
- Enhanced patient satisfaction
- Safer environment for healthcare consumers

Improving Team Engagement

Most healthcare organizations understand the positive impact that better team engagement has on patient care. Despite this, they struggle to implement the strategies on the ground.

Organizations can focus on the following key areas to improve their staff engagement.

Figure 2. Staff Engagement

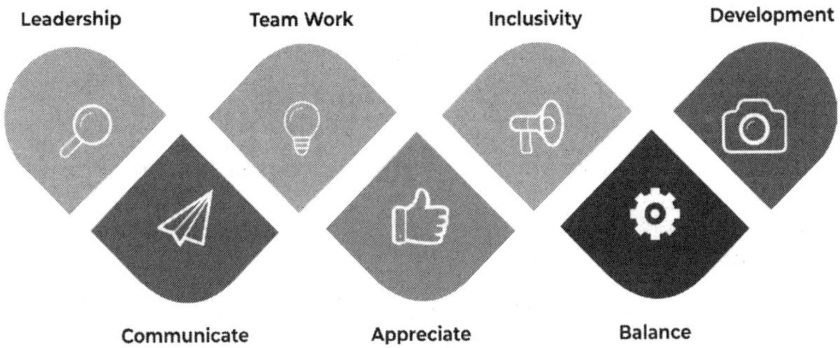

Leadership

Great leaders serve as inspirations to others. They can be role models and encourage, mentor, advise and motivate their team members. When the leadership of an organization becomes out of reach for its employees—most often due to poor people management skills—a negative or toxic culture is fostered at the workplace cascading down from the top. If this critical aspect of leadership is overlooked, most of the other efforts to boost morale and engagement will be wasted.

Communication

Measurable goals with clarity help employees understand how performance can drive an organization's success. Proactive and lucid internal communication of these goals ensures that the employees understand what they need to do to succeed. Internal communications are very critical in terms of giving instructions, sharing updates and important information, and aligning the employees with the organization's goals and telling them they can contribute to achieving them. Without this clarity in communication, the employees will effectively be working blindly in a directionless manner, without proper productivity or motivation.

Appreciation

If the focus is on improving employee morale in a healthcare setup, then one cannot miss the importance of rewards and recognition. Appreciation in the form of recognition, rewards or even simple feedback can make employees feel valued, while also successfully conveying the message that their contributions to the organization matter. Acknowledging the achievements of the team publicly not only shows the employees that they are being appreciated, but also showcases the organization's values to the other staff members. Celebrating successful performances with employees drives team building as well as team engagement.

Teamwork

Providing opportunities to the employees to come together and work as a team automatically enhances team engagement, eventually leading to a better workplace atmosphere, staff morale and brand loyalty. There are various ways to bring people across the organization together, helping them develop strong bonds among themselves. In addition to the formal approaches, such as corporate offsite events, this can also be achieved through casual or fun social events. Cooperative and cohesive teams work towards organizational goals in a focused way, since the team members know and understand each other well. This positively impacts the entire workplace.

Inclusivity

An inclusive and diverse work environment means that the employees feel more empowered that they are being taken care of and develop a sense of belonging. This also directly impacts patient care and satisfaction, since a diverse care-providing team would be more receptive to different cultural needs.

Development

Opportunities for continuous learning and development helps employees reach their full potential. Better career growth also translates into better loyalty towards the organization. Employees value the opportunities to gain new skills and succeed in their careers. Besides the obvious relationship between engagement levels and morale, the organization also benefits from having employees with up-to-date skills, which is a very worthwhile investment.

Balance

A positive work–life balance helps the employees be more engaged at work. When the organization strives to make this a priority in the form of trainings, communications and appropriate scheduling, the employees, too, take it in the right stride. This has become increasingly important with more millennials joining the workforce, who value a balance between their careers and personal lives.

Employee Engagement in Healthcare: The ROI

Hospitals and healthcare organizations most often run on tight budgets with slim margins. Thus, investing in employee engagement, while understandably important, is often moved down the organization's list of priorities. This is where many organizations get it wrong.

As evident from the discussion above—and backed up by numerous studies—there is a positive correlation between employee engagement and patient experiences. This, in turn, leads to various tangible and intangible financial benefits for the organization, making it necessary for the organizations to prioritize their employee engagement. According to a research conducted by Harvard Business Review, hospitals with higher levels of employee engagement are likely to have at least 5 per cent higher financial margins than those that don't.

There are numerous benefits of fostering greater employee engagement, both tangible and intangible. These include:

- Reduced hospital-acquired conditions and readmissions
- Lesser likelihood of negligence
- Preventable deaths decreased by as much as 50 per cent
- Lesser instances of defending lawsuits
- Reduced employee compensation claims
- Reduced absenteeism
- Decreased recruitment costs due to lower levels of staff turnover
- Positive experience and safety for both the staff and the patients
- Better patient outcomes (both clinical and non-clinical)
- Enhanced staff productivity with improved performance and effectiveness
- Better internal communication
- More cost-effective services for the community

- Improvement in the hospital's public perception and confidence

Ultimately, the knowledge that it is the right thing to do is simply PRICELESS.

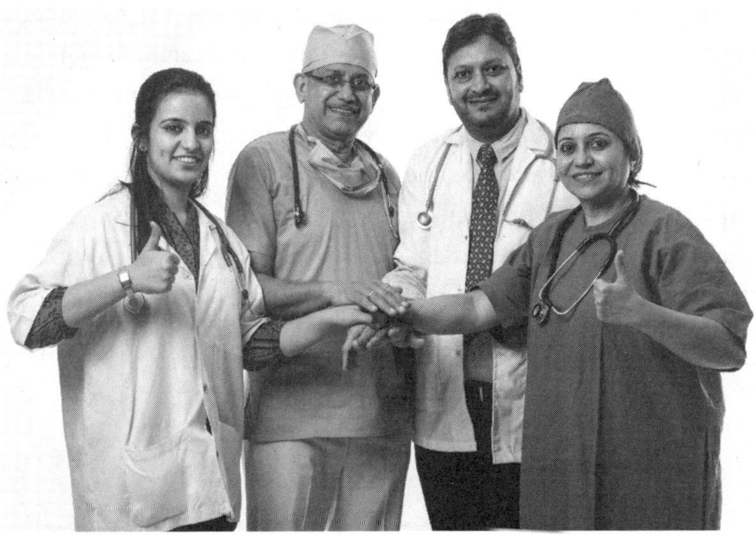

Courtsey: iStock by Getty Images

Team engagement is impactful

Building team engagement is not a seasonal or a one-time activity, but rather an effortful and time-consuming process. We cannot expect this change to happen overnight. Organizations need to make sustained efforts, keeping in mind that the ultimate goal is improved healthcare quality. Team engagement is more impactful as a slow and steady process. When the team is engaged, they like the work they do and feel connected. These emotions also result in better patient care. What needs to be ensured is proper investment of time, effort and resources to facilitate the changes, which will improve the organization's bottom-line by creating a happier workforce.

Improving team engagement also results in another important benefit. Many healthcare organizations struggle to find and retain people with critical skills, especially in clinical areas. Creating engagement among employees lowers the churn rate and helps retain skilled and exceptional practitioners.

While keeping up with the advancements in technology, developing partnerships within the care continuum, and building high-reliability organizations towards the transformation of service delivery, administrators should always keep in mind that, ultimately, patient care is delivered by their employees. Thus, engaging these employees around the behaviours and skills that drive clinical excellence and a positive patient experience will be a key determinant of whether a hospital thrives or not.

References:

1. G. Janes, T. Mills, L. Budworth, J. Johnson, R. Lawton. 'The Association Between Health Care Staff Engagement and Patient Safety Outcomes: A Systematic Review and Meta-Analysis', Journal of Patient Safety, vol. 17, no. 3, pp.207–216. DOI: 10.1097/PTS.0000000000000807. PMID: 33427792; PMCID: PMC7984750
2. Tammy Jones, 'Employee Engagement Reduces Mortality Rates Significantly, Especially in Nursing.', CA Short, 23 June 2017, https://www.cashort.com/blog/employee-engagement-reduces-mortality-rates-significantly-nursing
3. 'Study Suggests Medical Errors Now Third Leading Cause of Death in the U.S. Hopkins Medicine, 3 May 2016, https://www.hopkinsmedicine.org/news/media/releases/study_suggests_medical_errors_now_third_leading_cause_of_death_in_the_us.
4. 'State of the American Workplace', Gallup.com, https://www.gallup.com/workplace/238085/state-american-workplace-report-2017.aspx.
5. Lisa D. Ellis, 'How Increasing Employee Engagement Improves Your Environmental Health and Safety Efforts', Harvard Education, https://www.hsph.harvard.edu/ecpe/employee-engagement-improves-environmental-health-and-safety/.
6. Jim Harter, 'U.S. Employee Engagement Data Hold Steady in First Half of 2021', Gallup.com, https://www.gallup.com/workplace/352949/employee-engagement-holds-steady-first-half-2021.aspx.
7. Caroline Duncan, 'Best Employee Engagement Activities in Healthcare', Alert-software.com, 30 September 2021, https://www.alert-software.com/blog/employee-engagement-in-healthcare.

8. R. Sherwood, 'Employee Engagement Drives Health Care Quality and Financial Returns', Harvard Business Review, 30 October 2013, https://hbr.org/2013/10/employee-engagement-drives-health-care-quality-and-financial-returns.
9. Sarah Handzel, B.S.N., R.N, 'Correlations between staff, provider engagement, and culture of safety', Wolters Kluwer Health, 2 September 2020, https://www.wolterskluwer.com/en/expert-insights/correlations-between-staff-provider-engagement-culture-of-safety
10. 'Understanding Staff Engagement in Healthcare.' HSE.ie, https://www.hse.ie/eng/about/who/qid/staff-engagement/understanding-staff-engagement-in-healthcare.html.
11. J.L. Stone, 'The Importance of Employee Engagement in Healthcare', Blog.medicalgps.com, https://blog.medicalgps.com/the-importance-of-employee-engagement-in-healthcare/.
12. 'What's the Relationship Between Employee Engagement and Healthcare Quality?', Compass One Healthcare, https://www.compassonehealthcare.com/blog/whats-relationship-between-employee-engagement-and-healthcare-quality/.

6

Risk Management

Across healthcare organizations, risk and uncertainties cannot be avoided. Considering human nature, complicated processes and systems and the provision of intricate and multifaceted care lead to adverse circumstances. However, leveraging risk management tools mitigates these occurrences.

The risk management is becoming an integral component of hospital management that safeguards the healthcare organizations from numerous threats.

'Risk management is a more realistic term than safety. It implies that hazards are ever-present, that they must be identified, analyzed, evaluated and controlled or rationally accepted.'

—Jerome F. Lederer

Introduction

DESPITE DIFFERENT TYPES and sizes, all organizations face internal and external factors influencing their actions to achieve business objectives. The effect this uncertainty may have on an organization's objectives is called 'risk'. In recent times, all sectors of the economy have shifted their focus to the management of risk as the key to making an organization successful in delivering their objectives, while protecting the interests of their stakeholders.

What Is Risk?

Risk may be defined as an event or condition whose occurrence can negatively impact the organizational results. Thus, the exposure to the consequences of uncertainty constitutes a risk. There can be *good risks*, which are *value creating*, e.g., new products, new pricing models, or new markets, and *bad risks*, which are *value depleting*, e.g., penalties and fines, fraud, or disasters. The key is to manage the uncertainty to increase the probability of success and reduce the probability of failure. As the saying goes, 'Every dark cloud has a silver lining.'

Risk is inherent to any activity and has the potential to affect your success in both, a negative and positive way. Though traditionally seen in a negative light, risk also leads to opportunities for growth and development. Risk can be shaped but not entirely eliminated.

Across healthcare organizations, risk and uncertainties cannot be avoided. Considering human nature, complicated processes and systems and the provision of intricate and multifaceted care lead to adverse circumstances.

However, leveraging risk management tools mitigates these occurrences. Post the publication of Medicine (IOM) in 1999 highlighting that around 44,000–98,000 individuals were dying every year due to medical error, it became imperative to take every precautionary measure to save lives. In the US, accidental deaths due to medical errors account for 1,20,000 deaths, as compared to 43,649 motor vehicle deaths, 14,986 deaths from falls, 3,959 drowning deaths and 329 commercial aviation deaths (figures from the Philadelphia Inquirer). Even today, healthcare is categorized as more dangerous compared to airlines, chemical manufacturing, railroads and nuclear thermal power plants.

There is no denying that the healthcare industry is highly complex due to regular dealings with life and death situations, diseases, hope, and new learnings every day. Among all these, one must ensure that risk management is taken care of, since a sound risk management process will ensure better outcomes and help optimize the existing resources.

If we consider the practice of medicine in the last two decades, it was simple, comparatively ineffective but a lot safer! Remember the family physician of previous decades, who used to visit our household and distinctively remember each family member's health condition, medicine regime, allergy, etc.? But today's healthcare is an organizational system with complex embedded processes to deliver care. We call it complex because there are several people, processes, and equipment—and interdependencies between them.

For example, imagine a patient coming to the emergency department with severe chest pain. He will be attended by emergency doctors/nurses; referred to a cardiologist; assessed by a cardiology resident; directed with a plan of care to a senior cardiologist for further investigations; asked to wait for the lab results; shifted to Cath Lab for STEMI case for a Primary PTCA, where Cath lab technicians and nurses are available; shifted to HDU; then to ward; with a total ALOS of three days, which involves multiple caregivers round the clock. So, you have a scenario where one patient case is handled by approximately fifty different categories of caregivers. This is a very complex healthcare delivery model, which has made today's hospitals a risky environment.

The Joint Commission defines risk management in healthcare as 'clinical and administrative activities undertaken to identify, evaluate and reduce the risk of injury to patients, staff and visitors and the risk to the organization itself'. Risk management risk is a proactive function as it involves taking immediate actions to diminish the frequency and severity of unexpected incidents and impact of legal claims, and promotes reliable performance system design.

As we understand now, there is a possibility of things going wrong in every aspect of life and working. That is, *risk exists.* Take, for example, wrong patient identification, wrong site, wrong patient surgery, wrong medication indent or drug administration, etc. These are all incidents that do happen in a healthcare delivery system.

According to the Swiss Cheese model, at every step of a process, there are barriers to accidents at each level, such as leadership, SOP/Policies/Procedures, Resources, Communication, Training, etc. However, within each level of barrier, there are possibilities of failures in the system as well, which can cause latent errors during the process. These are nothing but potential risks to the process, which can cause harm to the patients, organization or other stakeholders.

In a recent development, all accreditation or certification standards focus on Pro-Active Risk Management, and subsequently, this has been included in all standards. The standards are now promoting the newer concept of Risk-Based Thinking, propagating that across the entire quality management system, risk is inherent. Arguable risks exist across all systems, processes and functions and risk-based thinking helps to identify and efficiently control the design and use of quality management systems. Leveraging risk-based thinking makes the consideration of risk an integral part. By early identification and action, it becomes proactive rather than reactive in preventing unwanted effects. Preventive action is built-in when a management system is risk-based.

Risk Management

It becomes essential for a hospital to focus on the identification and prevention of risk exposures within the organization that could:

- Cause injury to patients, visitors and employees
- Jeopardize the safety and security of the environment
- Result in claims with subsequent financial loss to the organization

The process of risk management must be defined clearly for better and sustainable results.

The hospital shall use the appropriate tools to mitigate the risks, and based on analysis, shall redesign or redeploy processes to reduce further risks to patients, family, staff and organization.

Investigation of adverse events shall be done through the following processes:

- Risk assessment
- Involvement of departments and analysing processes
- Identification of root causes
- Suggested action and education

Methodology for Risk Mitigation

Consistency: Same results on repeating the same tests/drills

Comparability: Different locations but same results with same methodology/controls

Validity: Real/acceptable results

Risk Assessment

Risk Identification

Risks cannot be managed unless they are first identified. Based on the context, the entire process/function needs to be screened, to identify as many risks as possible, through the use of data, institutional and industry knowledge, and by engaging everyone—patients, employees, administrators and payers. Risks can be identified in several ways:

- structured workshops;
- brainstorming sessions;
- incident reported including near miss event; and
- internal and external audits

It is also important that a specific process owner be identified as the 'Risk Owner', who will be tasked with periodically reviewing the risks within his/her department/process. All identified risks should be updated in a risk register, which should be regularly reviewed to ensure the pertinence of the risks listed.

The identification of the risks is done at the levels of different departments. These include:

- Discussion with different levels of staffs and brainstorming
- Accreditation and legal bodies survey reports
- Facility management and safety inspection reports
- Organization incident reporting system and sentinel events
- Infection control inspection, monitoring, compliance report and risk assessments
- Report on various safety committees such as hospital safety, radiation safety, laboratory safety, drug and therapeutic committee, etc.
- Reports of multidisciplinary clinical rounds and risk assessment
- Patient complaints and voice of customer survey reports
- International patient safety goals
- Various inspection, monitoring reports and quality indicator

Risk Analysis

Risk analysis is done by developing an understanding of the identified risks. In subjecting a risk to analysis, existing control measures must be considered for eliminating or reducing the risk. Existing control shall include:

- Plans, policies, standard operating procedures (SOPs), protocols, work instructions, guidelines
- Alarms and beeps
- Engineering controls
- Monitoring parameters, quality indicators, various test reports
- Various approaches to trainings
- Emergency response plans or contingency measures
- Preventative maintenance and schedule inspections

Adequacy, way of implementation, and effectiveness level of current control measures must be considered during their examination to reduce the risk to the lowest reasonably realistic level. During the risk identification step, the organization may have identified many risks, and it is often not possible to address all those identified. The risk analysis step will assist in determining which risks have a greater consequence or impact than others.

The analysis of risk involves:

- The risk drivers that would lead to the occurrence of the risks
- The positive and negative consequences of the risk, and the likelihood of the occurrence of the consequence
- The business, property and personnel impact or the severity

The main purpose of risk analysis is to identify the Key Risk Indicators (KRIs). KRIs are factors/drivers that could lead, directly or indirectly, to the occurrence of the risks. An event can have multiple consequences and can affect multiple objectives. Existing controls and their effectiveness and efficiency should also be taken into account.

Risk Prioritization

We can use various methods for risk prioritization.

- Hazard vulnerability analysis
- Hazard risk identification analysis and healthcare failure mode effects analysis tools
- Risk assessment matrix

Risk Reporting

The reporting of risks and incidents shall be done through the Incident Reporting System. All incident reports shall be submitted to the Quality Department for analysis. The incidents shall be analysed, and findings shall be shared with the department and staff to prevent recurrences.

Calculation of Risk Score

The risk score shall be calculated by multiplying the probability score with the severity of impact score as below:

Risk score (R) = Probability (P) × Severity of impact (S)

Table 1.

Probability Categories	Definitions	
	Frequency	**Probability**
Rare/Remote (1)	May occur every 5 - 10 years	More than 1%
Unlikely (2)	Occurs at some time in every 2-5 years	10%
Possible (3)	May happen every 1 or 2 years	50%
Likely (4)	Occurs bi-monthly or several times in years	75%
Frequent (5)	Occurs at least most weeks or monthly	99%

Table 2.

Score	Consequence / Impact
5	Catastrophe / Extreme
4	Major
3	Moderate
2	Minor
1	Negligible

**Source: HSE Integrated Risk Management Policy 2017*

Table 3. Consequence / Impact Table (Tool Kit)

IMPACT	Negligible (1)	Minor (2)	Moderate (3)	Major (4)	Catastrophic/ Extreme (5)
Injury/Harm to a Person	Adverse event that can lead to minor injury and doesn't need first aid.	Minor injury or illness, first aid treatment required <3 days absence. <3 days extended hospital stay	Significant injury requiring medical treatment, e.g. fracture and/or counselling. >3 days absence, 3-8 days extended hospital stay	Major injuries, long-term incapacity or disability (loss of limb) requiring medical treatment and/ or counselling	Incident leading to death or major permanent loss of function. Event that impacts a large number of patients.
Service User Experience	Diminished service quality experienced by user is directly connected to insufficient provision of information.	Unsatisfactory service user experience related to less-than-optimal treatment and/or inadequate information.	Unsatisfactory service user experience related to less than optimal treatment resulting in short-term effects (<1 week)	Unsatisfactory service user experience related to poor treatment resulting in long-term effects	Totally unsatisfactory service user outcome resulting in long term effects, or extremely poor experience of care provision.

IMPACT	Negligible (1)	Minor (2)	Moderate (3)	Major (4)	Catastrophic/ Extreme (5)
Compliance with Standards (Statutory, Clinical, Professional and Management)	Minor non-compliance with internal standards. A small number of minor issues requiring improvement.	Single failure to meet internal standards or follow protocol.	Repeated failure to meet internal standards or follow protocols.	Repeated failure to meet external standards. Failure to meet national norms and standards/ regulations.	Gross failure to meet external standards. Repeated failure to meet national norms and standards/ regulations.
Objectives/ Projects	Barely noticeable reduction in scope, quality or schedule.	Minor reduction in scope, quality or schedule.	Reduction in scope or quality of project; project objectives or schedule.	Significant project over–run.	Inability to meet project objectives. Reputation of the organization seriously damaged.

IMPACT	Negligible (1)	Minor (2)	Moderate (3)	Major (4)	Catastrophic/ Extreme (5)
Business Continuity	Interruption in a service that does not impact the delivery of service user care or the ability to continue to provide service.	Short-term disruption to service with minor impact on service user care.	Some disruption in service with unacceptable impact on service user care. Temporary loss of ability to provide service.	Sustained loss of service, which has a serious impact on delivery of service user care or service resulting in major contingency plans being involved.	Permanent loss of core service or facility. Disruption to facility leading to significant 'knock on' effect.

IMPACT	Negligible (1)	Minor (2)	Moderate (3)	Major (4)	Catastrophic/ Extreme (5)
Adverse Publicity/ Reputation	Rumours, no media coverage. No public concerns voiced. Little effect on staff morale. No review/ investigation is necessary.	Local media coverage, short-term. Some public concern. Minor effect on staff morale/public attitudes. Internal review is necessary.	Local media—adverse publicity. Significant effect on staff morale and public perception of the organization. Public calls (at local level) for specific remedial actions. Comprehensive review/ investigation necessary.	National media/adverse publicity, less than 3 days. News stories and features in national papers. Local media—long term adverse publicity. Public confidence in the organization was undermined.	National/ international media/adverse publicity, > 3 days. Editorial follows days of news stories and features in national papers Public confidence in the organization was undermined.

IMPACT	Negligible (1)	Minor (2)	Moderate (3)	Major (4)	Catastrophic/ Extreme (5)
Financial Loss (per Local Contact)	Rs 1,000	Rs 1,001–100,00	Rs 10,001–100,000	Rs 100,001–1,000,000	> Rs 1,000,000
Environment	Nuisance Release.	On site release contained by organization.	On site release contained by organization.	Release affecting minimal off-site area requiring external assistance (fire brigade, radiation, etc.)	Toxic release affecting off-site with detrimental effect requiring outside assistance.

Table 4.

Risk Category	Descriptor
Injury/Harm to a Person	Physical or psychological injury associated with a person, i.e., service user, staff member or member of the public.
Service User Experience	Negative service user experience that may have a negative impact on outcome, limit their engagement with a service or lead to a complaint.
Compliance with Standards (Statutory, Clinical, Professional and Management)	Failure to comply with standards, codes of practice or conduct set by professional regulators, relevant legislation, e.g., safety, health and welfare at work act, financial regulations, etc.
Objectives/Projects	Project slippage and failure to meet objectives of projects.
Business Continuity	Issues that would affect an organization's ability to provide service, e.g., deregistration, fire, flood, electric outage.
Adverse Publicity/ Reputation	Adverse publicity in the media, loss of public confidence in a service or the organization, e.g., poor service performance.
Financial Loss (per Local Contact)	Fraud, claims, budgetary overruns.
Environment	Release of substances that would have a detrimental environmental impact, e.g., chemical spills, poor waste management practices, radiological leaks.

Risk Score

Having established the probability and impact scores, the scores shall be plotted on the Risk Matrix to determine the score of the risk being assessed in terms of a colour and a numerical score for the risk.

- The high risks are scored between 15 and 25 and are coloured Red.
- Medium risks are scored between 6 and 14 and are coloured Amber.
- Low risks are scored between 1 and 5 and are coloured Green.

Table 5.

Risk Matrix	Negligible (1)	Minor (2)	Moderate (3)	Major (4)	Extreme (5)
Almost Certain (5)	**5**	**10**	**15**	**20**	**25**
Likely (4)	**4**	**8**	**12**	**16**	**20**
Possible (3)	**3**	**6**	**9**	**12**	**15**
Unlikely (2)	**2**	**4**	**6**	**8**	**10**
Rare/Remote (1)	**1**	**2**	**3**	**4**	**5**

Risk Assessment Worksheet

A sample worksheet is mentioned below, which helps to identify the risks associated with a particular area.

Table 6. Risk Register

Risk ID No.	Risk Category	Risk Statement	Risk Mitigation Strategies/ Existing Control	Probability Score (P)	Severity Score (S)	Total Score = (PXS)	Risk Owner

This exercise helps the team to define a Risk Matrix, also known as Hazard Identification and Risk Assessment (HIRA). Moreover, mitigation strategy is also designed based on the HIRA. Add solutions wherever you score more than 15 to minimize the risk.

Risk Evaluation

Quantify and Prioritize Risk

- Post identification, prioritizing risks based on their likelihood and impact of occurrence is imperative. Post this process, divide resources and allot tasks based on these parameters. Furthermore, risk matrices and heat maps can be deployed to accomplish this and they will also support to visualize risks and promote communication and collaborative decision-making. Risk evaluation involves the comparison of the level of risk identified during the analysis process with previously established risk criteria and deciding whether these risks require treatment.
- The result of risk evaluation is a prioritized list of risks that require further action.
- This step is about deciding whether risks are acceptable or need treatment.

The risks will be evaluated or assessed on qualitative twofold criteria. The two components of risk assessment are:

- The likelihood of occurrence of the risk events
- The magnitude of impact if the risk event occurs

In order to provide the inherent risk level, it is requisite to combine the likelihood of occurrence and the magnitude of impact. The magnitude of impact of an event, should it occur, and the likelihood of the event and its associated consequences, are assessed in the context of the existing controls. Impact and likelihood may be determined using statistical analysis and calculations. Alternatively, where no past data is available, subjective estimates may be made, which reflect an employer's or group's confidence relating to an event.

Impact and likelihood are combined to produce a level of risk. The risk should be classified into three zones based on the impact and likelihood score:

- Risk that scores within the red zone are considered 'Critical' or 'High' and require immediate action plans to close a significant control gap. (Average score of 12 or more, or where impact is very high
- Risks that score within the Yellow zone are considered "Cautionary" or "Moderate" where action steps to develop or enhance existing controls are also needed. (Average score in the range of 8 to 12, except where impact is very high)
- Risks that score within the green zone are considered "Acceptable" or "Low" in control. (Average score less than 8, except where the impact is very high)

The output of a risk evaluation is the prioritized list of risks for further action.

The objective of risk assessment and risk evaluation is to assist the organization in prioritizing risk to ensure that appropriate attention is given to risks based on their criticality, and that the hospital's resources are effectively utilized in managing these risks.

Risk Tolerance

This highlights the maximum quantum of risk that an organization is willing to accept.

Risk Treatment

1. **Avoiding the risk,** for example, means stopping the activity associated with the risk. This is not often an option for healthcare services. It is a proactive measure to ensure that the occurrence of the risky event/process is prevented.
2. **Mitigating the risk** means to reduce the severity of the loss or prevent such events from happening. Acknowledging the type of risk as positive or negative, and optimizing risks is necessary. It means looking for balance between negative risk and achievements from the operation or activity; and between mitigating risk and applying efforts.
3. **Transferring the risk,** for instance, involves outsourcing the activity to another agency, which will be responsible for the activity and attending to the risks.
4. **Retention** (accept and budget) involves acknowledging losses, and pros of achievements, from risk factors. Risk retention is an effective strategy for risks as insuring price against the risk would be more than the losses sustained. All risks that are avoided or transferred are retained by default.

If practicable, eliminate the risks altogether, or combat the risks at the source (for instance, use a secure substance rather than a dangerous one). If removing the risk is not possible, then try to minimize the risk at source. It can be done by substituting the material or process with the less hazardous, or try using additional equipment.

Finally, reduce the risk via administrative controls, strong protocols and safe systems of work. For instance, policies, procedures and guidelines for the safe use of sharp instruments and needles must be put in place to avoid any risk of injury.

Residual Risk

Residual risk is the level of risk leftover after we have implemented the action plan/additional controls or other risk treatment options. At this stage in the assessment and before we implement the actions, we have re-rated the risk using the same process.

Residual rating takes into account the effect of the totality of all controls that are in place and provides an indicator of the likely outcomes of the actions implemented.

Monitor and Review

Monitoring and reviewing are an essential and integral step in the risk management process. Process owners must monitor risks and review the effectiveness of the treatment plan, strategies and management system that have been set up to effectively manage risk. Risks and the effectiveness of control measured must be frequently analysed and ensure that evolving circumstances do not alter risk priorities. Few risks remain static. An ongoing review is essential to ensure that the management plans remain relevant. Factors that may affect the likelihood and impact of an outcome may change, as may the factors that affect the suitability or cost of the various treatment options.

- A risk review involves re-examination of all risks recorded in the Risk Profile and Risk Register, to ensure that the current assessments remain valid. Review also aims at assessing the progress of the risk treatment action plans. Risk reviews should form part of the agenda for every RMC meeting. The risk register should be reviewed, assessed and updated on a periodic basis.
- The Risk Coordinator is responsible for ensuring that the risk profile and risk register are reviewed and updated on a quarterly basis.

Sign Off

The risk profiles and risk register review report should be signed off by the respective risk owners.

Responsibility and Monitoring Procedures, including Additional Controls

The list of monitoring procedures that are in place to manage and monitor the risk have been documented, including any additional controls that:

a. Have a deliverable attached to it

b. Can be assigned to a named person

c. Can be assigned a due date

Risk assessments are reviewed if there is a change in the service and/or on an annual basis mandatorily.

Table 7. Risk Review Table

Risk ID No.: **Risk Category:** **Risk Statement:** **Risk Owner:** **Risk Review Team:**	**Document Reference No.:** **Review Date:**
Risk Mitigation Strategies /Action Taken	**Review Status**
Monitoring Data:	
Review Team	
Name	**Signature**

Conclusion

Risk management is a vital process and healthcare organizations must focus on it. It is inevitable to have risks in day-to-day activities of a healthcare organization, and hence, it should have better strategies to handle these risks. For an organization to survive in the long-term, the ability to manage these risks via an effective risk mitigation strategy is crucial.

References:

1. *Joint Commission International Accreditation Standards for Hospitals*, Joint Commission International, 7th Edition, https://store.jointcommissioninternational.org/assets/1/7/JCIH20_sample_pages_3_6_20.pdf
2. HSE Integrated Risk Management Policy, https://www.hse.ie/eng/about/who/riskmanagement/risk-management-documentation/hse-integrated-risk-management-policy-part-2-risk-assessment-and-treatment.pdf
3. 'Patient safety', World Health Organization, 9 March 2019, https://www.who.int/news-room/facts-in-pictures/detail/patient-safety
4. 'National Healthcare Quality & Disparities Reports', AHRQ, https://www.ahrq.gov/research/findings/nhqrdr/index.html
5. 'Patient Safety', IHI, http://www.ihi.org/PatientSafety
6. 'Risk Assessment Tool and Guidance - Health Service Executive', HSE, https://www.hse.ie/eng/about/who/riskmanagement/risk-assessment-tool-and-guidance-incl-application.pdf
7. 'ISO 31000 — Risk management', ISO, https://www.iso.org/iso-31000-risk-management.html
8. 'What Is Risk Management in Healthcare?', NEJM Catalyst, 25 April 2018, https://catalyst.nejm.org/doi/full/10.1056/CAT.18.0197
9. R. Carroll and S. Brown, *Risk Management Handbook for Health Care Organizations* (American Society for Healthcare Risk Management, 2009).

7

Importance of Surveys and How to Conduct Them

It is pivotal to ensure that workflows are simple and streamlined to help staff provide effective patient care. Hence, many healthcare organizations are using employee surveys to gather information on staff engagement and satisfaction. These surveys allow employees to be heard.

Surveys are an integral part of organizations, as they help improve processes and outcomes. Such surveys or audits must be done periodically, at regular intervals. The results can be used as a strategic improvement tool, to help the organizations improve their processes as well as management systems.

An internal surveyor team should be created within the organization according to the size of the hospital. They must be trained on assessment skills, possess an eye for detail, and be able to objectively assess the on-ground implementation of policies and procedures.

'Surveys are critical to know where we stand. Are we walking the talk?'

Introduction

HEALTHCARE IS COMPLEX, and every second matters in a hospital setting. Necessary processes need to be put in place to ensure that patients receive the best possible care, round the clock and in a safe environment. Healthcare process improvement also plays a major role in improving the quality of care while lowering costs. These processes include emergency care, admission, billing, transfer and patient flow within the hospital and outside the hospital to a different facility, medication, surgery, discharge—to name a few. All these processes impact daily operations and patient experience across the organization.

While every hospital has its own policies and processes in place, each hospital functions differently depending on specialties, patient population and regional challenges. Moreover, within a single hospital, not every part and/or process will be up to the expected standards. The hospital might be great in terms of the doctors' expectation, but not necessarily upto patients' experience, expectation and safety.

Ineffective processes and procedures interfere in daily hospital operations and incur cost. Doctors, nurses and other healthcare staff is involved in direct patient care. It is important to ensure that their workflows are simple and streamlined, to help them provide effective patient care. These days, many healthcare organizations—no matter how small or big—are using employee surveys to gather information on staff engagement and satisfaction. These surveys allow employees to be heard. It is on-ground staff who best understand which processes are working and which ones needs improvement. Therefore, the ideal starting point is asking employees to share their suggestions.

On the other hand, if there are gaps in hospital processes and functions, or if some needs are not being tended to, patients and their attendants would know the best. While not everyone may be ready to go the extra mile for material things, when it comes to their or their loved one's health, almost everyone will make the effort to go somewhere they can get the best of care. A hospital survey helps in identifying how your hospital is performing compared to other hospitals in terms of services, outcomes, processes and patient experience as well as satisfaction.

Surveys are an integral part of organizations, as they help improve processes and outcomes. Such surveys or audits must be done periodically, at regular intervals. The results can be used as a strategic improvement tool, to help the organizations improve their processes as well as management systems. There are various hospital standards—Joint Commission International (JCI), National Accreditation Board for Hospitals (NABH), International Organization for Standardization (ISO), etc.—and hospitals may need to ensure compliance with all of them.

To assess a hospital's performance, two types of audits are conducted: internal survey and external.

Internal Survey

This is a scheduled and impartial assessment of the organization's policies, procedures and processes conducted by selected members within the organization. The purpose is to identify inaccuracies, eccentricities or any performance issues in the processes and procedures, and suggest necessary action points to resolve the gaps.

An internal surveyor team should be created within the organization according to the size of the hospital. They must be trained on assessment skills, possess an eye for detail, and be able to objectively assess the on-ground implementation of policies and procedures.

Internal audits are conducted at regular intervals, for example, monthly, quarterly and biannually, or as predefined by the organization. Some, however, can also be conducted as 'surprise audits', to encourage healthcare organizations to ensure that they provide safe, high quality of care at all times and not just in the lead up to a scheduled survey.

The internal audit team develops a checklist to be referred to during these audits. A scoring methodology should also be included in the checklist to check for compliance and non-compliance.

Table 1. Internal Audit Checklist [Sample]

	INTERNAL AUDIT CHECKLIST (Radiology and PET CT)				
	Name of the Unit:	**Date Audited:**			
	Name of the Department:				
Topic	**Policies & Protocols**	**Com**	**NC**	**NA**	**Remarks**
General Concerns	Staff are wearing ID cards and proper uniform				
	Staff effectively communicate with patients, attendants and walk-ins				
	Patients and attendants are being taken care of properly in case of delays/waiting				
	Phone calls are attended on time and appropriate guidance and responses are given				
	Patients' queries are addressed immediately or escalated to seniors				
	Patients' queries are given proper responses				
	Security is available 24*7				

	INTERNAL AUDIT CHECKLIST (Radiology and PET CT)				
	Name of the Unit:	Date Audited:			
	Name of the Department:				
Topic	Policies & Protocols	Com	NC	NA	Remarks
General Concerns	Proper network is available for billing and other investigations reporting				
	Backup documents are maintained for dashboard entries				
	Refrigerator temperature monitoring is done every day and recorded				
	Glucometer records are maintained and updated				
	Crash carts are sealed & checked				
	Imprest stocks are checked daily				
	LASA stored separately				
	Contrast marked & labelled				
	Lead aprons are marked/numbered and PM updated				

	INTERNAL AUDIT CHECKLIST (Radiology and PET CT)				
	Name of the Unit:	**Date Audited:**			
	Name of the Department:				
Topic	**Policies & Protocols**	**Com**	**NC**	**NA**	**Remarks**
General Concerns	Lead aprons are never stored in a folded manner				
	Staff and consultants wear TLD badges				
	Chemicals are labelled and stored in HAZMAT cupboard				
	Drinking water available and signages are mentioned				
	Washrooms are clean and hygienic				
	Tissue rolls and hand driers are available at every handwash sink				

	INTERNAL AUDIT CHECKLIST (Radiology and PET CT)				
	Name of the Unit:	Date Audited:			
	Name of the Department:				
Topic	Policies & Protocols	Com	NC	NA	Remarks
Infection Control	All six steps of handwashing are followed				
	Technicians are wearing gloves and masks				
	Adequate hand wash sinks, tissue rolls and hand driers are available				
	Biomedical waste management protocols are followed				
	Sharps disposed of in an approved puncture-proof container				
	All colour bins are with lids and correct bags				
	BMW Posters are available and in good condition				
	Cleaning protocols are available for all equipment				
	Disinfection of equipment is done after each procedure				

	INTERNAL AUDIT CHECKLIST (Radiology and PET CT)				
	Name of the Unit:	**Date Audited:**			
	Name of the Department:				
Topic	**Policies & Protocols**	**Com**	**NC**	**NA**	**Remarks**
Facility Safety	PM check for all equipment is done by the concerned department (biomedical, maintenance, IT) immediately after information				
	Work areas, storerooms and corridors free from clutter or obstruction				
	Adequate space and lighting to work is available				
	False ceiling is in good condition, without seepage/fungus/ broken tiles				
	Shafts and electrical panel doors are locked				
	All defective equipment are red tagged and taken out of use				
	No safety concerns				
	No broken, chipped or missing tiles				

	INTERNAL AUDIT CHECKLIST (Radiology and PET CT)				
	Name of the Unit:	**Date Audited:**			
	Name of the Department:				
Topic	**Policies & Protocols**	**Com**	**NC**	**NA**	**Remarks**
Fire Safety	Adequate fire exit signs are provided where required & are properly illuminated				
	Minimum of two fire exits are available & not blocked				
	Fire extinguishers are mounted on the hook and not obstructed				
	Suitable signage/numbering is found above the extinguishers				
	Fire sprinklers and smoke detectors available and functioning				
	MRI-compatible extinguisher is available				
	PPE are located at every strategic location				
	Staff aware of RACE and PASS (ask 2 staff)				
	Fire orders (RACE) located in all staff areas				
	Emergency fire floor plans located				

	INTERNAL AUDIT CHECKLIST (Radiology and PET CT)				
	Name of the Unit:	**Date Audited:**			
	Name of the Department:				
Topic	**Policies & Protocols**	**Com**	**NC**	**NA**	**Remarks**
Staff Awareness	Incident reporting				
	Job responsibilities				
	IPSGs				
	Critical values reported and documented				
	Radiology SOPs				
	Quality indicators				
	BLS				
	Radiation safety *(TLD Badges / Lead Aprons)*				
	HAZMAT safety / spill management				
	Unit binders and manuals, MSDS				
	Patient rights & responsibilities				
	Hospital policies				
	5S				
	Codes and drills				

	INTERNAL AUDIT CHECKLIST (Radiology and PET CT)				
	Name of the Unit:	Date Audited:			
	Name of the Department:				
Topic	Policies & Protocols	Com	NC	NA	Remarks
% Compliance	Total Observations (A)				
	Total Compliances (B)				
	Total Non-Compliances				
	Percentage Compliance (B/A)* 100				
Any Other Observations					

External Survey

This is an independent assessment of the organization's processes and procedures conducted by an appointed team from a recognized and accredited external body such as JCI or NABH. Such a survey minutely analyses the organization's processes, procedures, policies to determine their implementation on ground, and the consistency and adherence to a given standard or a measurable element.

Certificates issued after an external survey establish the fact that the organization is performing efficiently, validating that there are no risks in any areas of patient care and management processes. It provides reassurance for patients, attendants, staff and visitors that the hospital is complying with the applicable laws and regulations, and standard requirements.

One important aim of conducting an external audit is to publicly demonstrate your organization's performance or compliance record—like the 'Gold Seal' for all JCI-accredited hospitals.

An external survey audit is usually conducted when an organization is expecting a certification and/or recertification from JCI, NABH, ISO or some other accreditation standard. These surveys are carried out at regular intervals, e.g., annually or every three years.

Survey Preparation: Best Practices

1. Gap Study

Gap study should be undertaken by the hospital at the initial stage, when it decides to go for an accreditation. This assessment compares the organization's current services and processes to the accreditation standards, to identify areas of partial or no compliance.

Figure 1. Factors to deliberate prior to initiating the survey process

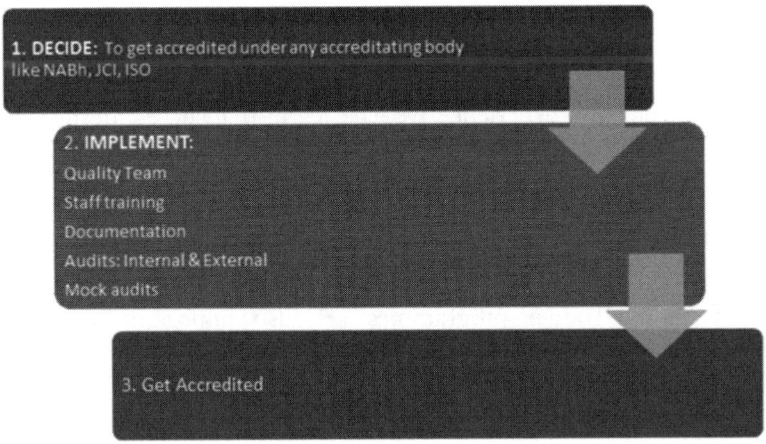

2. Leadership Involvement and Support to Staff

The leaders should support the staff and reassure them that survey preparation is a team effort, and not any individual's sole responsibility for any area of concern. Leadership, along with the Quality Department, must establish a plan with a timeline for all survey preparation activities, along with assigning responsibilities for each standard.

3. Survey Co-ordinator

Appoint one person as a survey co-ordinator, preferably the Quality Head of the organization, who will gather the team together, take the lead in discussing the standards, and guide the team for the survey.

4. Staff Training

If there is one area that has a substantial impact on accreditation and reaccreditation, it is the training of staff. Hence, while preparing for any kind of survey, staff training plays a vital role.

From our own experience, we have learnt that successful training of all the staff in any organization, specifically in healthcare, is easier said than done. There are multiple reasons, but *attrition* tops it all. To address this concern, organizations should have a training calendar. Regular training sessions for staff is important.

Train-the-Trainer programmes are also important, where a pool of trainers is created from existing team members in the organization. You can identify individuals with good knowledge on hospital policies and protocols, and who have good communication skills. These individuals can be trained as 'trainers', who will then train other staff and new recruits on the standards, policies and procedures that the hospital must meet.

Training records must be kept up to date. Pre- and post-training evaluation for all training modules is critical.

5. Focused Weekly Internal Audits

Weekly internal audits must be conducted, following patient journeys in the hospital through medical record and process compliance checks. Documentation is key. During these internal audits, medical record compliance must be checked. Everything from ceiling tiles to floor conditions must be noted and issues discussed in daily morning huddles with the relevant department heads. Close follow up may be required by the Quality Team in closing all the issues identified during tracers. Team members should be quizzed on policies and processes, and where to find them.

6. Mock Audit

A mock audit is a simulation of the final survey process, and it identifies the gaps in compliance to the standards. It is done prior to the accreditation survey and serves as a final checkpoint in survey preparation and readiness. Mock audits provide an ideal opportunity to engage senior leadership and prepare the staff for the final survey.

Conclusion

Motivational speaker Zig Ziglar once said, '*Success occurs when opportunity meets preparation.*' The opportunity to achieve accreditation or reaccreditation can be seized with adequate groundwork and preparation at all levels.

Periodic surveys help gauge the effectiveness of the organization's improvement initiatives. Over time, hospital leadership has realized the role of surveys and how to use survey data to better engage doctors, staff and patients.

References:

1. 'The Power of Hospital Surveys', National Business Research Institute, https://www.nbrii.com/blog/the-power-of-hospital-surveys/
2. 'What's the Difference Between an Internal Audit & External Audit', Compliance Help Consulting, LLC, https://www.quality-assurance.com/blog/learn-whats-the-difference-between-an-internal-audit-and-external-audit.html
3. Suzanne C. Watson, 'A Primer in Survey Research', Appstate Edu, *Journal of Continuing Higher Education* (Winter 1998) pp. 31–40, http://www.appstate.edu/~steelekm/classes/psy3100/Documents/PrimerOnSurveys.pdf
4. E. D. de Leeuw, 'Data Quality in Mail, Telephone and Face to Face Surveys', ERIC Document Reproduction Service No. ED 374 136, 1992.
5. P. Salant, and D.A. Dillman, *How to Conduct Your Own Survey* (New York: Wiley, 1992).
6. J.C. Sherblom, C.F. Sullivan and E.C. Sherblom, 'The What, the Whom, and the Hows of Survey Research', *Bulletin of the Association for Business Communication* vol. 56 No. 4, pp. 58–64.

8

Clinical Pathways

With a clinical pathway in place, patients of a common type are treated with a single process defined by the clinical pathway, potentially eliminating all wastages and avoiding duplication of efforts. It is applied as an active management tool that facilitates quality management and focused outcomes.

A clinical pathway is seen as one of the main tools used to manage clinical quality by standardizing the patient care processes. It is a powerful tool and concept, which provides guidelines, protocols, and widely agreed, evidence-based, patient-centred best practices applied to everyday use for individual patients.

'The true compass of how to treat a patient is to enhance clinical outcomes and improve overall clinical and safety standards.'

Introduction

TWO PATIENTS WITH similar clinical history and manifestations underwent a total knee replacement surgery with significantly different surgical outcomes. Even their length of hospital stays varied, with a difference of more than four days. The only difference in both these surgeries was a different surgeon.

Healthcare outcomes largely depend on comorbid condition of patient and other clinical factors, however the outcomes would not vary much if standardised clinical processes are followed. The course of antibiotics, education and diagnostics can be standardized to a large extent in order to prevent larger variations in clinical outcomes. The aim is to realign the focus on the patient's overall care, rather than the contribution of each specialty or caring function independently.

Let's understand this a bit more in detail.

Medical care that doctors or healthcare professionals deliver is based upon tradition, their training, and personal anecdotal experience. As a result, patients with a common condition are treated differently by different physicians resulting in differing outcomes. Variation in care often obscures the effect of a particular intervention on that care. With a clinical pathway in place, patients of a common type (e.g., total knee replacement) are treated with a single process defined by the clinical pathway, potentially eliminating all wastages and avoiding duplication of efforts.

Evidence-based healthcare practices can effectively be guided through these tools, i.e., clinical pathways—also known as care pathway, integrated care pathway, critical pathway or care map. The use and implementation of clinical pathways has been considered very old, dating back to the 1980s. A clinical pathway is considered one of the main tools used to manage clinical quality by standardizing the patient care processes. It is a powerful tool and concept, which provides guidelines, protocols, and widely agreed, evidence-based, patient-centred best practices applied to everyday use for individual patients.

The implementation of pathways reduces the variability in clinical practice to a large extent and significantly improves patient safety and clinical outcomes. They can be implemented in any area of healthcare, i.e., preventive, acute, chronic, or palliative care. Clinical pathways aim to promote organized and efficient patient care based on evidence-based practices (from the best evidence to the best practice by implementing clinical pathways). A clinical pathway improves patient care by adopting standard clinical processes. It is applied as an active management tool that facilitates quality management and focused outcomes.

Clinical pathways are not the same as guidelines. A primary difference between the two is that pathways provide definite treatment recommendations based on multiple criteria, while guidelines provide a set of rational treatment options, without specific recommendations. It should be noted that since clinical pathway recommendations are developed and tested on a specific set of a similar patient groups, they may vary based on the patients' profiles.

Figure 1. Clinical Pathway

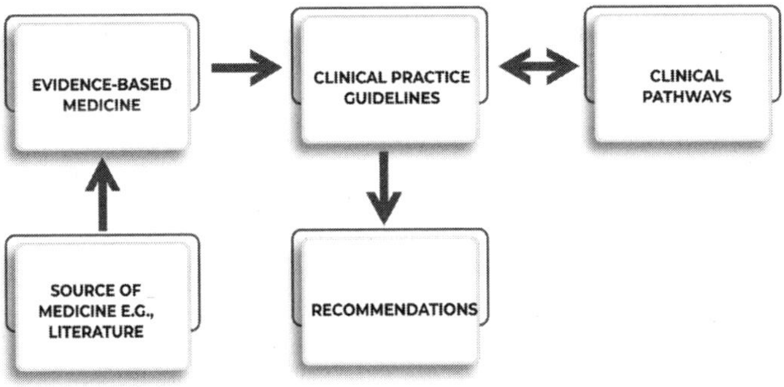
EVIDENCE-BASED MEDICINE
CLINICAL PRACTICE GUIDELINES
CLINICAL PATHWAYS
SOURCE OF MEDICINE E.G., LITERATURE
RECOMMENDATIONS

Clinical pathways are usually formulated based on the best available resources and clinical evidence, i.e., clinical practice guidelines or systematic research and reviews. Hence, with the help of clinical pathways, it is possible to restructure and standardize the clinical practices for a specific patient group, a specific diagnosis, or for a specific surgery or clinical procedure.

Figure 2. Clinical Pathway Benefits

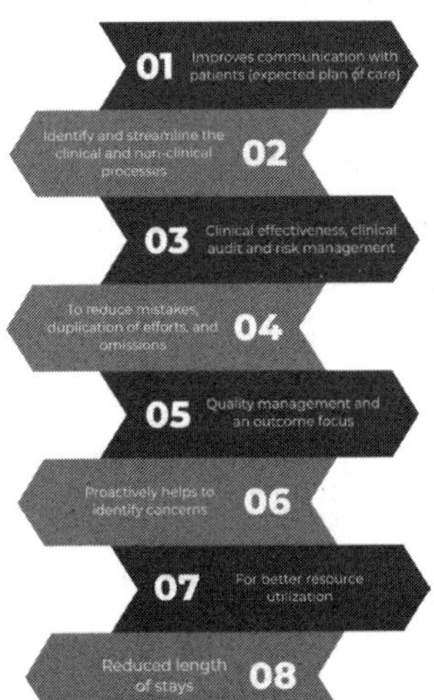
01
Improves communication with patients (expected plan of care)
Identify and streamline the clinical and non-clinical processes
02
03
Clinical effectiveness, clinical audit and risk management
To reduce mistakes, duplication of efforts, and omissions
04
05
Quality management and an outcome focus
Proactively helps to identify concerns
06
07
For better resource utilization
Reduced length of stays
08

Implementation of Clinical Pathways

Implementing a clinical pathway is one of the most challenging tasks for quality teams across the world. It is not easy, but it is also not impossible!

We should have the 'right' strategy in place and follow the 'right' methodology. The clinical pathway implementation methodology is typically divided into four phases: selection, development, implementation and evaluation.

Figure 3. Implementation Process

1
Selection
Applicability
Benefits Vs Challenges
Mandate
2
Evaluate
Context
Relevance
Adjust
3
Approval
Clinical Leadership
Clinicians
Support Systems
4
Training
Clinical staff
Support staff
5
Monitor
Consistent use
Outcomes
Effectiveness
Areas of
Improvement

These phases may further be divided as under:

1. Identifying the Topic

It is difficult to have clinical pathways for every disease or surgery. Ideally, you should focus on a topic that is likely to impact most of your patients. Evaluate your patient population, the volumes of surgeries/patients that are cared for, or the areas where concerns are noted. Ensure that it is based on a scientific criterion.

Prioritization Grid: It is important to develop your internal mechanism to prioritize the diagnosis/surgery/procedure. We developed one, and you could refer to the same in the example provided towards the end of this chapter.

2. Getting Clinicians on Board

It is always preferable to pick a pathway where a smaller number of clinicians are involved. The success of this can help more people see the benefits and adopt. Meet clinicians, share the benefits, and request their support.

3. Finalizing

The pathway should be finalized based on the inputs from clinicians, dieticians, physiotherapists and the nursing team. Evidence-based guidelines need to be considered, along with the current outcomes at the hospital. The patient populations and their course of care should also be evaluated and considered before finalizing. A 'sign-off' by multiple and relevant stakeholders is important.

4. Team Formation

A multidisciplinary team needs to be created to ensure emphasis on the implementation. It is requisite to clearly define the roles and responsibilities of each discipline and team member. It is important to stress the need for consensus meetings. A multidisciplinary team must reach agreements by performing a critical analysis of various functionalities of the care process and enhancements must be introduced.

5. Pilot Implementation

The date of pilot rollout should be announced in advance. The individuals who are expected to be a part of this pilot should be informed, trained and followed up. Close monitoring of implementation is a critical step. The observations should be noted along with identified challenges and areas for improvement.

For example, how long did the patient spend at each stage of the treatment process, and how has this changed after the beginning of the pilot project? Variance analysis can be used as a tool. How do the results deviate from the expected care path and why? Based on the analysis, we can make further improvement plans.

6. Further Implementation

The report on the pilot should be discussed with the forum/ interdisciplinary team. The final format should be designed along with the plan of implementation. All stakeholders should be informed and trained on usage. This should also clearly list the expectations of every member. The final rollout should happen on the finalized rollout date.

7. Monitoring

Implementation could only be effective if we know the status of the same. To do so, it is critical to have a set of well-articulated measures of Quality Indicators (QIs). These should have a set baseline (before the implementation of the pathway) and a target measure (an expected value that we aim to achieve). Clinicians can also help in identifying the inclusions and exclusions to the pathway. While pathways may not fit every patient, it is prudent that we monitor the variations as well. A separate process should be implemented to monitor variations and their causes. Such an analysis will help continuously modify the pathway or identify focus areas for improvement.

It is an important requisite to update the care pathway and its documents regularly, based on the publication of new scientific evidence. The updates must comprise the recent variances, with a focus on achieving its objectives. One specific feature for analysis and evaluation of the care pathway is the variance report, which provides information on the analysis of variance sheets of the clinical pathway. Variances (or deviations) may infuse actions that were undertaken but not elaborated in the care pathway. Hence, they need to be defined or included in the care pathway. Patient condition, family issues and organizational conditions may cause variations.

Another necessary document required for the evaluation of care pathways is the 'follow-up report', including the complete follow-up of the new record documentation, the variance report, and the assessment of the results via the predefined parameters (quality indicators), which are related to the agreed/defined objectives of the pathway.

8. Governance

A committee/focus group should be set up to meet at a defined interval (at least once a quarter is suggested). This group should evaluate the outcomes, review the data, and decide on the next course of action for a more powerful impact. The group should also focus on continuous sustenance practices.

Next Steps

- Establishing dates for periodic reviews (recommended every three months post-official implementation)
- Conducting a systematic and ongoing audit
- Tracking the new record documentation and its completion (It is considered important in the initial 12 months as a reminder call for all the professionals.)
- Monitoring of variances with a fixed periodicity
- Assessment and evaluation of the results from the records recorded in the care pathway documentation

- Impact analysis on the care process of the care pathway implementation
- Providing feedback to managers and staff regarding the follow up of indicators/outcomes and variances (essential to incentivize staff to continue working on care pathways)

Figure 4. Pathway development process

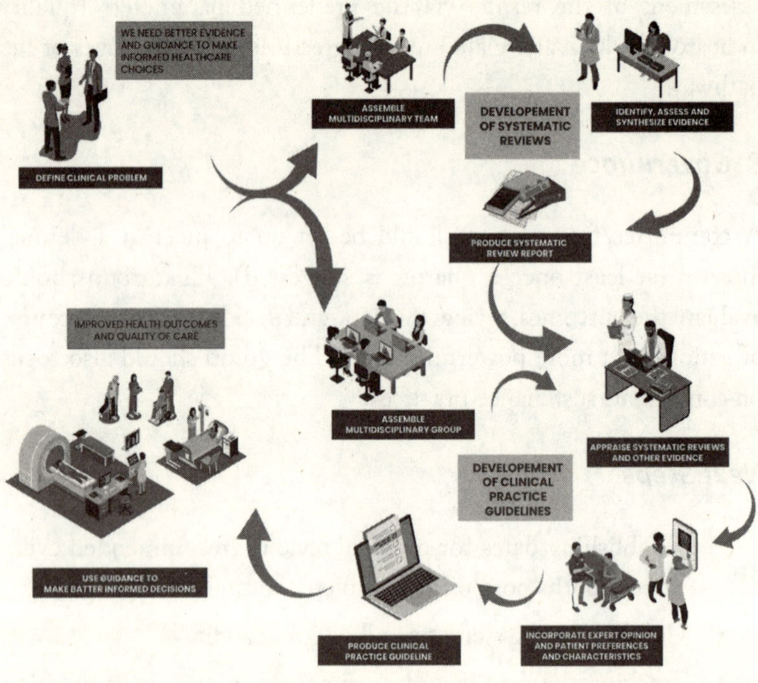

With the advancement in computers and internet technology, clinical pathways have led to advancements in dynamic knowledge-based management tools. Integrated with existing tools such as Clinical Information Systems (CIS) and Hospital Information

Systems (HIS) for activities such as diagnostic tests, medication and surgeries, the clinical pathway provides comprehensive methods of planning, delivering and monitoring different healthcare services provided to patients.

The organizational culture of quality and patient safety plays a pivotal role in the development and implementation of a clinical pathway. Invariably, there are many hurdles when such initiatives are implemented. Some of these issues include general reluctance among clinicians, a lack of consensus among the clinical team members, difficulty monitoring data/results and accepting the deviations and variances, reluctance to change the practices, etc. Such problems must be anticipated and addressed appropriately as and when necessary, as they may become roadblocks in the successful implementation of clinical pathways.

Sample Pathway

Now, let us look at one example of a clinical pathway that was implemented in our Group Hospital. This pathway is on 'Acute Coronary Syndrome in Adults', which has been adapted from the American Heart Association.

The first phase is to select the pathway. Clinicians (ER physicians, cardiologists) were brought on board, and they were taken through the process of the clinical pathway.

A prioritization grid was used to understand the risk and to get a score. A high score of 24 was achieved, and it was also established that the topic has relevance to the major population. A publication by *BMJ* revealed that 4.6 per cent of the study population had a family history of premature CAD. The overall prevalence of diabetes was 16 per cent (5.6 per cent diagnosed during the study and the remaining 10.4 per cent already on medication). Hypertension was present in 21 per cent of subjects. The prevalence of dyslipidaemia was significantly high, with 45.6 per cent of study subjects having a high total cholesterol/high-density lipoprotein ratio. Overall, 78.6 per cent of subjects had two or more risk factors for CAD. The study showcases that the Indian Urban Population has a high prevalence of CAD risk factors. Therefore, there is a need to initiate measures to raise our clinical standard by implementing the guideline to improve the clinical outcome and patient experience.

Table 1. Priority Grid

Criterion / Score	Priority Level (3)	Priority Level (2)	Priority Level (1)	Priority Level (0)
Patient population affected	3			
Relevance to identified patient population, diagnosis, disease	3			
Resources available to provide care	3			
Patient risk	3			
Patient outcome	3			
Cost to implement	—		1	
Patient needs/ expectations		2		

Criterion / Score	Priority Level (3)	Priority Level (2)	Priority Level (1)	Priority Level (0)
Impact on quality of care	3			
Impact on safety	3			
TOTAL SCORE	**24**			

Courtesy: Apollo Hospitals

Score >18: Top priority | Score 14–18: Moderate priority | Score 10–14: Low priority | Score <10: Not a priority

Then, the team decided to formulate the ACS pathway with the following objectives:

- To implement comprehensive care for ACS patients coming to Emergency and to ensure a multidisciplinary approach for all ACS patients.
- To enhance the patient's experience, quality of care, and efficiency of the guideline and ensure uniform care for all ACS patients needing care.

A Clinical–Multidisciplinary Committee (doctors, nurses, technicians, and other clinical and nonclinical staff) approach was taken to developing the ACS pathway. All the documents for the pathway were designed and finalized for implementation. Description for inclusion and exclusion criteria was finalized.

Acute Coronary Syndrome in Adults Clinical Pathway:

Figure 5.

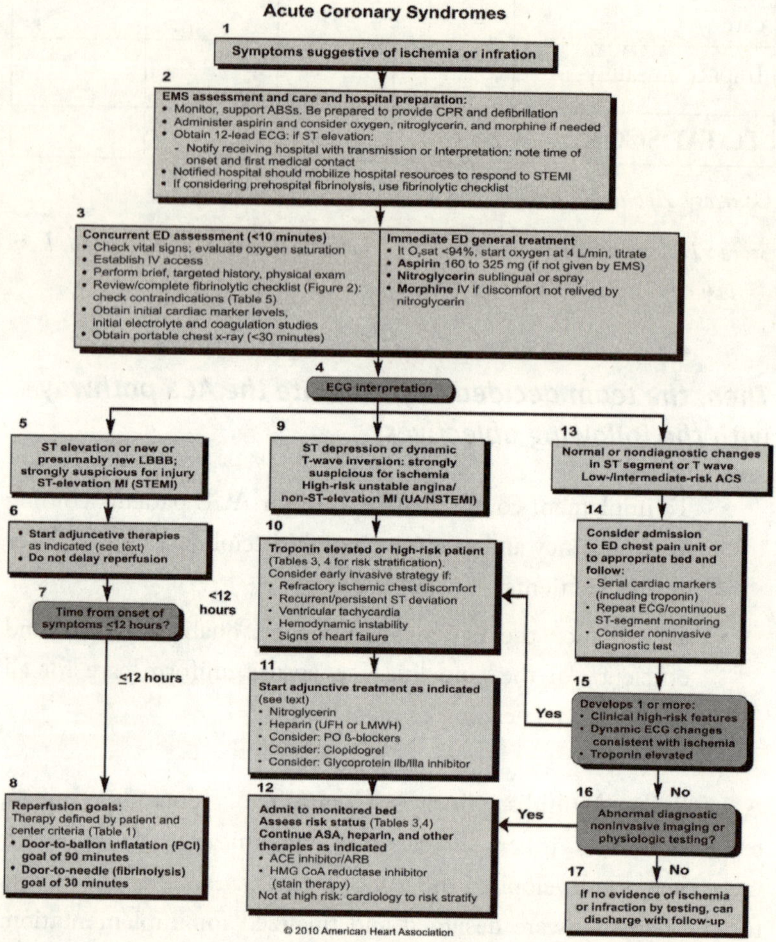

Soure: Adopted from American Heart Associations and re-drafted in Apollo Hospitals

Sample ACS Sheets:

- Patient Identification Data
- Timeline of Symptoms
- Co-morbidity Risk Factors
- CVS Investigation and Examination
- Management Plan
- Drug Chart
- ST Elevation ACS Management
- ST Depression ACS/Unstable Angina Management
- If Nondiagnostic Chest Pain
- Patient and Family Education
- Medication Reconciliation

Figure 6. ACS Sheets

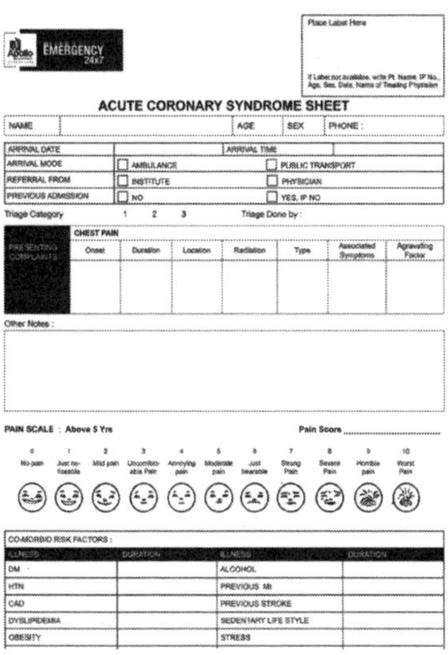

ACUTE CORONARY SYNDROME SHEET

NAME | AGE | SEX | PHONE :

ARRIVAL DATE | ARRIVAL TIME

ARRIVAL MODE: AMBULANCE / PUBLIC TRANSPORT

REFERRAL FROM: INSTITUTE / PHYSICIAN

PREVIOUS ADMISSION: NO / YES, IP NO

Triage Category 1 2 3 — Triage Done by :

PRESENTING COMPLAINTS — CHEST PAIN: Onset | Duration | Location | Radiation | Type | Associated Symptoms | Agravating Factor

Other Notes :

PAIN SCALE : Above 5 Yrs — Pain Score

CO-MORBID RISK FACTORS :

ILLNESS	DURATION	ILLNESS	DURATION
DM		ALCOHOL	
HTN		PREVIOUS MI	
CAD		PREVIOUS STROKE	
DYSLIPIDEMIA		SEDENTARY LIFE STYLE	
OBESITY		STRESS	

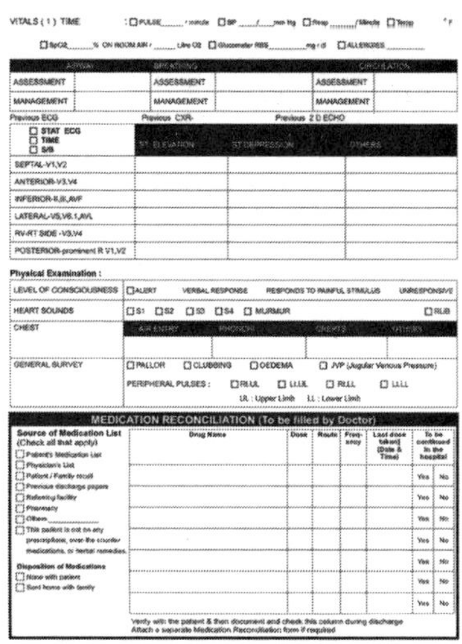

VITALS (1) TIME

AIRWAY | BREATHING | CIRCULATION — ASSESSMENT / MANAGEMENT

Previous ECG | Previous CXR | Previous 2 D ECHO

STAT ECG / TIME / S/B — ST ELEVATION | ST DEPRESSION | OTHERS

SEPTAL-V1,V2; ANTERIOR-V3,V4; INFERIOR-II,III,AVF; LATERAL-V5,V6,1,AVL; RV-RT SIDE -V3,V4; POSTERIOR-prominent R V1,V2

Physical Examination :

LEVEL OF CONSCIOUSNESS: ALERT / VERBAL RESPONSE / RESPONDS TO PAINFUL STIMULUS / UNRESPONSIVE

HEART SOUNDS: S1 / S2 / S3 / S4 / MURMUR / RUB

CHEST

GENERAL SURVEY: PALLOR / CLUBBING / OEDEMA / JVP (Jugular Venous Pressure)

PERIPHERAL PULSES :

MEDICATION RECONCILIATION (To be filled by Doctor)

Source of Medication List — Drug Name | Dose | Route | Frequency | Last dose taken (Date & Time) | To be continued in the hospital

Disposition of Medications

Courtesy: Apollo Hospitals

Working Diagnosis :

ACS : Unstable Angina ☐ STEMI ☐ NSTEMI ☐ Non Cardiac Chest Pain ☐

Associated Issues :

Management Plan :

1) If STEMI refer page 4
2) NSTEMI / Unstable Angina refer page 5
3) Non Diagnostic Chest Pain refer page 6

Cardiologist Informed	**Time**
Proposed care plan briefed	Y / N
Patient prognosis explained	Y / N
Proposed cost explained	Y / N

Investigation	Adv. Time	Report Time	Report
Blood			
Imaging			

TREATMENT ADVISED :

☐ OXYGEN @ ____ / MIN ☐ IV ACCESS ☐ LT ARM ☐ RT ARM ☐ CARDIAC MONITOR

DRUG CHART

Name of drug	Dose	Route	Site*	Freq.	Ordered by	Given by	Time
ASPIRIN (DISPRIN)	325 mg	PO					
CLOPIDOGREL	4 X 75 mg	PO					
MORPHINE							
SORBITRATE	5 mg						
NTG							
BETA BLOCKER							
HEPARIN							
STATINS							

FOR ST ELEVATION ACS : (STEMI)

REPERFUSION STRATEGY ☐ PRIMARY PTCA ☐ THROMBOLYSIS

IF PRIMARY PTCA
Cath Lab informed at ____________ Cardiologist seen at ____________ Shifted to Cath Lab at ____________

* Angio Findings
* Door to Balloon Inflation time
* Shifted out of Cathlab at

*to be filled in cathlab

If Thrombolysis

Checklist For Thrombolytic Therapy

INDICATIONS	CONTRAINDICATIONS
☐ Chest Pain Suggesting MI	**Absolute :**
☐ St Elevation > 0.1 Mv (0.1Mm) In 2 Or More Continuous Leads	☐ Previous Hemorrhagic Stroke ☐ CVA Within 1 Year ☐ Active Internal Bleeding (Menses Excluded) ☐ Suspected Aortic Dissection
☐ Or New Lbbb , Strongly Suspicious Of Injury	**Relative :**
☐ Time Of Therapy <12 Hrs	☐ Severe Uncontrolled Hypertension On Presentation (Bp > 180 / 110 Mm Hg), H / O Severe Chronic Hypertension
☐ Age < 75 Yrs	☐ Current Use Of Anticoagulation (Inr > 2.5) ☐ Known Bleeding Disorder ☐ Recent Trauma (Within 2 – 4 Wks) , Including Head Injury And Traumatic Cpr Or Major Surgery Within 3 WEEKS ☐ Recent (Within 2 – 4 Wks) Internal Bleeding , Active Peptic Ulcer Disease ☐ Pregnancy ☐ For Streptokinase : Allergy Or Prior Exposure (5 Days – 2 Years)

Thrombolytic Drug	Dose	Route	Administered By	Time
		IV		

Door to Needle Time : ________ Mins

Post Thrombolysis ECG - 90 Mins

Other Notes :

Referred to Speciality / Consultant ____________ Time ________ Seen at ________
Transferred to ____________
Vitals at time of transfer ____ Temp ____ Pulse ____ Resp ____ BP ____ SPO2 ____ PAIN SCORE ________
ER Physician Name ____________ Signature ________ Date ________ Time ________

4

FOR ST DEPRESSION ACS : (NSTEMI) / UNSTABLE ANGINA

INVESTIGATION	IMAGING		BLOOD
ADV. TIME		☐ TROP – I	☐ OTHERS
REPORT		☐ CPK-MB	

Name of drug	Dose	Route	Site*	Freq.	Ordered by	Given by	Time
ASPIRIN (DISPRIN)	325 mg	PO					
CLOPIDOGREL	4 X 75 mg	PO					
SORBITRATE	5 mg						
NTG							
BETA BLOCKER							
( )							
HEPARIN / LMWH (Low Moldecular Weight Heparin)							
GP IIB/IIA INHIBITORS ( )							
STATINS							

*Site to be written in case of IM injection & Transdermal Patches

Other Notes :

TIMI Score - High risk
Low risk
Intermediate risk

Repeat ECG

Referred to Speciality / Consultant ____________ Time ________ Seen at ________
Transferred to ____________
Vitals at time of transfer ____ Temp ____ Pulse ____ Resp ____ BP ____ SPO2 ____ PAIN SCORE ________
ER Physician Name ____________ Signature ________ Date ________ Time ________

5

If Non Diagnostic

☐ Admission ☐ Observation In ER for ________ Hrs (From ______ AM / PM to ______ AM /PM)

Vitals at Time of Transfer :

Temp ____ Pulse ____ Resp ____ BP ____ SPO_2 ____ Room Air ____ Lit O_2 ____ PAIN SCORE ____

☐ **Repeat ECG** ____________ Seen by ________ Time ________ AM /PM

☐ **Lab Report if any**

Investigation	Adv. Time	Report Time	Report
Blood			
Imaging			

Name of drug	Dose	Route	Site*	Freq.	Ordered by	Given by	Time

*Site to be written in case of IM injection & Transdermal Patches

Disposal :

Referred To Speciality/Consultant ____________ Time ________ Seen At ________
Transferred To ____________
Conclusions at Termination of Treatment ____________

Condition Of The Patient At Discharge ____________
Follow Up Instructions ____________

ER Physician Name ____________ Signature ________ Date/Time ________

6

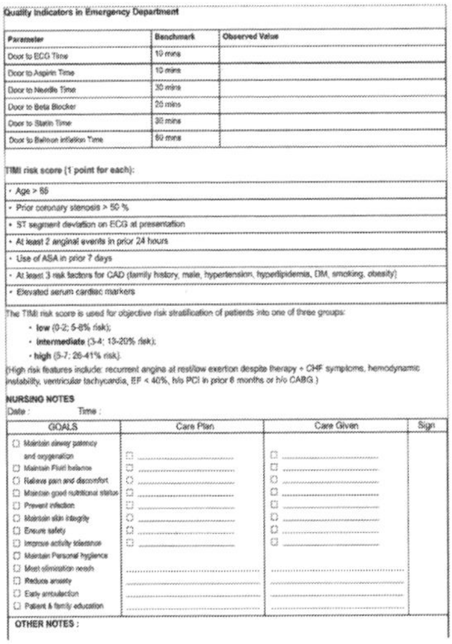

Quality Indicators in Emergency Department

Parameter	Benchmark	Observed Value
Door to ECG Time	10 mins	
Door to Aspirin Time	10 mins	
Door to Needle Time	30 mins	
Door to Beta Blocker	20 mins	
Door to Statin Time	30 mins	
Door to Balloon inflation Time	60 mins	

TIMI risk score (1 point for each):

- Age > 65
- Prior coronary stenosis > 50 %
- ST segment deviation on ECG at presentation
- At least 2 anginal events in prior 24 hours
- Use of ASA in prior 7 days
- At least 3 risk factors for CAD (family history, male, hypertension, hyperlipidemia, DM, smoking, obesity)
- Elevated serum cardiac markers

The TIMI risk score is used for objective risk stratification of patients into one of three groups:

- **low** (0-2; 5-8% risk);
- **intermediate** (3-4; 13-20% risk);
- **high** (5-7; 26-41% risk).

(High risk features include: recurrent angina at rest/low exertion despite therapy + CHF symptoms, hemodynamic instability, ventricular tachycardia, EF < 40%, h/o PCI in prior 6 months or h/o CABG.)

NURSING NOTES

Date : Time :

GOALS	Care Plan	Care Given	Sign
☐ Maintain airway patency and oxygenation			
☐ Maintain Fluid balance			
☐ Relieve pain and discomfort			
☐ Maintain good nutritional status			
☐ Prevent infection			
☐ Maintain skin integrity			
☐ Ensure safety			
☐ Improve activity tolerance			
☐ Maintain Personal hygience			
☐ Meet elimination needs			
☐ Reduce anxiety			
☐ Early ambulation			
☐ Patient & family education			

OTHER NOTES :

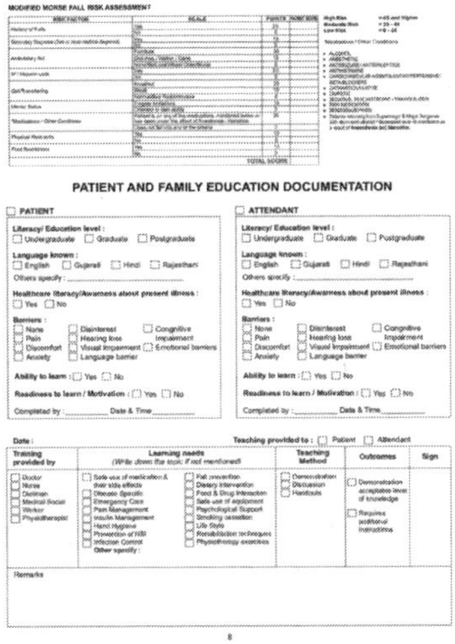

MODIFIED MORSE FALL RISK ASSESSMENT

PATIENT AND FAMILY EDUCATION DOCUMENTATION

☐ **PATIENT**

Literacy/ Education level : ☐ Undergraduate ☐ Graduate ☐ Postgraduate

Language known : ☐ English ☐ Gujarati ☐ Hindi ☐ Rajasthani

Others specify : ________

Healthcare literacy/Awarness about present illness : ☐ Yes ☐ No

Barriers : ☐ None ☐ Pain ☐ Discomfort ☐ Anxiety ☐ Disinterest ☐ Hearing loss ☐ Visual Impairment ☐ Language barrier ☐ Congnitive Impairment ☐ Emotional barriers

Ability to learn : ☐ Yes ☐ No

Readiness to learn / Motivation : ☐ Yes ☐ No

Completed by : ______ Date & Time ______

☐ **ATTENDANT**

Literacy/ Education level : ☐ Undergraduate ☐ Graduate ☐ Postgraduate

Language known : ☐ English ☐ Gujarati ☐ Hindi ☐ Rajasthani

Others specify : ________

Healthcare literacy/Awarness about present illness : ☐ Yes ☐ No

Barriers : ☐ None ☐ Pain ☐ Discomfort ☐ Anxiety ☐ Disinterest ☐ Hearing loss ☐ Visual Impairment ☐ Language barrier ☐ Congnitive Impairment ☐ Emotional barriers

Ability to learn : ☐ Yes ☐ No

Readiness to learn / Motivation : ☐ Yes ☐ No

Completed by : ______ Date & Time ______

Date : **Teaching provided to :** ☐ Patient ☐ Attendant

Training provided by	Learning needs (Write down the topic if not mentioned)		Teaching Method	Outcomes	Sign
☐ Doctor ☐ Nurse ☐ Dietician ☐ Medical Social Worker ☐ Physiotherapist	☐ Safe use of medication & their side effects ☐ Disease Specific ☐ Emergency Care ☐ Pain Management ☐ Insulin Management ☐ Hand Hygiene ☐ Prevention of NRI ☐ Infection Control Other specify :	☐ Fall prevention ☐ Dietary intervention ☐ Food & Drug Interaction ☐ Safe use of equipment ☐ Psychological Support ☐ Smoking cessation ☐ Life Style ☐ Rehabilitation techniques ☐ Physiotherapy exercises	☐ Demonstration ☐ Discussion ☐ Handouts	☐ Demonstration acceptable level of knowledge ☐ Requires additional instructions	

Remarks

8

Since mainly emergency room physicians, nurses and cardiologists are involved in cases of ACS, it was easy to train the staff on the identification and management of such cases. Patient education brochures were also developed (heart attack, angiography and angioplasty) for the same and is displayed for reference.

Method of Implementation

- Stakeholder interviews between the programme leader and stakeholders from each of the two sites, and sensitization towards the use of clinical guidelines were conducted.
- The roles and responsibilities of each discipline and team member were defined clearly.
- Staff was trained on the adoption of the clinical pathway.
- Draft versions of the pathway were presented and deliberated upon in closed group meetings, including members from major disciplines involved in the care process and comments

Figure 7. Education Material

responding to insulin properly — causes your body's blood sugar levels to rise. Diabetes, especially uncontrolled, increases your risk of a heart attack.

- **Family history of heart attack.** If your siblings, parents or grandparents have had early heart attacks (by age 55 for male relatives and by age 65 for female relatives), you may be at increased risk.
- **Lack of physical activity.** An inactive lifestyle contributes to high blood cholesterol levels and obesity. People who get regular aerobic exercise have better cardiovascular fitness, which decreases their overall risk of heart attack. Exercise is also beneficial in lowering high blood pressure.
- **Obesity.** Obesity is associated with high blood cholesterol levels, high triglyceride levels, high blood pressure and diabetes. Losing just 10 percent of your body weight can lower this risk, however.
- **Stress.** You may respond to stress in ways that can increase your risk of a heart attack.
- **Illegal drug use.** Using stimulant drugs, such as cocaine or amphetamines, can trigger a spasm of your coronary arteries that can cause a heart attack.
- **A history of preeclampsia.** This condition causes high blood pressure during pregnancy and increases the lifetime risk of heart disease.
- **A history of an autoimmune condition,** such as rheumatoid arthritis or lupus. Conditions such as rheumatoid arthritis, lupus and other autoimmune conditions can increase your risk of having a heart attack.

How to prevent heart attack?

- Our lifestyle affects your heart health. The

- **Control your blood pressure and cholesterol levels.** If one or both of these is high, your doctor can prescribe changes to your diet and medications. Ask your doctor how often you need to have your blood pressure and cholesterol levels monitored.
- **Get regular medical checkups.** Some of the major risk factors for heart attack — high blood cholesterol, high blood pressure and diabetes — cause no symptoms early on. Your doctor can perform tests to check for these conditions and help you manage them, if necessary.
- **Exercise regularly.** Regular exercise helps improve heart muscle function after a heart attack and helps prevent a heart attack by helping you to control your weight, diabetes, cholesterol and blood pressure. Exercise needn't be vigorous. Walking 30 minutes a day, five days a week can improve your health.
- **Maintain a healthy weight.** Excess weight strains your heart and can contribute to high cholesterol, high blood pressure and diabetes.
- **Eat a heart-healthy diet.** Saturated fat, trans fats and cholesterol in your diet can narrow arteries to your heart, and too much salt can raise blood pressure. Eat a heart-healthy diet that includes lean proteins, such as fish and beans, plenty of fruits and vegetables and whole grains.
- **Manage diabetes.** High blood sugar is damaging to your heart. Regular exercise, eating well and losing weight all help to keep blood sugar levels at more-desirable levels. Many people also need medication to manage their diabetes.
- **Control stress.** Reduce stress in your day-to-day activities. Rethink workaholic habits and find healthy ways to minimize or deal

Patient Information

HEART ATTACK
(MYOCARDIAL INFARCTION)

Apollo HOSPITALS
TOUCHING LIVES

Appointment: 079 6670 1880, 76988 15003

Apollo Hospitals International Limited
Plot 1A, Bhat GIDC Estate,
Gandhinagar, Gujarat - 382428

What is heart attack?

A heart attack occurs when the flow of blood to the heart is blocked, most often by a build-up of fat, cholesterol and other substances, which form a plaque in the arteries that feed the heart (coronary arteries). The interrupted blood flow can damage or destroy part of the heart muscle.

A heart attack, also called a myocardial infarction, can be fatal, but treatment has improved dramatically over the years. It's crucial to call 1066 emergency medical help if you think you might be having a heart attack.

Common heart attack signs and symptoms include:

- Pressure, tightness, pain, or a squeezing or aching sensation in your chest or arms that may spread to your neck, jaw or back
- Nausea, indigestion, heartburn or abdominal pain
- Shortness of breath
- Cold sweat
- Fatigue
- Lightheadedness or sudden dizziness

Classic Heart Attack Symptoms

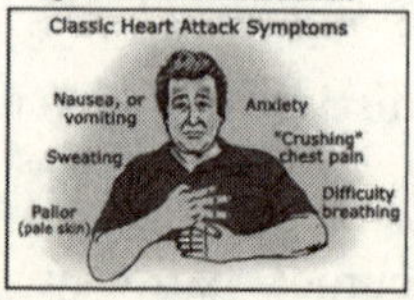

Some heart attacks strike suddenly, but many people have warning signs and symptoms hours, days or weeks in advance. The earliest warning may be recurrent chest pain (angina) that's triggered by exertion and relieved by rest. Angina is caused by a temporary decrease in blood flow to the heart.

A heart attack differs from a condition in which your heart suddenly stops (sudden cardiac arrest, which occurs when an electrical disturbance disrupts your heart's pumping action and causes blood to stop flowing to the rest of your body). A heart attack can cause cardiac arrest, but it's not the only cause.

When to see a doctor?

Act immediately. Some people wait too long because they don't recognize the important signs and symptoms. If you suspect you're having a heart attack, don't hesitate. Immediately call 1066 or your local emergency number. If you don't have access to emergency medical services, have someone drive you to the nearest hospital.

What to do if you see someone having a heart attack?

If you encounter someone who is unconscious, first call for emergency medical help. Then begin CPR to keep blood flowing. Push hard and fast on the person's chest — about 100 compressions a minute. It's not necessary to check the person's airway or deliver rescue breaths unless you've been trained in CPR.

What are the causes of heart attack?

- A heart attack occurs when one or more of your coronary arteries become blocked. Over time, a coronary artery can narrow from the buildup of various substances, including cholesterol (atherosclerosis). This

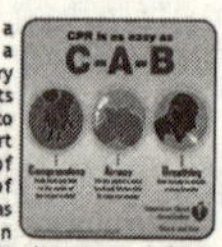

- Another cause of a heart attack is a spasm of a coronary artery that shuts down blood flow to part of the heart muscle. Use of tobacco and of illicit drugs, such as cocaine, can cause a life-threatening spasm. A heart attack can also occur due to a tear in the heart artery (spontaneous coronary artery dissection).

What are the risk factors of heart attack?

Certain factors contribute to the unwanted buildup of fatty deposits (atherosclerosis) that narrows arteries throughout your body. You can improve or eliminate many of these risk factors to reduce your chances of having a first or subsequent heart attack.

Heart attack risk factors include:

- **Age.** Men age 45 or older and women age 55 or older are more likely to have a heart attack than are younger men and women.
- **Tobacco.** Smoking and long-term exposure to secondhand smoke increase the risk of a heart attack.
- **High blood pressure.** Over time, high blood pressure can damage arteries that feed your heart by accelerating atherosclerosis. High blood pressure that occurs with obesity, smoking, high cholesterol or diabetes increases your risk even more.
- **High blood cholesterol or triglyceride levels.** A high level of low-density lipoprotein (LDL) cholesterol (the "bad" cholesterol) is most likely to narrow

Courtesy: Apollo Hospitals

received were reviewed by the working group for discussion, and when appropriate, for incorporation into the pathway.

- The guideline was then taken up for implementation.
- Close monitoring of pilot implementation was done for three months.
- Post pilot phase, evaluated the new documentation.
- Started the care pathway implementation officially post initial evaluation of the documentation.

Evaluation/Follow-Up

- In this phase, the care pathway was controlled, analysed and updated.
- They are best-in-class tools to be periodically reviewed and adapted.
- In this last phase, the first activity was to appoint a dedicated resource for tracking the care pathway. Who is suited for the job, a doctor or a nurse? The involvement of professionals from both medical and nursing fields is recommended to avoid discontinuation of the pathway compliance through concerned physicians and nurses.
- Periodic reviews were conducted every three months.
- A systematic clinical audit was conducted.
- Follow up on completion of medical record documents.
- Monitoring of variances with a fixed periodicity.
- Outcomes were assessed and evaluated from the information recorded in the care pathway documentation.
- Analysis of the impact of the care pathway implementation on the care process.

- Feedback was provided to managers and staff regarding the follow-up of indicators/outcomes and variances.

Figure 8. Quarter ACS Pathway Evaluation

QUARTERLY – ACS PATHWAY EVALUATION

Guideline: ACS Clinical Pathway - AHA
Evaluation Duration: Jan'16 to March'16
Sample Evaluated: 75% of Total Cases
Evaluation Done By: ER Head

Sl No.	Particular	Compliance %
1	Basic Assessment o Triage o Identification Data	 100% 100%
2	Assessment Sign & Symptoms Co-morbid Risk Factors	 100% 100%
3	Concurrent ED Assessment in < 10mins	100%
4	ECG Assessment <10mins	Average 5.2mins (Highest 15mins and Lowest 1min)
5	X-Ray <30mins	0%
6	Clopidogrel, Aspirin on Arrival	100%
7	Beta Block on Arrival (Whenever indicated)	100%
6	Medication Reconciliation with Source	100%
7	Treatment Plan & Diagnosis	100%
8	Door to Balloon Inflation Time	Average Time - 142mins
9	Nursing Care Plan	100%
10	Fall Risk Assessment	100%
11	Patient & Family Education Charting	100%

REVIEW COMMENTS:

- In ACS case ECG is key measure based on results for assessment and deciding the line of treatment. In couple of records review it was evident it took > 10mins to take ECG.
- It was decided during implantation of pathway x-ray will be not considered for measuring Pathway Compliance as it is not routinely done at AHIL until it is clinical indicated.
- Significant no. of patient has cross the door to balloon inflation time, however in March'16 it has reduced marginally but still lagging behind 90mins benchmark.
- Rest all key component of pathway has almost 99% of compliance.

Courtesy: Apollo Hospitals

Evaluation Parameters (Expected Values)

- Door to ECG time (10 min)
- Door to aspirin time (10 min)
- Door to needle time (30 min)
- Door to beta-blocker (20 min)
- Door to balloon inflation time (60 min)

Figure 9.

Door to balloon inflation time in acute coronary syndrome (ACS)

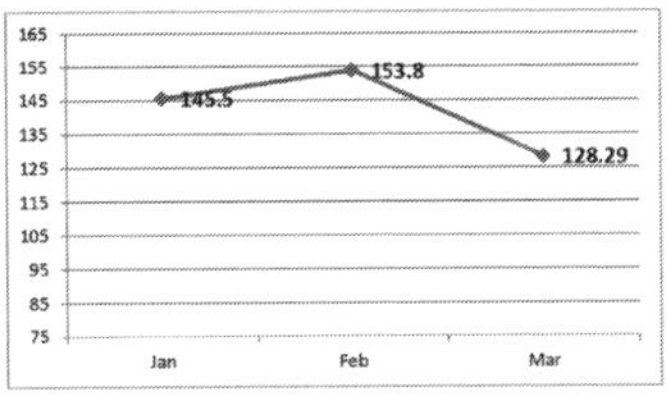

Particulars	Jan	Feb	Mar
Total time from arrival of patients with ACS in ER to balloon inflation in cathlab	2910	2000	3977
Total number of patients with ACS	20	13	31
Avg. Time in Minutes	145.5	153.8	128.29
Benchmark (90mins – AHA Guideline)			

Aspirin on Arrival AMI Case

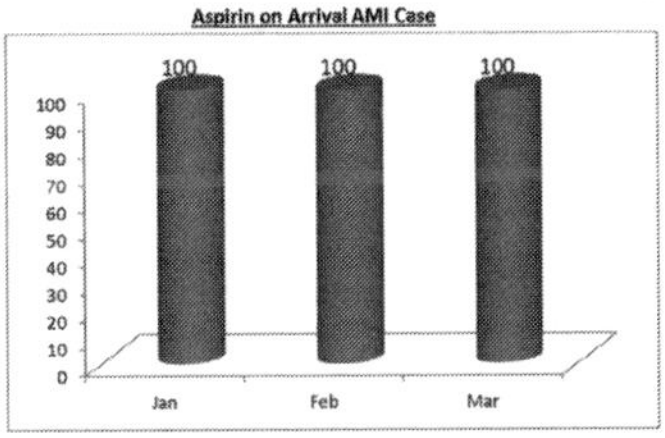

Particulars	Jan	Feb	Mar
Number of AMI patients receiving aspirin at arrival	11	9	22
Number of AMI patients who age is >= 18 years	11	9	22
Compliance in %	100%	100%	100%
Benchmark 100%			

Aspirin in Acute coronary syndrome (ACS) patients

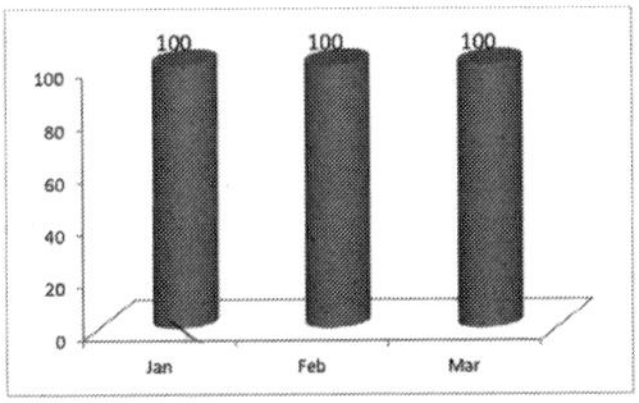

Particulars	Jan	Feb	Mar
Number of patients with ACS receiving aspirin at arrival	20	13	31
Number of ACS patients	20	13	31
Avg. Time in Minutes	100%	100%	100%
Benchmark 100%			

Door to EGC Time

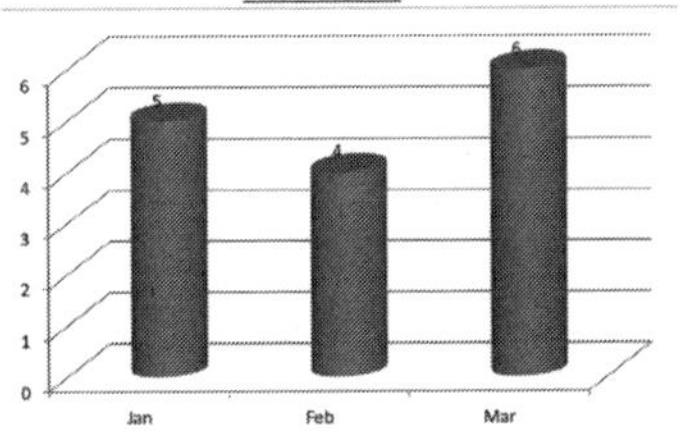

Particulars	Jan	Feb	Mar
Time in minutes	5	4	6
Benchmark 10mins			

Courtesy: Apollo Hospitals

Updating the care pathway and documentation of its records is mandatory and should be done based on the publication of new scientific evidence, the information collected about the most frequent variances, and considering the achieved objectives.

Conclusion

A clinical pathway is a roadmap for a patient as well as for the treatment team, which supports structured, efficient and effective patient care. Clinical pathways are disease-specific and individually customized to account for the specific environment, reputation and experience in the implementing hospital.

They detail the essential steps in the care of patients with a specific clinical problem and describe the expected progress of the patient; they ease the introduction into clinical practice of clinical guidelines and systematic, continuing audit of clinical practices; they can act as a link between the establishment of clinical guidelines and their use; they help in communication with patients by giving them access to a distinctly written summary of their expected care plan and progress over time.

References:

1. American Heart Association: ACS Guidelines 2010
2. British Medical Journal Open; 'Prevalence of risk factors for coronary artery disease in an urban Indian population', *BMJ*, Vol. 4, No. 12, doi: 10.1136/bmjopen-2014-005346
3. T. Rotter, R. Jong, et al, 'Clinical pathways as a quality strategy', National Library of Medicine, https://www.ncbi.nlm.nih.gov/books/NBK549262/
4. 'Constipation: Clinical Pathways', John Hopkins All Children's Hospital, https://www.hopkinsallchildrens.org/Health-Professionals/Clinical-Pathways/Constipation
5. 'Clinical Pathways: What They Are & How They Impact Patient Care', Telligen, 17 April 2018, https://www.telligen.com/recent-news/clinical-pathways-what-they-are-how-they-impact-patient-care/
6. T. A., *The Role of Clinical Pathways in Improving Patient Outcomes*, Academia.edu, https://www.academia.edu/6850634/The_Role_of_Clinical_Pathways_in_Improving_Patient_Outcomes
7. Ricard Rosique, 'Care Pathways: The Basics', Asian Hospital and Healthcare Management, https://www.asianhhm.com/healthcare-management/care-pathways-basics
8. A. Lawal, T. Rotter, et al., 'What is a clinical pathway? Refinement of an operational definition to identify clinical pathway studies for a Cochrane systematic review', *BMC Medicine* (2016) Vol. 14, No. 35.
9. C. Wells and J. Forrester, *Acute Care Management of the Older Adult*, *Clinical Nursing* (February 2011), Vol. 20.

10. Mona Gupta, 'Improved health or improved decision making? The ethical goals of EBM', *Journal of Evaluating Clinical Practice* (October 2011), Vol. 17, No. 5.
11. J. Heffner, 'Does Evidence-Based Medicine Help the Development of Clinical Practice Guidelines?', *CHEST* (1998, March).
12. William Charles Watters III, 'Clinical guidelines strengthened by evidence-based practice', *AAOS Now*, 1 January 2007, https://www.aaos.org/aaosnow/2007/janfeb/research/research4/
13. M. De Allegri, et al, 'Which factors are important for the successful development and implementation of clinical pathways? A qualitative study', *BMJ Quality and Safety* (March 2011) 2, Vol. 20 No. 3.
14. M. Dawsey, 'Clinical pathways in hip and knee arthroplasty: a prospective randomised controlled study', *Medical Journal of Australia* (January 2018), Vol. 17, No. 2.
15. M. Gomez, et al., 'An emergency department-based protocol for rapidly ruling out myocardial ischemia reduces hospital time and expense: Results of a randomized study (ROMIO)', *Journal of American College of Cardiology* (July 1996), Vol. 28, No.1.
16. T. Rotter, et al., 'Clinical pathways: effects on professional practice, patient outcomes, length of stay and hospital costs', *Cochrane Database Systematic Reviews* (March 2010), Vol. 17, No. 3.
17. 'International experiences in the use of care pathways', *Journal of Care Services Management* (2013), Vol. 7 Issue 4, https://www.tandfonline.com/doi/abs/10.1179/1750168714Y.0000000028
18. L. Kinsman, E. James and J. Ham, 'An Interdisciplinary, Evidence-Based Process of Clinical Pathway Implementation Increases Pathway Usage', Lippincott's Case Management (Jul–Aug 2004) Vol. 9, No. 4.

9

Quality Indicators: What Gets Measured Gets Improved

There are many norms, standards, and other qualitative and quantitative measures used in determining the quality of healthcare. They are used to determine and monitor the quality of a healthcare organization's performance. These indicators are measurable and relate to the outcome of patient care or service performance.

Quality Indicators (QIs) are standardized, evidence/standard-based measures of quality that can be used as a tool to monitor the care/service provided and further improve the quality and patient safety in hospitals.

All departments and services, clinical and non-clinical, must select measuring indicators related to their priorities. After setting priorities for improvement and selecting what is to be measured, how to collect, validate and analyse the data becomes yet another important step in the process.

'Process improvement programs are like teaching people how to fish. Strategy maps and scorecards teach people where to fish.'

—Robert S. Kaplan

Introduction

ORGANIZATIONS MUST HAVE a specific framework to support the ongoing quality improvement and patient safety efforts. A comprehensive approach to quality improvement and patient safety encompasses the measurement and analysis of quality data, followed by the implementation of necessary measures and interventions to enhance, reinforce and sustain the results.

The approach includes:

- Departmental level inputs and active participation;
- Use of objective and validated data to measure how well processes work;
- Effectively using tools and techniques for further analysis; and
- Comparing results with available and relevant benchmarks, to initiate and implement systemic changes that result in improvement.

As clinical staff assesses the patient's needs and provides care, key clinical indicators can help them understand how to make real improvements that can help patients and reduce the risks. Similarly, non-clinical staff monitors key indicators relevant to their daily work to understand how the processes can be more efficient, how resources can be used more wisely, and how physical risks can be reduced.

All departments and services, clinical and non-clinical, must select measuring indicators related to their priorities. In larger hospitals, there is some opportunity for similar measures to be selected in more than one department. For example, the pharmacy and infection control department may each set priorities related to rationalizing antibiotic usage in the hospital. These measures may then be integrated and considered as 'hospital-wide Indicators'.

After setting priorities for improvement and selecting what is to be measured, how to collect, validate and analyse the data becomes yet another important step in the process. Reliability and validity of measurement and quality of the data must be established through the data validation process. The aggregated data and resultant analysis provide the hospital with an effective tool for identifying opportunities for further improvement, and allow the comparison of the hospital's performance with other hospitals.

Quality Indicators

What Are Quality Indicators?

There are many norms, standards, and other qualitative and quantitative measures used in determining the quality of healthcare. They are used to determine and monitor the quality of a healthcare organization's performance. These indicators are measurable and relate to the outcome of patient care or service performance.

Quality Indicators (QIs) are standardized, evidence/standard-based measures of quality that can be used as a tool to monitor the care/service provided and further improve the quality and patient safety in hospitals.

Why Do We Need Quality Indicators?

QIs play a major role in measuring the quality of the healthcare and services provided by the organization. The timely and accurate collection of QIs ensures continuous improvement in any healthcare organization. We can only improve what we can measure, as it difficult to verify improvements in any qualitative way.

How to Form Quality Indicators?

Quality Indicators are developed based on various professional standards or evidence-based concepts. It also includes the voice of customers, personal experiences, literature reviews, and discussions with experts from within and outside the organization.

After identifying a particular QI, we should define the numerator and denominator, along with the inclusion and exclusion criteria, if any. We should also ascertain the data collection timelines/duration, source of data, sampling methods, and calculation formula beforehand. Quality indicators, including trend tracking and deviation detection, should be continuously monitored, and the analysis should be periodically shared with the respective stakeholders.

How to Select and Prioritize Quality Indicators?

We can use many tools to select a particular QI. The best way to decide QIs is to draw on customer feedback (both internal and external), feedback from various stakeholders, own experiences, and frequently raised incidents including near-misses and sentinel events. We can also adopt a better and more objective method to decide a QI: using a formal prioritization grid that can help evaluate quantitatively the importance and necessity of a specific QI.

Based on predefined criteria, the multidisciplinary team may decide whether to select a particular indicator or not. There are many advisories and models available in current times that depict such priorities and help us to select specific indicators. However, the matrix given below summarizes the overall concept of selection and prioritization of quality indicators.

The Next Steps

QIs are more effective when used to promote the changes in the quality of patient care, than only as a tool to assess performance. Now, let's understand how one should proceed.

How to Collect?

Generally, a predesigned checklist is used for data collection that may have a few mandatory fields to capture all the relevant raw data. The checklist can be modified as per the requirement of the organization/department. Data on a few QIs may also be obtained through various observations, audits, feedback, interviews, etc.

Who Should Collect?

The responsibility for data collection is assigned to the respective department member, who is a part of the process on the ground and can collect the data as desired.

The data collector should be aware of the entire process flow, how and from where to capture the data, and how to collate and document the data. Having an automated system is the best way to avoid any ambiguity or erroneous data. In any case, the staff member responsible for the data collection must be well-trained and should have thorough knowledge about the same.

How to Validate?

A *data validation must be conducted by the Quality Department, or departmental leaders, through a proper statistical method. Validation should be done whenever there is:

- A new measure
- Data to be made public/put on the website
- A change in data collection tool
- Change in data resulting from the existing measure, in an unexplainable way
- Change in data source
- Change in the subject of data collection

When to Collect?

Although we generally collect and aggregate the data on a monthly basis, the frequency of data collection varies from indicator to indicator. The indicators that are directly related to patient care outcome and safety (patient falls, hospital-acquired infections, etc.) need to be monitored frequently, or as and when it happens. Employee and organization-centric outcomes often need to be monitored regularly. It completely depends on the organization to define the periodicity of data collection and further analysis and distribution of results.

What to Do with the Data?

The raw data collected needs to be converted into meaningful information. The same can be done using various analytical and statistical tools. Data is systemically aggregated and analysed with appropriate statistical tools and techniques. Some of the analytical tools are as under:

1. Flow charts
2. Control charts
3. Histograms
4. Pareto charts
5. Cause-and-effect or fishbone diagrams
6. FMEA analysis
7. Scatter diagrams

These tools can help organize the collected information understandably. It is also important to remember that different tools and techniques must be used for different problems.

Types of Quality Indicators

As first proposed by Avediinto Donabedian (1966), QIs can be categorized into three types:

1. **Outcome**: 'Outcome' measures attempt to describe the effects of care on the health status of patients and populations. Improvements in the patient's knowledge and salutary changes in the patient's behaviour may be included under

a broad definition of the outcome, and may represent the degree of the patient's satisfaction with care. For example, the mortality rate of all in-patients, surgical mortality.

2. **Process**: Process denotes what is done in giving and receiving care, i.e., the doctor's activities in making a diagnosis, recommending or implementing treatment, or other interaction with the patient. For example, Discharge summary compliance, and the average length of stay in ICU.
3. **Structure**: For example, nurse-to-bed ratio, or the average years of experience of nursing staff.

How to Use Quality Indicators

One should strive to incorporate comparisons with themselves over time, as well as with other comparable organizations, with regard to standards and best practices.

Benchmarking in healthcare is a great tool to improve clinical and operational QIs. It is the process of comparing one's indicators, outcomes and performance metrics to other best indicators, outcomes and performance metrics, or to best practices from other healthcare organizations. It helps organizations to develop plans on how to make improvements or adapt specific best practices, usually to improve some aspects of performance.

Benchmarking could be external or internal benchmarking. Some of the sources for comparison that we generally use are:

- Performance compared to the performance of similar processes in other organizations
- Performance compared to external sources of information

- Recent scientific, clinical and management literature
- Well-formulated practice guidelines or parameters
- Performance measures
- Standards that are periodically reviewed and revised
- JCI/NABH/NABL published data

Undesirable patterns or trends in performance are intensively analysed if the comparisons show that:

- Important single events, levels of performance, patterns or trends vary significantly from those expected
- Performance varies significantly and undesirably from other organizations
- Performance varies significantly and undesirably from recognized standards or practice guidelines
- When a critical or sentinel event occurs

This process of comparison with the benchmark and analysing patterns involves the necessary departments and their team members to conclude the need for further intensive measurement and collection of further data.

A systematic analysis process is used to assess collected data, to determine whether specifications for newly designed processes have been met; the level of quality and stability of important existing processes; priorities for possible improvement of existing processes; actions taken to refine the quality improvement processes; and whether changes in the processes resulted in improvement.

Table 1. An Example of a Prioritization Matrix

Criterion	Score 3	Score 2	Score 1	Score 0	SCORE
Patient needs/ expectations	Indicated by the survey/complaints	Possible high positive effect	Possible moderate effect	Minimal or no effect	2
Patient outcome	Important improvement	Some improvement	Little improvement	No improvement	3
Strategic plan related to cost efficiency	Strong relationship	Moderate	Minimal	None	3
Regulatory compliance	Required (payment of bills on time)	N/A	N/A	Not required	0
Cost to implement	No cost/budgeted item	One time, <5% of operating budget	5-10% of operating budget	The ongoing increase in costs	3

Criterion	Score 3	Score 2	Score 1	Score 0	SCORE
Impact on efficiency/ budget	Reduction of 1 FTE or >10% reduction	Reduction of 0-1 FTE or 1-10% red.	No impact	Increase in staff or operating costs	0
Patient volume affected	100% of patients	50-75% of patients	25-50% of patients	0-25% of patients	3
Patient risk	May cause death	Permanent serious complications	Temporary serious complications	Temporary or no risk	1
Problem-prone	Increased risk to staff or patients	Moderate risk	Low risk (with high costs)	No risk	3
				TOTAL	**18**

Courtesy: Apollo Hospitals

Prioritization Matrix: An Example

Hand hygiene is a very crucial process indicator, which describes the status of implementation of infection control practices in a hospital. The data is collected by an Infection Control Nurse and shared with the quality team for analysis.

The total score is 18, so it should be considered a priority indicator.

Definition: Hand hygiene is defined as any method that removes or destroys microorganisms on hands. It is well-documented that effective hand washing is the most important measure for preventing the spread of pathogens.

Indicator Calculation: Total number of compliance/Total number of opportunities*100

Data Collection Methodology: Surveillance and audits by Infection Control Nurse.

Data Source: Manual and Digital

Exclusion Criteria: All the staff that were not present at the time of the audit.

Data Validation: Infection Control convenor, medical administration, and quality.

Standard Deviation: It is a measure of the distribution of a set of data from its mean. The more spread apart the data, the higher the deviation.

Mean: It is an average of the numbers. To calculate mean, just add up all the numbers, then divide by the total number.

Upper Control Limit: A value that indicates the highest level of quality acceptable for service. The upper control limit is used in conjunction with the lower control limit to create the range of variability for quality specifications.

Lower Control Limit: It is the opposite of upper control limit. It is defined as the bottom limit in quality control for data points being analysed below the control (average) line in a control chart.

Interpretation: The graph clearly describes that the hand compliance among the healthcare workers is on average 93 per cent. The desired benchmark is 80 per cent as per the internal data source. Hence, the caregiver team must focus on sustaining this trend.

Corrective Action: The corrective action should include on-the-job training by the Infection Control Team on the missing steps or other concerns, e.g., not following five moments of hand wash, all the steps of hand hygiene not being done properly, or lack of knowledge.

Preventive Action: Preventive action should focus on on-the-job training for all the healthcare workers, providing brochures and posters across all the wash basins that act as a reminder, and spy checks at regular intervals to keep a close watch on the adherence.

Conclusion

Each QI is a storyboard that denotes the quality of a certain process/outcome. The corrective and preventive steps guide the organization to improve compliance and sustain good practices. All these efforts eventually lead to better patient outcomes and processes.

QIs measure the extent to which set targets are achieved. They are expressed as numbers, rates, percentages or averages that can provide a basis for organizations, doctors, administrators and planners aiming to achieve improvement in the standard of care, and thereby improvising the processes by which patient care is delivered.

Hence, every organization must stress on proper data collection and analysis. The interpretation and result will impact the overall patient, employee and organization outcome/satisfaction.

References:

1. R. Nair, P. Babu Anne, et al., 'Quality improvement interventions for Bedside Transfusion safety: An experience from a tertiary healthcare center of Western India,' *ISBT Science Series*, https://www.semanticscholar.org/paper/Quality-improvement-interventions-for-Bedside-An-a-Nair-Anne/be397d71f827af3af9039ed08bb6050fdbf6ba00
2. *JCI Accreditation Standards for Hospitals, 7th edition*, Joint Commission International, https://store.jointcommissioninternational.org/jci-accreditation-standards-for-hospitals-7th-edition/
3. J. Mainz, 'Defining and classifying clinical indicators for quality improvement.'
4. T. Vuk, et al., 'Quality Monitoring and Risk Management in Blood Transfusion Services,' *ISBT Science Series* (2018), Vol. 13, pp. 284–289, https://scirp.org/(S(czeh2tfqyw2orz553k1w0r45))/reference/referencespapers.aspx?referenceid=3092291
5. L. Chadwick, et al., 'Senior staff perspectives of a quality indicator program in public sector residential aged care services: A qualitative cross-sectional study in Victoria, Australia.'
6. W. Arkaravichien, A. Wongpratat, and S. Lertsinudom, 'Quality indicators to compare accredited independent pharmacies and accredited chain pharmacies in Thailand', 2016, *International Journal of Clinical Pharmacy*, Vol. 38, No. 4, pp. 899–907, doi: 10.1007/s11096-016-0307-4.
7. T. Vuk, 'Vuk Implementation of ISBT quality indicators in the quality management and hemovigilance systems', *ISBT Science Series* (2015), Vol. 10, No. S1, pp. 371–375, doi: 10.1111/voxs.12149; https://onlinelibrary.wiley.com/doi/pdf/10.1111/voxs.12149.
8. Y. Ayob, 'Monitoring transfusion practice,' *ISBT Science Series* (2014), Vol. 9, No. 1, pp. 72–79, doi10.1111/voxs.12089; https://onlinelibrary.wiley.com/doi/full/10.1111/voxs.12089.

10

Incident Reporting: Report It to Stop It

Incident Reporting has an imperative influence on improving patient safety. It offers valuable insights into how and why patients can be harmed at the organizational level.

The purpose of the adverse event reporting is to prevent further incidents, events or near misses and/or their occurrences. Investigating and dealing with incidents, events and near misses enables lessons to be learnt and corrective and preventive measures to be taken to improve patient safety.

Furthermore, it is critical to establish a robust mechanism to capture an incident: a tool that is not only just user-friendly but also allows the user to keep their identity anonymous. The idea is to encourage a culture of safety among various healthcare workers.

'An incident is just the tip of the iceberg, a sign of a much larger problem below the surface.'

—Don Brown

Introduction

IT WAS A busy morning for the ABC hospital's nursing team as they had just taken the handover from the night shift team. While trying to make a list of her tasks, one of the nurses noticed a small needle thrown in the dustbin in the nursing station. She ignored it, as she was rushing to administer a medication. While returning and in a rush to discard waste, she got herself pricked from the same needle.

She panicked and immediately rushed to the emergency department of the hospital. This entire incident could have been avoided, provided she had taken the situation seriously rather than ignoring it. We, as healthcare professionals, often come across many such incidents, near misses, and serious adverse events in our day-to-day activities. It is quite crucial to raise an alarm for all such incidents.

An incident is an event that has unintentionally happened, but it may or may not result in damage, harm or injury. Adverse events could be errors, acts of omission or commission, near misses or sentinel events. An incident report should be supported by facts and be objective rather than biased. Reporting of all near misses, adverse incidents and sentinel events is the mainstay and most important tool for risk management. Re-occurrence of any adverse event carries certain risks, the severity of which depends upon the likelihood and impact of consequences. To minimize the associated risks, such as untoward happenings, these must be intensely examined by a Root Cause Analysis (RCA). Based on the findings of a RCA, a preventive action plan can be formulated and implemented to avoid recurrence.

It is also extremely crucial for an organization to promote a culture of safety that enables its employees to report any adverse incidents objectively, without the fear of retribution. Such a culture seeks to create an environment that encourages individuals to report mistakes and submit honest reports, so there is no blame and fear. The staff is empowered to take accountability and be more vigilant in the future.

Rationale of Incident Reporting

The purpose of the adverse event reporting is to prevent further incidents, events or near misses, and/or their occurrences. Investigating and dealing with incidents, events and near misses enables lessons to be learnt and corrective and preventive measures to be taken to improve patient safety. It also encourages a culture of patient safety and continuous quality improvement. Incident reporting aims to document the exact details of such occurrences while they are fresh in the minds of those who witnessed the event.

This information may be useful in the future when dealing with similar issues. If incidents are meticulously reported and documented, it is possible to conduct RCA and re-engineer processes to avoid repeated occurrences of similar incidents. By compiling a database of such adverse events, it is also possible for the organization to understand the trends related to a particular area, personnel, or types of incidents, and to decide appropriate measures needed to prevent such incidents in the future. Additionally, it is possible to assess the effects of process management by studying these trends of occurrence of incidents, obtained by collating available data.

It is important to ensure that initiating an adverse event report does not lead to any disciplinary action except where acts of omissions are malicious, criminal or constitute gross or repeated professional negligence or misconduct.

Reportable Incidents

An incident is any event that jeopardizes the safety of a patient, employee safety or an organization. While the list of reportable incidents is substantial, a few of them are illustrated below.

1. **Facility-related issues**: Any issues related to the infrastructure or facility that needs attention can be raised as an incident.

   Example: A malfunctioning lift or empty fire extinguisher is identified by staff. An incident is raised, addressed to the maintenance team. This is a classic example of a 'near miss'.

2. **Injuries:** Any bodily injury to a staff, patient, visitor or another person in the hospital vicinity can be picked up to raisc an alarm.

   Example: A sharp edge of the stretcher is protruding, causing an accidental injury to a patient. Immediately after stabilizing the patient, the concerned staff available should raise an incident that needs to be addressed by the respective biomedical/maintenance team.

3. **Medication errors:** In a healthcare facility, the most common incidents are those related to any medication error. An organization can decide whether all medication errors, such as prescription errors, transcription errors, dispensing errors and administration errors, need to be raised as incidents

or only the actual incidents that have reached the patients should be raised.

Example: A missed dose by a nursing staff must be escalated, and an incident should be raised to avoid such incidents in the future.

4. **Equipment failure:** An equipment failure can be fatal in a healthcare organization. Hence, apart from regular preventive maintenance, it is very crucial to pick up any other equipment failure. Such alertness shall help to prevent any untoward incident.

   Example: A non-working monitor (even after proper preventive maintenance) in the ICU must be immediately addressed by the biomedical team, and hence an alert has to be raised at the earliest to fix the issue.

5. **Adverse reactions to drugs or treatments:** Any adverse drug reaction to a drug or treatment is a concern, and an incident must be raised to create awareness among healthcare workers and patients and/or family members.

   Example: If a patient is developing an allergy to an antibiotic, the antibiotic must be immediately stopped and an incident must be raised, so that the doctor, nurse, pharmacy, as well as the patient can get informed about the reaction.

6. **Fall:** In healthcare organizations, there must be zero tolerance for falls. Adequate measures must be taken 365*24*7 days to ensure that no patient slips or falls in the hospital.

   Example: A patient who went to the washroom and slipped on the floor will have concerns. So, the team must raise an incident and understand the reason for the fall, so that in the future such an incident can be avoided.

7. **Blood transfusion reactions or errors in patient care:** Any reaction to a patient post blood transfusion or any other error in patient care must be highlighted and brought to the notice of the relevant stakeholder.

   Example: A patient admitted for a total knee transplant receives four units of whole blood after surgery. Then the nurse notice rashes and itching all over the patient's body. The nurse should immediately stop the transfusion and inform the doctor. After the patient gets stabilized, they should raise an incident to help the team analyse the probable causes and how such a situation can be avoided in the future.

Some other reportable incidents are mentioned in the figure below.

Incident Reporting and Management Methods

An organization must define the process flow for raising any incident. The relevant staff members must be trained regularly on the process. The reporting mechanism may be online or paper-based. The organization should also enable its employees to report incidents with appropriate anonymity, to generate a greater number of incidents.

An incident should be reported as soon as possible after the adverse event occurs, but only after the situation has been stabilized. The reporter should objectively narrate the whole incident with the date/time/location of the incident, details of immediate actions taken to stabilize the situation, and their own remarks. If any medicine or equipment is involved, then it must be identified, retained, and not used until inspected and passed as safe and reusable by an appropriate qualified technical professional.

Figure 1. Category of Reportable Incidents

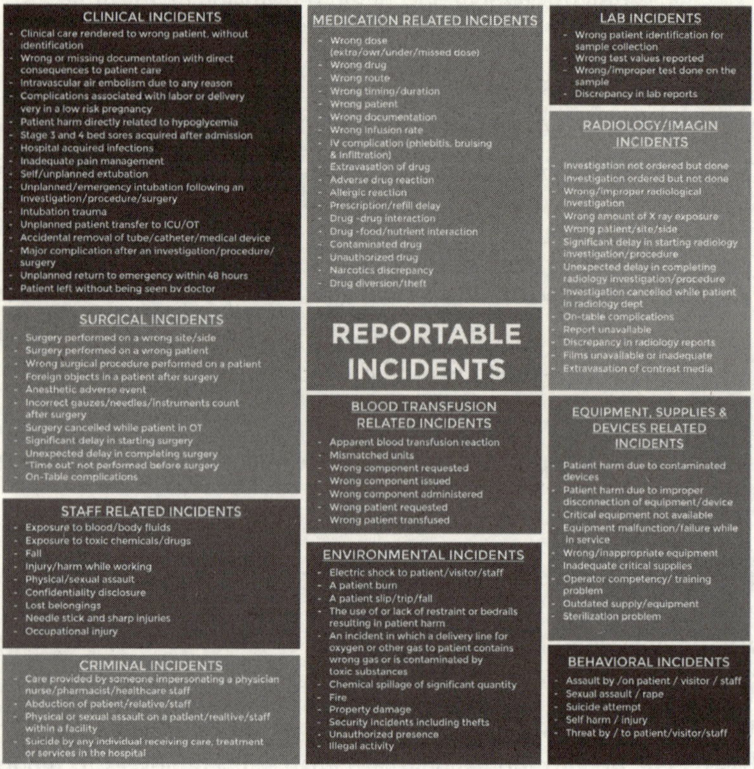

After an incident is reported, the Quality Department (or its equivalent) should review the same and assign a score based on its severity. It can then be forwarded to respective departmental heads(s) for appropriate investigations and RCA, which may jointly be conducted by the concerned departmental staff and quality team. Comments should be endorsed before closing the incident with information to all the concerned team members.

An improvement plan based on the closure of the incident should be implemented on the ground to prevent such incidents in the future. The whole process for closure of any incident and improvement made thereof should be done within an agreed time frame (suggested: three to seven days).

Figure 2. Incident Reporting Process Flow

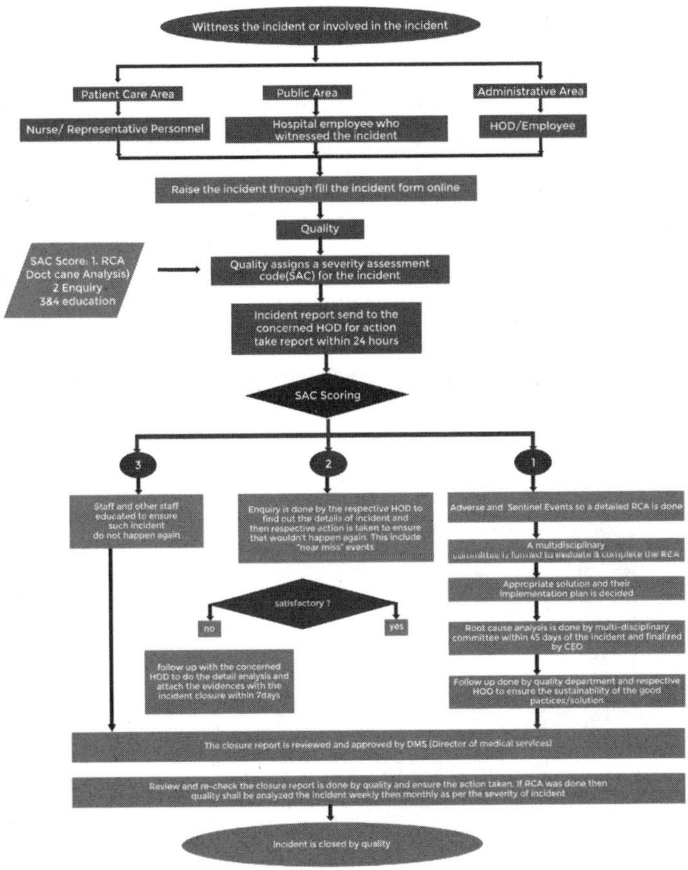

***Courtesy: Apollo Hospitals*

**Definitions adopted from the Joint Commission International 7th edition standards.*

Incident Analysis

Since we encourage the healthcare staff to raise a red flag every time anything goes wrong, there lies a bigger challenge and responsibility to analyse these incidents regularly. The results of the analysis must be shared with the leadership and respective stakeholders to minimize them in the future.

Periodically consolidated incidents should further be analysed to uncover risk levels and severity trends. The analysis can be done with different statistical tools, such as cause and effect diagram, scatter diagram, Pareto analysis or control charts. This analysis should be discussed with core committee members and further corrective and preventive actions should be envisaged.

Figure 3. Incident Patient Safety Incidents

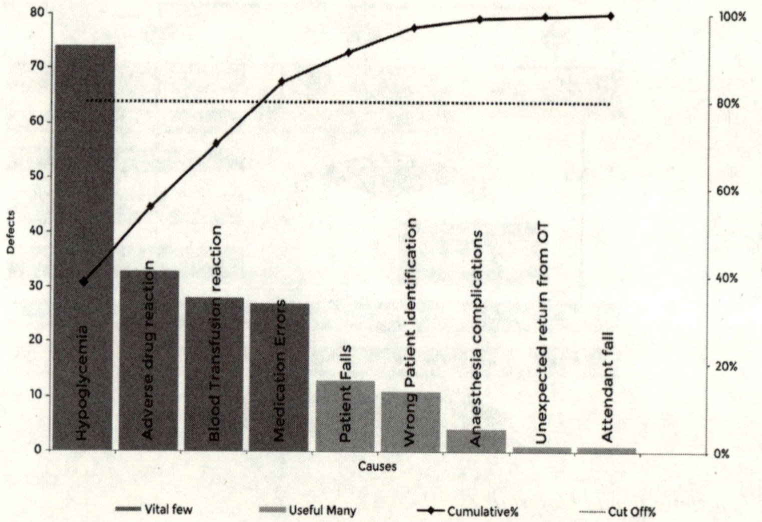

Figure 4. Severity Assessment Code

	Serious	Majcr	Moderate	Minor	Minimum
Patient*	Patients with **death** unrelated to the natural course of the illness and differing from the immediate expected outcome of the patient management **A national sentinel event** (refer to the national sentinel events list)*.	Patient suffering a **Major permanent loss of function** (sensory, motor physiologic or psycho-logic) unrelated to the natural course of the illness and differing from the expected outcome of patient management Suffering significant disfigurement as a result of the incident	Patient with **permanent reduction in bodily functioning** (sensory, motor, physiologic, or psycho logic) unrelated to the natural course of the illness and differing from the expected outcome of patient management **Any of the following:** Increased length of stay as a result of the incident Surgical intervention required as a result of the incident	Patient requiring **increased level of care** including:Review and evaluation Additional investigations Referral to another clinician	Patient with No injury or increased Level of career length of stay
Staff	Death of staff member related to work incident or suicide Hospitalization of 3 or more staff.	Permanent injury to staff member Hospitalization of 2 staff Lost time or restricted duty or illness for 2 or more staff Pending or actual prosecution Threatened or actual physical or verbal assault of staff requiring external or police intervention	Medical expenses, lost time or restricted duties or injury / illness for 1 or more staff	First aid treatment only with no lost time or restricted duties	No injury or review required
Visitor	Death of visitor or hospitalization of 3 or more visitors	Hospitalization of up to 2 visitors related to the incident Pending or actual prosecution	Medical expenses incurred or treatment of up to 2 visitors not requiring hospitalization	Evaluation and treatment with no expenses	No treatment required or refused treatment
Service	Complete loss of service or output	Major loss of agency / service	Disruption to users due to agency problems	Reduced efficiency or disruption	No loss of service
Financial	Loss of assets replacement value due to damage, fire, etc.>$1M Loss of cash, investments, assets due to fraud, over payment or theft>$100K Work cover claims>$100K	Loss of assets replacement value due to damage,fire,etc.$100K-$1M Loss of cash, investments, assets due to fraud, over payment or theft $10K-$100K Work cover claims $50K-$100K	Loss of assets replacement value due to damage,fire,etc.$50K to $100 K Loss of cash, investments,assets due to fraud,over payment or the $10K	Loss of assets replacement value due to damage, fire, etc. up-to $50K	No financial loss
Environmental	Toxic release off-site with detrimental effect. Fire requiring-evacuation	Off-site release with no detrimental effects Fire that grows larger than an incipient stage	Offsite release contained with outside assistance Fire incipient stage or less	Off-site release contained without outside assistance	Nuisance releases

An important role is played by the Quality Department members in grading these incidents based on the severity, and later with the help of various stakeholders, analysing them for outcomes.

All the incidents are primarily analysed based on:

1. Probability and Severity Scores
2. Outcomes
3. Category

1. Probability and Severity Scores

The probability score enables us to assess the likelihood of the incident's occurrence or recurrence while the severity score helps understand the extent to which an incident has had an impact on the organization.

Figure 5. Probability Categories

Probability	Definition
Frequent	Is expected to occur again either immediately or within a short period of time (likely to occur most weeks or months)
Likely	Will probably occur in most circumstances (several times a year)
Possible	Possibly will recur-might occur at sometime (may happen every 1to2 years)
Unlikely	Possibly will recur-could occur at sometime in 2to 5years
Rare	Unlikely to recur-may occur only in exceptional circumstances (may happen every 5 to30years)

Figure 6. Actions Required

	Action Required*
1	**Extreme risk** - Immediate action required - Notify Organization Director. Summary report for all SAC 1 incidents must be forwarded to Organization Director and Q&AD within 48 hours. Confidential **Root cause analysis (RCA)** Investigation must be under taken.
2	**High risk**-Notify Organization Director-**Detailed investigation required.** Ongoing monitoring of trended aggregated incident data may also identify and prioritize issues requiring a practice improvement project.
3	**Medium risk-Concise analysis** must be undertaken-Aggregate data analysis may also bed one for practice improvement purposes.
4	**Low risk-Concise analysis** must be undertaken -Aggregate data analysis may also bed one for practice improvement purposes.

Source: *NSW Health, November 2005.*

2. Outcomes

Outcome-based events may be no-harm events, near-miss events, adverse events, hazardous events or sentinel events (definitions adopted from the Joint Commission International 7th edition standards).

No-Harm Event: A no-harm event is a patient safety event that reaches the patient but does no harm.

Near-Miss Event: A near miss, or close call, is a patient safety event that was averted before it reached the patient.

Adverse Event: An adverse event is a patient safety event that results in harm to a patient.

Hazardous (or 'Unsafe') Event: Hazardous (or 'unsafe') event(s) are circumstances and conditions (not including a patient's disease condition) that increase the probability of an adverse event.

Sentinel Event: A sentinel event is a patient safety event (not primarily related to the natural course of the patient's illness or underlying condition) that reaches a patient and results in one of the following:

1. Death
2. Permanent harm
3. Severe temporary harm

3. Category

Incidents are categorized based on the nature/type of occurrences, such as, patient safety related, infection control related, process related, policy related, product/device related, facility related.

Let's look at an example to see how the above mechanism can be used to analyse the incidents over some time in a hospital.

Figure 7. Patient Safety Incidents

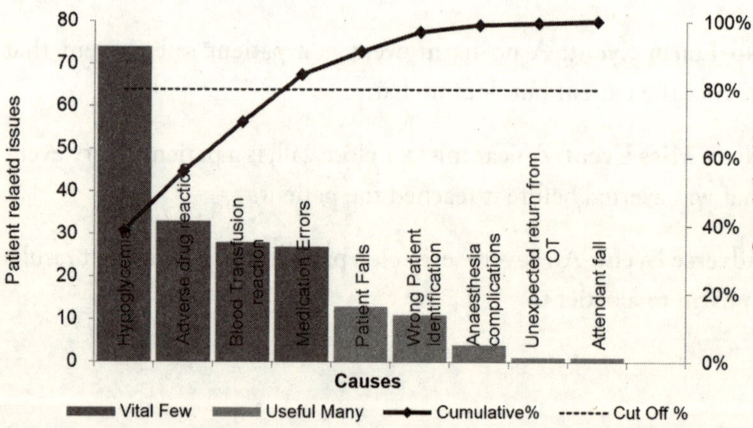

This is the analysis of patient safety incidents illustrated through a Pareto Chart. The Pareto Principle states that 80 per cent of the total incidents are responsible for 20 per cent of the total patient-related issues. Hence, by focusing on those factors, the administration can ensure a better and safer place for the patients and employees.

Figure 8. Sample Cause and Effect Analysis

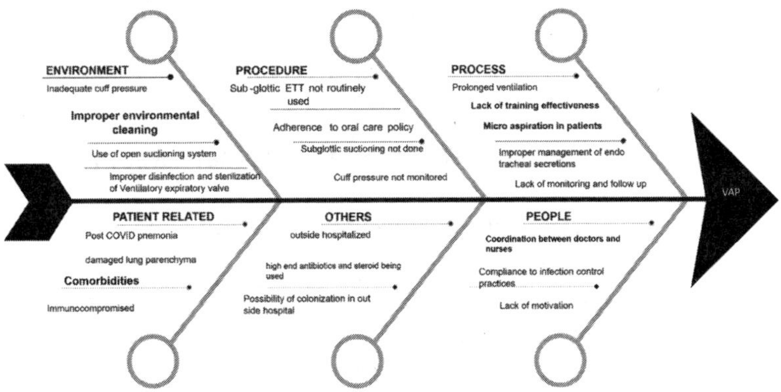

A Cause-and-Effect Analysis has been used here to find out the cause and effect of needle-stick injuries in a hospital over some time. Thus, raising the incidents related to needle-stick injuries helps the teams to understand the actual reasons, circumstances and scenarios, enabling them to devise an action plan to avoid such injuries in the future.

Trends are shared with the hospital leadership and the staff regularly to help other team members stay alert. Actions are taken as per recommendations.

Conclusion

It is important to not only act on an issue but also to escalate it—every time it occurs. Hence, for a safer healthcare system, we must ensure that all the staff is aware of the incident reporting system. They should be empowered to escalate any issue, feel accountable for the events, and be more vigilant in the future.

Raising an alarm over incidents that can jeopardize the safety of a patient, staff, or the organization is a responsibility of the healthcare workers. Encouraging a culture of safety that promotes such activities is highly needed and appreciated. To this end, it is the primary responsibility of the management to ensure that the staff is well aware of the culture of safety and feel empowered to raise an incident.

Figure 9. Sample Format of the Incident Report

EMPLOYEE INCIDENT REPORT FORM

Use this form to report accidents, injuries, medical situations, criminal activities, traffic incidents, or student behavior incidents. If possible, a report should be completed within 24 hours of the event.

Date of Report: ______________, 20___

PERSON INVOLVED

Full Name: ______________ Address: ______________________

Identification: ☐ Driver's License No. __________ ☐ Passport No. ________
☐ Other: ______________

Phone: (___) ___-____ E-Mail: __________

THE INCIDENT

Date of Incident: ______________, 20___ Time: ___:___ ☐ AM ☐ PM

Location: ______________________

Describe the Incident: ______________________

INJURIES

Was anyone injured? ☐ Yes ☐ No

If yes, describe the injuries: ______________________

WITNESSES

Were there witnesses to the incident? ☐ Yes ☐ No

If yes, enter the witnesses' names and contact info: ______________________

Page 1 of 2

References:

1. Andy Marker, 'Free Incident Report Templates', Smartsheet, 3 January 2017, https://www.smartsheet.com/free-incident-report-templates.
2. OSHA Training, Incident/Accident Analysis Program management, https://www.oshatrain.org/pdf/otn702w.pdf.
3. 'What is an Incident Report?', Safeopedia, 27 September 2021, https://www.safeopedia.com/definition/3310/incident-report
4. 'What is just culture? Changing the way we think about errors to improve patient safety and staff satisfaction', Brigham and Women's Faulkner Hospital, https://www.brighamandwomensfaulkner.org/about-bwfh/news/what-is-just-culture-changing-the-way-we-think-about-errors-to-improve-patient-safety-and-staff-satisfaction
5. Victoria Clarke, 'How to Write an Incident Report [+ Templates]', Venngage, 18 October 2021, https://venngage.com/blog/incident-report
6. 'Writing Effective Incident Reports', NFIC, https://www.nfic.org/docs/WrittingEffectiveIncidentReports.pdf
7. *JCI Accreditation Standards for Hospitals*, 7th edition (Joint Commission International, 2020), https://store.jointcommissioninternational.org/jci-accreditation-standards-for-hospitals-7th-edition/
8. T. Fetherston, 'The importance of critical incident reporting – and how to do it', *Community Eye Health* (2015), Vol. 28, No. 90, https://www.ncbi.nlm.nih.gov/pmc/articles/PMC4675258/
9. L. Donaldson, *An Organisation with a Memory: Report of an Expert Group on Learning from Adverse Events in the NHS Chaired by the Chief Medical Officer* (London, UK: The Stationery Office, 2000),

https://psnet.ahrq.gov/issue/organisation-memory-report-expert-group-learning-adverse-events-nhs-chaired-chief-medical

10. T. Fukami, M. Uemura and Y. Nagao, 'Significance of incident reports by medical doctors for organizational transparency and driving forces for patient safety', *Patient Safety in Surgery* (2020) Vol. 14, No. 13.

11

Collaborative Governance in Hospitals

Collaborative governance is an effective way of leading to mutual learning and shared experiences. Additionally, it clears the directions for institutional capacity building inside and outside agencies and organizations.

Integrated care is a goal of many healthcare systems. However, operationalizing and implementing integrated care remains challenging, especially in continuously evolving policy environments.

This chapter outlines the structure of collaborative governance in a hospital, its significance, communication flow, and other major aspects for strengthening collaborative governance by analysing challenges associated with it.

'Leadership is about making others better as a result of your presence, and making sure that impact lasts in your absence.'

—Sheryl Sandberg

Introduction

ALL THE PROCESSES of managing the organizations and their core business activities can effectively be accounted for in the collective governance. This framework of interlinking governing board and organizational leadership helps in constantly improving processes and performance pertaining to clinical and non-clinical operations, safety, as well as financial performance.

Collaborative Governance

What Is Collaborative Governance?

This is a very important process in decision-making, which puts the accountability and authority for various key clinical and administrative functions with doctors, leaders of supporting functions, and administrators.

It is an established belief that common goals and a shared vision can lead to a highly dedicated and dynamic workforce, that participation is empowering, and that people will make suitable decisions when adequate information is known and communicated.

In a healthcare setting, collaborative governance involves governing board, hospital leadership, clinical staff (doctors, nurses, paramedics), and administrative functions communicating with each other in an identified forum (committee) and coming together to work and achieve the manifold that an individual could achieve on its own.

Support, leadership and a forum are requisite for Collaborative Governance. Policy issue to be resolved is identified by the support. Bringing personnel together from multiple disciplines into the forum is taken care by the leadership. Then, the forum's members collaborate to curate policies, procedures and solutions.

Figure 1. Collaborative Governance

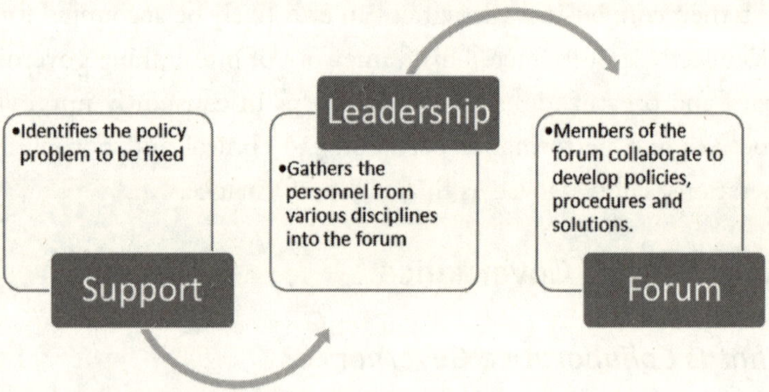

Advantages of Collaborative Governance

To improve the effectiveness and overall practice of hospital functioning is the intent of collaborative governance.

The pros of effective collaborative governance are that it promotes a seamless understanding of complex issues involving multiple stakeholders and allows them to work together and agree on solutions.

Hospital policymakers are benefitted as they are able to identify and target problems and act more effectively.

Stakeholders involved in creating solutions are likely to accept directions given or decisions made.

Thus, it can serve as a path to detect policy solutions having greater resistance and contribute to new perspectives on issues and policy solutions. It offers enhanced ways to implement strategies for change.

For officials attached to administration and management, collaborative governance serves as a genuine way in the policy making process by allowing a wider array of ideas and suggestions. Before implementation, it can be leveraged for testing ideas and analysing responses. For uninvolved personnel in formal administration and management, it allows a better understanding of the inner workings of administration and carries impact in the decision-making process.

It also enables them to see beyond healthcare institutions being merely a means for patient care service delivery. They have a sense of ownership of the system, further empowering them to be agents within the institution's decision making.

A collaborative commitment drives organizational change for the healthcare institution and affects resource reallocation.

Combining relevant skills and capacities and allowing specialization are some of the other benefits.

Overall, collaborative governance is an effective way of leading to mutual learning and shared experiences. Additionally, it clears the directions for institutional capacity building inside and outside agencies and organizations.

Figure 2. Advantages of Collaborative Governance

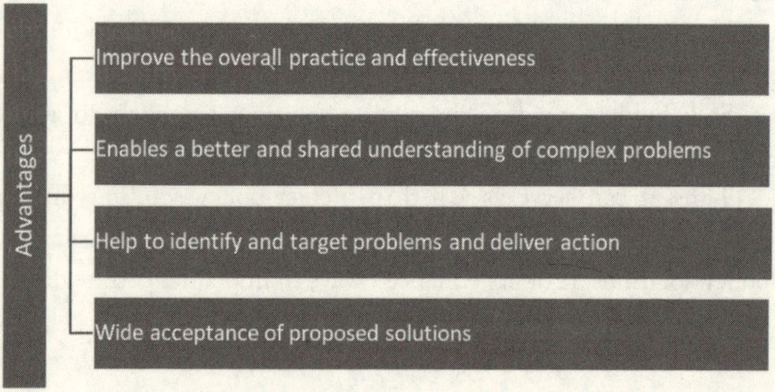

Disadvantages of Collaborative Governance

In relation to complex problems, collaborative governance is a time-consuming process, it may not result in an agreement to solutions, and the relevant departments/individuals may not implement the agreed-upon solutions.

Moreover, in a complex structure with many entities working together, individual roles can become unclear and confusing. Some individuals act largely in a personal capacity, while others may act on behalf of department/unit.

Powerful stakeholder groups may seek to manipulate the process. Sometimes, stakeholders can also begin to feel 'stakeholder fatigue'—a feeling they get when they are repeatedly consulted by different individuals/departments on similar issues. This kind of dynamic can be burdensome and time-consuming.

Structural issues can also affect agendas and outcomes. Open structures with loose leadership allow multiple participants to gain access to a fast-expanding agenda. Achieving the goals of such a wide agenda becomes more difficult as an increasing number of players struggle to resolve differences and coordinate the desired actions.

Furthermore, challenges arise for implementation when representatives are allowed to come and go with no real obligations to other collaborators. Accountability of participating members, unequal or hidden agendas, trust between members, power imbalances, language and cultural barriers are all issues that can arise in collaborative governance.

Collaborative Governance used in a Hospital: Sample Structure

Figure 3. Collaborative Governance Structure

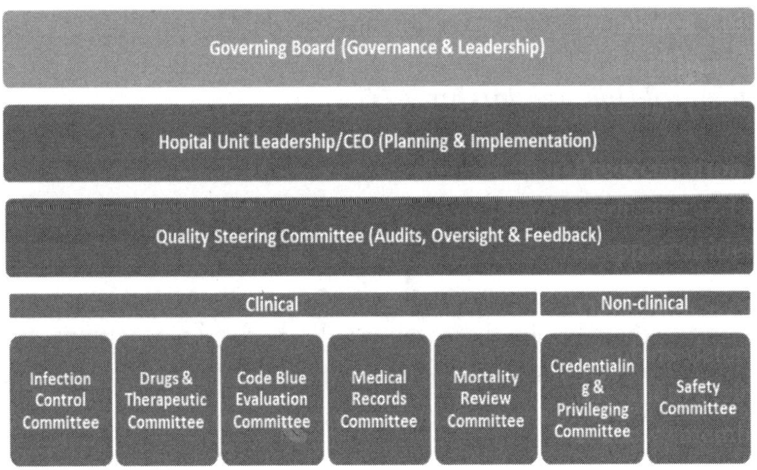

Courtesy: Apollo Hospitals

Governing Board

The governing board of the hospital develops and reviews the overall mission and strategy of the hospital and guides to attain long-term goals by designing strategic plans and taking crucial decisions.

The board doesn't get involved in managing the hospital's activities; rather, it oversees them. As part of their oversight duties, the board sets the job description for the hospital unit leadership and is responsible for hiring, firing and monitoring the unit leadership. It typically sets clear goals and expectations for the unit leadership, in keeping with strategic planning. The governing board assists and supports the unit leadership with input about management policies, procedures and decisions.

The board is responsible for approving the annual capital and operating budget; the strategic and operational plan; expansion, diversification, borrowings, acquisition, etc.; the Annual Quality Improvement; and the Patient Safety Programme. Further, the board should receive quarterly reports regarding the quality and patient safety programme—details on sentinel events or adverse events, IPSG compliance etc.—and use these to take further actions.

Hospital Unit Leadership/CEO

The CEO of a hospital is the highest-ranking executive position in the hospital's infrastructure. The CEO manages the day-to-day activities of the hospital and works with the governing board to develop and implement the hospital's strategies. The CEO is the highest leader that oversees the hospital's operations and programmes. The governing board receives regular summaries of the hospital's work, along with proposals for changes, from the CEO.

Communications Flow

Under collaborative governance, the communication flow is always bidirectional or to-and-fro. Thus, communications or directions are received from the board of directors and first passed on to the unit leadership/CEO. The CEO then disseminates the same information downwards to the other stakeholders. Similarly, in the reverse order, the communications, the reports and other information from different committees/programmes flows towards the governing board through the CEO.

Figure 4. Communication Flow

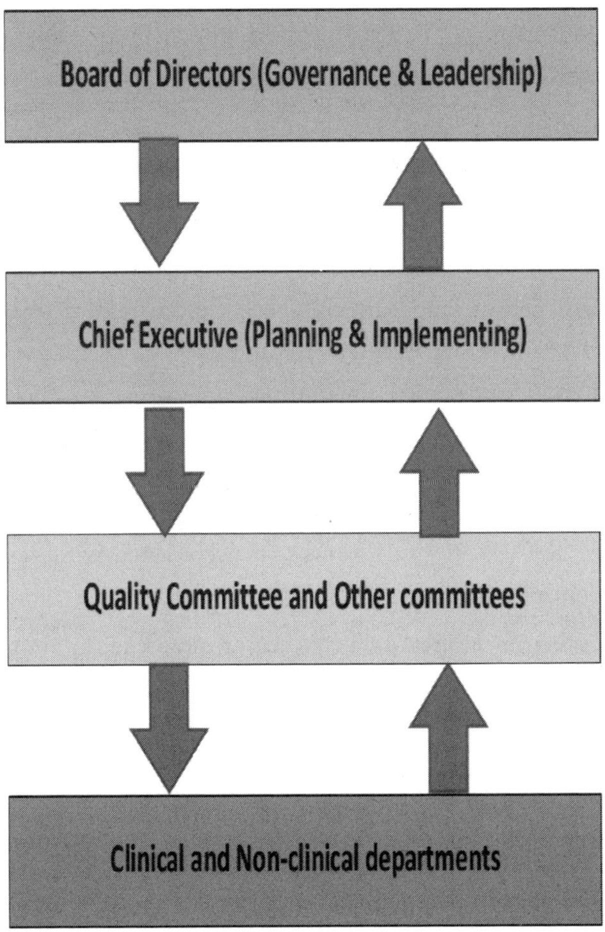
Board of Directors (Governance & Leadership)
Chief Executive (Planning & Implementing)
Quality Committee and Other committees
Clinical and Non-clinical departments

Courtesy: Apollo Hospitals

Important Committees and their Terms of Reference (TOR)

1. Drugs and Therapeutic Committee

This Drugs and Therapeutic Committee oversees the entire activities of the pharmacy and related functions, including the capture of medication errors. It is also involved in the preparation of drug formulary for the hospital.

Constitution of the Committee

The committee is composed of members drawn from among the employees of the hospital. The committee has representation from both medical and surgical specialties, a clinical pharmacist, pharmacist, nurse representative, purchase representative and a representative from the administration.

Responsibilities

- Periodically developing and reviewing a formulary or drug list for use in the hospital, in accordance with regulatory requirements and accreditation standards.
- Evaluating clinical data concerning new drugs or preparations requested for use in the hospital and presenting the same at committee meetings for decision-making.
- Performing analysis of Adverse Drug Reactions within a reasonable period of time, communicating the outcome to all stakeholders and periodically auditing adverse drug reactions in the hospital to make appropriate recommendations for corrective and preventive actions.
- Organizing prescription audit teams to conduct day-to-day audits in the outpatient, in-patient and emergency areas,

and present the outcomes of the audits during committee meetings.

- Evaluating periodically the medication management practices across the organization and initiating corrective and preventive actions based on the evaluation.
- Serving as an evaluative, educational and advisory capacity to the medical staff, pharmacy and administration in all matters pertaining to the purchase, stocking, distribution, prescription and use of drugs.
- Ensuring a proper system for storing, prescribing and dispensing of narcotics and controlled drugs.
- Establishing programmes and procedures that promote rational prescribing practices and cost-effective drug therapy.
- Initiating and directing drug use evaluation programmes and studies, and reviewing the results of such activities.
- Recommending policies and procedures for drug evaluation and clinical trials, and considering requests for such drug trials on hospital patients.

2. Code Blue (Cardiac Resuscitation) Evaluation Committee

The Code Blue (Cardiac Resuscitation) Evaluation Committee is responsible for analysing all cardiac arrests in which cardiopulmonary resuscitation (CPR) has been initiated. The analysis generally includes the cause for arrest, response time of the team, appropriateness of steps taken to resuscitate, outcome of the resuscitation and any equipment/infrastructure related issues that negatively influenced the process or the outcome of the resuscitation.

The goal of the committee is to identify preventable causes of cardiac arrest. It also identifies factors that were responsible for unsuccessful resuscitation, wherever applicable.

Constitution of the Committee

The committee is a multidisciplinary committee. This should have at least one senior Anaesthetist/Critical care specialist, one senior physician, emergency department physician and one senior nurse.

Responsibilities

- Developing and implementing the code blue protocol.
- Documenting requirements for resuscitation, ensuring organization-wide availability, and standardizing the design and content of crash carts across the organization.
- Identifying the processes for accessing and managing code blue.
- Providing efficient and effective basic life support measure in the event of a cardiac arrest.
- Evaluating the code blue responses and analysing immediately, or within reasonable time, all cardiac arrests where cardio-pulmonary resuscitation (CPR) was initiated across the hospital.
- Initiating appropriate corrective and preventive actions depending on the findings of the post-event analysis.
- Conducting the code-blue mock drills periodically.
- Providing training and orientation to code-blue team members.
- Evaluating the preparedness to notice early warning signs and arresting conversions of these calls to code blue.
- Educating and training the staff in Basic Life Support in accordance with the latest guidelines.
- Identifying training requirements in Advanced Cardiac Life Support based on the findings of the post-event analysis.

3. Infection Control Committee

The Infection Control Committee is the most important governing body of any hospital. This body is responsible for ensuring that the patients, visitors and employees of the hospital are prevented from any hospital-acquired infection through proper practice of the established asepsis and sanitation protocols. The committee also ensures that proper biomedical waste management is practised across the organization.

Constitution of the Committee

The committee generally consists of head of the hospital, head medical services, head quality, head nursing services, head emergency, intensivists, paediatric heads, paediatricians, paediatric intensivists, infectious disease physicians, clinical pharmacologists and infection control teams. In addition, the committee can also have members from different support departments such as CSSD, Laundry, Housekeeping, Engineering, Food & Beverages, OT, ICU and Microbiology, in order to ensure wider representation.

Responsibilities

The responsibilities of the Infection Control Committee include, but are not limited to:

- Ensuring proper implementation of infection control practices across the hospital, including proper biomedical waste management.
- Developing a hospital-wide infection control programme and maintaining surveillance over the programme.
- Regularly visiting and liaising with hospital departments, especially the following:

    - Engineering Department (equipment, water supply, air conditioning and environmental hygiene)
    - Catering Department (food hygiene)
    - Pharmacy (Antibiotics and Disinfectant policies)
    - Wards, Clinics, ICU, OT
    - Housekeeping (cleaning, waste disposable policies)
    - Laboratory Department (laboratory hazards, waste disposals)
- Developing a system for reporting, identifying and analysing the incidence and cause of nosocomial infections, including assignment of responsibility for the ongoing collection and analytic review of such data, and follow-up activities.
- Developing and maintaining a practical system for reporting, evaluating and recording infections among patients and personnel.
- Developing and implementing a preventive and corrective programme designed to minimize infection hazards, including establishing, reviewing and evaluating aseptic, isolation and sanitation techniques.
- Reviewing plans for renovation of existing facilities and new construction to ensure incorporation of infection control principles.
- Coordinating action on findings from the medical staff's review of the clinical use of antibiotics.
- Reviewing sensitivities of organisms specific to the facility and developing antibiotic assistance accordingly.
- Establishing policy criteria for distinguishing between nosocomial and community-acquired infections.

- Monitoring and following up on needle-stick injuries, bedsores, immunization of employees, hand-washing compliance, etc.
- Conducting regular auditing of housekeeping services, laundry services, engineering services for critical areas.
- Liaising with concerned consultants in case of proposed action, which may have implications for infection control in the hospital.
- Requesting an urgent meeting of the infection control committee in the event of major incidents/outbreaks.
- Organizing the relevant education of healthcare staff and encouraging reflexive practising of infection control measures.

4. Safety Committee

The Safety Committee undertakes proactive risk assessment, of both clinical and non-clinical nature, and executes necessary corrective and preventive actions. The committee also undertakes periodic training in safety aspects for all staff of the institution.

Constitution of the Committee

The committee consists of the head of the hospital, head of medical services, head of nursing services, quality head, head operations, and head engineering. In addition, it could also have members from different departments to ensure wide representation.

Responsibilities

- Developing and implementing a hospital-wide safety programme.
- Formulating and implementing proactive safety measures throughout the organization.

- Updating the safety programme at least once a year based on identified needs.
- Coordinating, supervising and implementing safety activities within the hospital. This is done by the Safety Officer, in consultation with the Safety Committee.
- Overseeing the safety programme, in addition to the duties outlined in the various safety policies. This is primarily the responsibility of the Safety Officer.
- Undertaking safety rounds, implementing changes as required, and conducting periodic and need-based training for all staff. These tasks are assigned to all members of the committee.
- Undertaking rounds of the hospital, identifying areas/ processes to be improved, and taking appropriate decisions. All members of the committee carry out these responsibilities, and their activities result in actions. Following up should be the responsibility of the committee.
- Addressing occupational health issues of employees and staff.

Committee Outcomes

Discussions of any committee should be documented in the form of minutes and circulated among its members and relevant stakeholders, who will be required to action-out the decisions made in the committee. These minutes should be circulated within a defined timeframe, as decided by the hospital leadership.

The convenor/executive officer should also maintain the tracker of action items of the committee and its status, which must be presented during the start of the next committee meeting.

Table 1. Sample Format for Meeting Minutes

<table>
<tr><td colspan="2">Committee Name:</td><td colspan="3"></td></tr>
<tr><td colspan="2">Date of Meeting: (DD/MM/YYYY)</td><td></td><td colspan="2">Time:</td></tr>
<tr><td colspan="2">Location:</td><td></td><td>Start:</td><td></td></tr>
<tr><td colspan="2">Minutes Prepared By:</td><td></td><td>End:</td><td></td></tr>
<tr><td colspan="2">Chairperson by:</td><td></td><td>Meeting No.</td><td></td></tr>
<tr><td colspan="5">1. Attendance at Meeting (add rows as necessary)</td></tr>
<tr><td colspan="5"></td></tr>
<tr><td colspan="5">2. Meeting Agenda</td></tr>
<tr><td colspan="5"></td></tr>
<tr><td colspan="5">3. Previous Meeting Discussions/Follow Ups (if any)</td></tr>
<tr><td colspan="5"></td></tr>
<tr><td colspan="4">4. Action Items/Decision Tracker (add rows as necessary)</td><td></td></tr>
<tr><td>Agenda</td><td>Discussions & Decisions</td><td>Responsibility</td><td>Due Date</td><td>Follow up</td></tr>
<tr><td></td><td></td><td></td><td></td><td></td></tr>
<tr><td></td><td></td><td></td><td></td><td></td></tr>
</table>

Signed by (Chairperson):
Date:

Courtesy: Apollo Hospitals

Review of Committee Effectiveness/Performance

A review of performance can be very helpful in enabling a committee to be constructively critical of its own operations, and thereby enhance its effectiveness, though monitoring can be a conscious activity at every meeting by the chair and members. The chair can encourage members from the outset to comment on or suggest improvements in the committee's operations at any time. Such comments should preferably be in writing to the chair or be made in face-to-face discussions.

When to Review

It is advisable to conduct reviews annually, but they can be scheduled more frequently as decided by the hospital leadership.

How to Review

Probably the simplest way to conduct a review is to produce a performance review survey document that all members of the committee complete and return by a set date.

While there are certainly other ways of undertaking a review (interviews of members, discussions at meetings, review by the leadership and the like), a good survey document is comprehensive and cost-effective, and gives all members the chance to make their views known.

Survey documents normally comprise several specific statements with which respondents indicate their level of agreement or disagreement.

For example:
Agenda papers have been well organized and easy to follow:

- strongly agree
- agree
- disagree
- strongly disagree

The kinds of information a survey document would usually cover include:

- (For any new members) whether the information package and induction session provided a satisfactory and timely introduction to the committee's work;
- whether the committee's business in the survey period has been consistent with its role as stated in the constitution/terms;
- whether committee time has been used efficiently and effectively to consider significant matters;
- the fitness of the membership as a group (in terms of skills, experience and other attributes) to deal with the committee's business;
- whether all members have come to meetings prepared, and have actively participated;
- whether members feel they can get any information/help they need from the chair, deputy chair or executive officer;
- whether agendas have been received within the deadline;
- whether agendas have been clear and sufficiently comprehensive and detailed to allow members to understand the issues and make well-informed decisions;

- whether the minutes have been accurate and clear;
- whether the minutes have been received within the deadline;
- whether the meetings have been efficiently chaired;
- whether the chair has given all members the chance to participate in meetings;
- whether the chair has ensured that the time spent on items at meetings has generally been appropriate to their significance;
- whether the atmosphere at meetings has been conducive to open and productive debate; and
- whether the behaviour of all members at meetings has been courteous and professional.

The list above is not exhaustive, and you may wish to add to it. You'll probably want to allow space in the survey document for members to make any additional comments or suggestions they have, or to elaborate on or explain responses already made.

Administering the Survey

Ideally, every member of the committee should complete the survey so that its outcomes reflect the full range of views. However, practices vary from committee to committee. Give respondents a reasonable time to complete and return it and be prepared to allow a little extra time to remind those who have not returned it by the closing date.

Analysing and Reporting on the Outcomes of the Survey

Once you've received the responses to your survey, you'll need to analyse them, write up a brief report and present it to the committee at the earliest opportunity. The same should also be submitted to the hospital leadership.

References:

1. 'Collaborative governance', Wikipedia, https://en.wikipedia.org/wiki/Collaborative_governance
2. Collaborative Governance, https://www.mghpcs.org/ipc/programs/committees/index.asp
3. The University of Western Australia, https://www.governance.uwa.edu.au/committees
4. 'Implementing collaborative governance: models, experiences, and challenges', Taylor & Francis, https://www.tandfonline.com/doi/full/10.1080/14719037.2021.1878777
5. 'Collaborative Governance', Participedia, https://participedia.net/method/150
6. Innovations in American Government Awards (2022), https://www.innovations.harvard.edu/sites/default/files/workingpaper_2_donahue.pdf
7. 'Collaborative governance as a policy strategy in healthcare', *Emerald Insight*, https://www.emerald.com/insight/content/doi/10.1108/JHOM-10-2018-0313/full/html#:~:text=%E2%80%9CCollaborative%20governance %E2%80%9D%20is%20seen%20as,several%20policy%20fields%20including%20healthcare.&text=Instead%2C%20collaborative%20governance%20builds%20on,Ulibarri%20and%20Scott%2C%202017)
8. D. Gordon, S. McKay, et al, 'Collaborative Governance for Integrated Care: Insights from a Policy Stakeholder Dialogue'.
9. Jeanette Ives Erickson, et al, 'The Value of Collaborative Governance/Staff Empowerment', *The Journal of Nursing Administration* (March 2003), Vol. 33 No. 2, pp. 96–104, https://www.researchgate.net/publication/10903310_The_Value_of_Collaborative_GovernanceStaff_Empowerment

10. H. Warsono, 'Collaborative Governance Framework in Health Care: A Qualitative Exploration of Hospital Pharmacy Management Reform at Hospital Setting in Indonesia', *Systematic Reviews in Pharmacy* (2020), Vol. 11 No. 4, pp.337–341, https://www.bibliomed.org/?mno=101619

11. Ted Ball, 'Designing and Aligning Collaborative Governance Strategies, Structures, Cultures and Skills', Quantum Transformation Technologies, http://quantumtransformationtechnologies.com/what-is-the-current-environment-within-your-lhinhealth-link-community/

12. L. Eisenstein, 'The Role of Governance in Healthcare Organizations', Board Effect, 28 June 2019, https://www.boardeffect.com/blog/role-governance-healthcare-organizations/

13. N. Price, 'Roles & Responsibilities of a Board of Directors for a Hospital,' Board Effect, 31 January 2018, https://www.boardeffect.com/blog/roles-responsibilities-board-directors-hospital/#:~:text=The%20board%20of%20trustees%20is,making%20strategic%20plans%20and%20decisions

12

Measuring Reliability in Healthcare: Think–Plan–Act Differently

Healthcare is inherently interdependent and increasingly complex. In healthcare delivery, the implementation of high reliability principles is considered as an effective strategy for minimizing any sort of harm to patients and staff. Hence, the High Reliability framework encompassing the functionalities of high-risk yet secure systems curated via in-depth research is required.

Implementation of high-reliability methods includes multiple strategies to anticipate and mitigate threats such as simulation and observation of practices; development of Standard Operating Procedures (SOPs), checklists, diligent reporting of errors, near-misses and hazards, and empowerment of team members to work to the full scope of their capabilities.

'Something is wrong if workers do not look around each day, find things that are tedious or boring, and then rewrite the procedures. Even last month's manual should be out of date.'

—Taiichi Ohno

Introduction

A HIGH-RELIABILITY ORGANIZATION (HRO) is defined as an organization with reliable systems and processes that support consistent operations while identifying and correcting potentially catastrophic errors before they happen.

The High Reliability framework elaborates the functionalities of high-risk yet secure systems curated via in-depth research conducted in non-healthcare systems such as nuclear submarines, aircraft carriers, and aviation; healthcare shares the complex and high-risk nature of these industries, where a small error or miss can lead to a disastrous situation.

Aviation safety expert John Nash in his book *Why Hospitals Should Fly* notes that healthcare organizations can achieve high reliability if leaders embrace the lessons learnt in other high-risk organizations. As per Joint Commission International (JCI), 'High reliability in healthcare means maintaining consistently high levels of safety and quality over time and across all services and settings.'

With the surge in the number of healthcare providers over the last twenty years, numerous organizations have been striving to become HRO delivering effective and efficient quality care.

Foundational Elements of an HRO

HROs are based on six foundational elements:

Sensitivity to Operations: HROs work quickly to detect problems and potential errors, to reduce the actual number of errors. Regular interactions with staff and patients improve operational awareness at the top of the organization, concerning the issues that may be present.

Reluctance to Simplify: HROs avoid overly simple explanations for failures. This does not depict that HROs are against streamlining or simplifying processes; rather, they don't attribute failure to any particular cause.

Preoccupation with Failure: Instead of reacting, HROs focus on predicting and eliminating catastrophes. 'Near misses' are considered as opportunities to enhance existing systems and processes.

Deference to Expertize: HROs promote a culture where team members defer to individuals with more knowledge or experience relevant to a critical situation, irrespective of any rank, title or position. It allows members to question others about safety practices, such as washing hands or properly completing a patient chart, without the fear of anyone's position in the hierarchy.

Commitment to Resilience: In case of any unexpected turn of events, HROs continue to operate. A commitment to resilience helps team members improvise and quickly develop plans to respond to any unanticipated situations.

Collective Mindfulness: Collective mindfulness is operating 'mindfully' and making necessary amendments in a timely manner to manage the unexpected in a challenging and extremely competitive environment. It creates a safety culture and sustains high reliability in the organization. Collective mindfulness also enables leaders to continuously identify potential errors and unsafe conditions before they can pose a risk to the organization.

Figure 1. Elements of HRO

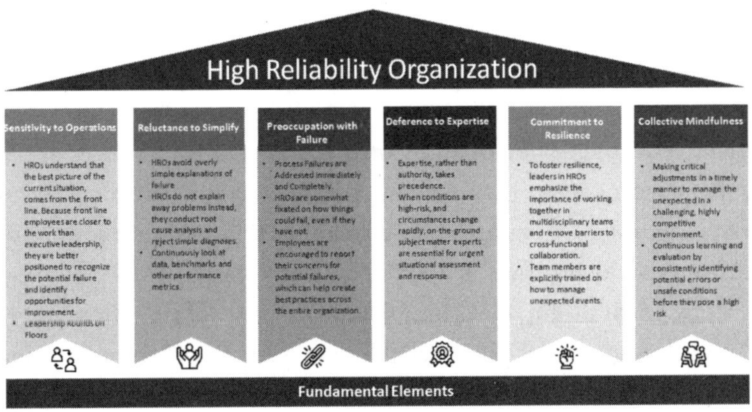

These six elements serve as the foundational principles for developing an HRO strategy for any organization. In healthcare, the high-reliability framework focuses on improvements in patient safety through the elimination of variation in care delivery, while improving clinical results and reducing cost. Reaching this level of clinical and operational excellence often requires a transformation of culture, organically changing the attitudes, beliefs, goals and ethics of an organization.

Measuring Reliability

Reliability is defined as error-free operation over time. The effectiveness of the processes and occurrence of failures is the key to measuring the reliability of the system.

Reliability = Number of actions that achieve the intended result ÷ Total number of actions taken

It is convenient to use failure rate (calculated as 1 minus Reliability) as an index, expressed as an order of magnitude. Thus, 10^{-1} means one defect per 10 attempts, 10^{-2} is one defect per 100 attempts, 10^{-3} is one defect per 1,000 attempts, and so on.

In terms of healthcare, a process measuring 10^{-1} fails to be effectively applied for one out of every 10 patients. For example, if 90 per cent of surgery patients get their prophylactic antibiotic within an hour of surgical incision, the reliability of that process as measured by defect rate is 10^{-1}.

The Institute for Healthcare Improvement (IHI) uses a three-tiered strategy for designing reliable care systems, with processes and procedures in place intended to:

1. **Prevent failure** (a breakdown in operations or functions) using strategies to ensure that patients receive the standardized process of care. More emphasis is given to determining whether individual doctors or nurses adhere to defined policies and processes. This typically results in 10^{-1} performance.
2. **Identify and mitigate failure** by 'error-proofing', and removing uncertainties in the way work is being done, diminishing the need for 'workaround' solutions.

To give few examples of such strategies:

- Reminders: Calling patients the day before their admission appointments to reduce no-shows and late arrivals.
- Differentiation: To minimize scepticism when actions, parts or numbers are alike segregating the Look Alike & Sound Alike (LASA) drugs by colour coding, Tall-Man Lettering, etc.
- Intelligent restrictions: Implementing computer auto-pops or alerts when two contraindicated medications are prescribed together, or a medication is prescribed to which the patient is allergic.
- Discharge scheduling
- Use of safe surgery checklist before any invasive procedures.

These strategies can help in hard-wiring the reliability of a process to or towards 10^{-2}.

3. **Redesigning the process** based on the critical failures identified: Performance at 10^{-3} and beyond involves identifying the failure modes of the standardized process. At this level, Failure Modes and Effects Analysis (FMEA) is a pivotal tool. It is a systematic way to evaluate a process in order to identify where and how it might fail and to assess the relative impact of different failures. The Healthcare FMEA (HFMEA) is applied when:

    - A new process, function or service with an associated hazard has not yet been implemented.

- A current process, function or service undergoes modifications/changes due to past failure or sentinel events.
- A current process, function or service is being used in a new or similar location.

Interventions for Hardwiring High Reliability within the Organization: *The Apollo Model*

Identify High-Risk Areas and Processes

The first step in creating an HRO is to conduct an assessment to evaluate how your current processes work within your organization and where errors are likely to occur. The crucial tasks involve identifying high-risk areas that could cause harm to all the stakeholders—patients, visitors, employees.

You can filter the identified events through a grid SAFER™ Matrix, designed by the JCI, which clarifies the significance and exigencies to rectify the problem and evaluate the risk of any undesirable outcomes.

Learn from Safety Events

> **'To err is human, to cover up is unforgivable, and to fail to learn is inexcusable.'**
>
> —Prof. Liam Donaldson, WHO Envoy for Patient Safety

Nobody is perfect, and we all make mistakes. Healthcare being a complex system, some degree of error is inevitable. Recording safety events, whether they have resulted in harm or not, offers an important insight into what can backfire, and how to prevent such events. If we do not know what kind of problems are happening, how often it is happening, the pattern of occurrence, it is impossible to design an 'error-proof' system that makes healthcare safer.

For example, if there are no reports of medication errors, no one will know if there is a problem with the medication transcription process. Therefore, the first step in improving patient safety is to put in place an open incident reporting system for reporting all adverse incidents and near misses.

At Apollo Hospitals, all our staff has been encouraged to report problems, failures and mistakes. Safety is everyone's responsibility, no matter how junior or senior they are. No one is criticized or punished for reporting a problem. Non-punitive culture is embedded in the fabric of organizational values and beliefs. The safety events analysis is shared with the staff on a regular basis. We discuss why any process doesn't perform up to the mark and what changes were introduced considering the analysis.

Evaluate the Culture of Safety Regularly

A safety culture assessment provides an organization with a basic understanding of the safety-related perceptions and attitudes of its staff. For HROs, the safety culture is emphasized and prioritized throughout all levels of the business, from frontline workers to managers, administrators and executives.

When it comes to becoming an HRO in healthcare, the JCI has developed a framework for healthcare organizations to follow:

1. The leadership must be committed to the goal of zero harm.
2. There should be a culture of safety, wherein all staff feel that they can speak up and bring attention to issues or challenges that may reflect negatively on the organization without fear of retribution.

3. The workforce must be empowered to employ Robust Process Improvement (RPI) tools to address any improvement opportunities that could result in significant change. (RPI is a combination of Lean Six Sigma and change management that addresses performance improvement, including efficiency, empowerment, quality and behaviour.)

Trust is the cornerstone of a safety culture. Trust motivates staff to be cautious, report risks and analyse opportunities for improvement. When leadership responds positively to these improvement opportunities rather than blaming the staff, employees are motivated to report, which in turn results in system-wide improvement. This builds even greater levels of trust between the employees and the leadership.

For hospitals, creating a safety culture has many benefits. It makes the work environment healthier for all staff members while improving the patient experience. When employees feel safe, supported and cared for at work, they provide better and safer care to patients; and when patients receive better care, they report higher satisfaction levels overall—indicating a clear, reciprocal relationship between the patient experience and the employee experience.

Many organizations utilize the survey tool by the Agency for Healthcare Research and Quality (AHRQ) to create their patient safety scores. The survey tool has a set of questionnaires to evaluate staff perceptions of patient safety. These survey tools offer valuable insights to leaders regarding specific dimensions of a culture of safety, like hand-off communication, teamwork, reporting of errors, and management support of patient safety. If any particular area like hand-off communication is detected as a challenge within your organization, focus on curating standardized systems to enhance the process. For example, purposeful communication techniques such as SBAR (Situation Background Assessment Recommendation) and interdisciplinary rounds may be used to enhance the process of hands-off communication in between shifts and staff.

In the chapter on safety culture, a detailed guide is given on how to conduct a safety culture survey in your organization.

Ameliorate Teamwork

For achieving high reliability, particularly in healthcare organizations, teamwork is essential. Clear communication, management of conflict, seeking information from team members—these are all important to efficient team functioning in a healthcare setup.

Healthcare is inherently interdependent and increasingly complex. No one individual can assure the highest standard of care for a patient or protect the patient from all potential harms stemming from complex treatment or procedures. It involves a multitude of professional roles, configured in different structures and completing varied tasks.

For example, transitions of care between care areas or shift changes in healthcare settings are susceptible to communication failures that can directly cause harm to the patient. In these high-risk interactions, critical information about the patient's status and plan of care can be miscommunicated, leading to delays in treatment or resulting in an adverse event. Hierarchy (e.g., between professional roles and over occupational tenure) can hinder the assertive communication necessary for safe patient care. By strengthening teamwork and coordination, we will be able to deliver a better patient outcome in a complex healthcare system.

Rather than using status or member rank, HROs encourage their staff to use expertize as a source of power to determine value to the group. It recognizes the value of knowledge, regardless of the position of the team member within the organization. HROs recognize that the knowledge and actions of one team member are important to consider in decision-making regarding safety.

Be an Advocate for Patient Safety and Speak Up

Everyone plays an important role in making healthcare safe. That includes doctors, nurses, healthcare technicians and healthcare executives. Make sure you convey about the unsafe practices to your manager as it can prevent patients from any risk. Any staff member can prevent a potentially unsafe process or adverse event by just ensuring accuracy of the process before proceeding.

There are many such run by WHO, JCI and IHI (Institute for Healthcare Improvement) to encourage all the patients and relatives, as well as the healthcare staff, to speak up when there is a potential threat to the safety of the patient. The 'Speak Up™' programme, sponsored by JCI, encourages patients to be involved in their own healthcare. The campaign advises patients that they have the right to receive information about care in their preferred language, know the name(s) of the caregiver(s), receive treatment for pain, be informed about the care they should expect. Their concerns will be heard, and they will receive an up-to-date list of their current medications and be treated with respect.

Apollo HRO Model: An Example

Combating the Menace of COVID-19 Pandemic through a High-Reliability Blueprint

As the second wave of the pandemic unfolded, India moved from being the 'pharmacy of the world' by dispatching medicines and vaccines to numerous countries to becoming the 'epicentre of the coronavirus pandemic'. India reported over 30 million cases of COVID-19 as of June, 2021, with more than 2.9 million recoveries and about 402,000 fatalities. After a relatively controlled first wave, the country had been reporting record numbers of new infections and deaths since April 2021 as it experienced the second wave.[1]

In this war field of COVID-19 pandemic, bullets had been replaced by a deadly virus and bulletproof jackets by Personal Protective Equipment (PPEs), and war soldiers by frontline healthcare staff. End results were loss of human lives, suffering, uncertainty and economic disruption. The healthcare industry had never seen such a significant disruption of its clinical and business processes in its day-to-day operations.

Under these circumstances, it was very difficult to understand what strategy to follow. Preparing for an unpredictable pandemic is a big challenge and a difficult exercise. In healthcare delivery, implementation of high reliability principles is considered as an effective strategy for minimizing any sort of harm to patients and staff.

Apollo Hospital's HRO strategy to handle the COVID-19 pandemic in India deployed several strategies. The HROs recognize that humans are fallible; therefore, they create systems to recognize failure at early stages in the processes and contain damage.

With the pandemic upon us, our hospitals were facing an unprecedented safety threat. The severity of the disease in those with the infection overwhelmed healthcare systems and frontline healthcare providers, and exhausted resources—both human and material. We present an outline of how Apollo Hospitals was prepared for this pandemic in advance in many ways, compared to others healthcare organizations.

Figure 2. Our Preparedness Measures for Management of Epidemic

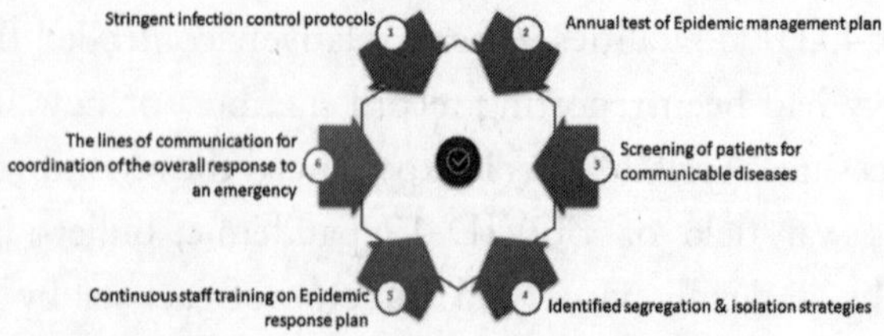

Courtesy: Apollo Hospitals

The six fundamental elements of the HRO model discussed above are vital for any improvement. In the context of pandemic preparation and implementation of high-reliability methods in our hospital, we included multiple strategies to anticipate and mitigate threats such as simulation and observation of practices; development of Standard Operating Procedures (SOPs), checklists, diligent reporting of errors, near-misses and hazards, and empowerment of team members to work to the full scope of their capabilities.

Figure 3. Apollo Hospitals: High-Reliability Framework

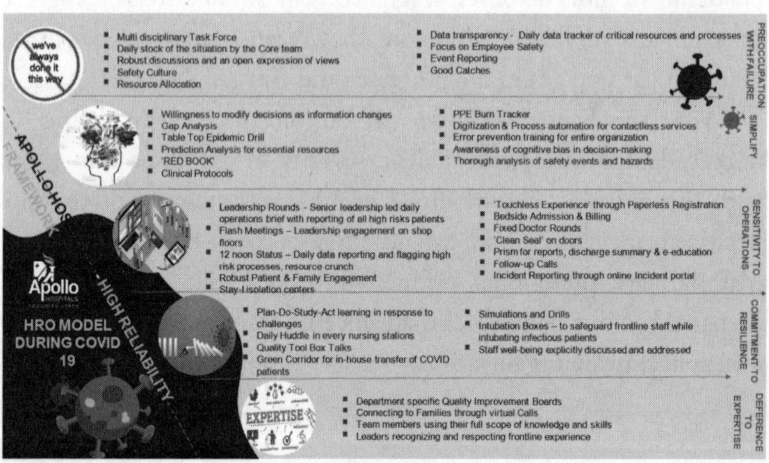

Courtesy: Apollo Hospitals

Preoccupation with Failure

Teams that are preoccupied with failure identify that even the best-in-class plans are at risk of failing and they vigilantly monitor for potential lapses in reliability. Keeping this in mind, a multidisciplinary task force was created, which consisted of the individuals from senior leadership, Quality, Operations, Medical, Nursing, Infection Prevention and Control, Information Technology, Innovation, Facility Safety, Service Excellence, to name a few. The core team met daily through virtual forums to discuss and review the policies, any active issues, and provide real-time multidisciplinary resolutions. Robust discussions were held, and an open expression of views and ideas was welcomed without fear of repercussions. This team also was responsible for resource allocation, managing admission and discharge including bed shortages, staff allocation, etc.

Figure 4. Governance

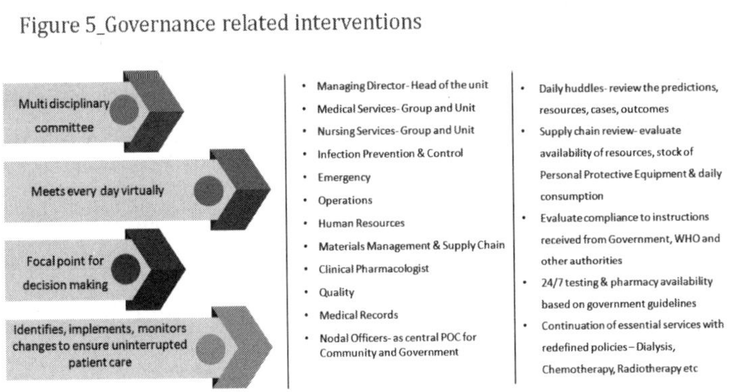

Courtesy: Apollo Hospitals

Reluctance to Simplify

The pandemic has proven that systems may fail in ways that have never happened before.

When the first case of COVID-19 was reported, we initiated a gap analysis, keeping in mind hospital-related risks. Tabletop drills were conducted to assess the status of our resources (PPEs, ventilators, pulse oximeters, thermal scanners, etc.); staff training and process automation to ensure safe and minimal patient contact and staff experience.

Demand for PPEs, and essential supplies such as oxygen, ventilators and critical medications increased significantly and created an increased pressure on our hospitals. To meet this challenge, predication analysis was done for all essential supplies, consumables and PPEs to forecast the demand. It helped in close monitoring and ensuring availability of adequate end-to-end supply chain. A PPE Burn tracker was put in place to keep a tab on consumption and ensure availability across all units.

A *Red Book* was designed that included everything from the screening criteria and protocols to infection control protocols and clinical algorithm to guide judicious testing and treatment, PPE usage as per the function of the area, and PPE consumption tracking to area-specific protocols. The *Red Book* was reviewed and revised frequently, with updated guidelines and processes. Twenty versions of the *Red Book* were released, with updated guidelines and modified processes.

Clinical protocols for adults, paediatric and neonates were developed, reviewed and updated as and when required. Forty versions of updated guidelines have been released as of now.

Sensitivity to Operations

In operations, we closely understand the potential failure modes and anticipate how changes in one aspect can affect another.

Daily Leadership Rounds were conducted by senior leadership. Leaders visited the shop floors, observed the work, and engaged with the staff. This helped a lot in boosting staff morale, especially during these difficult times. Frontline staff were able to speak up about the challenges they were facing and offer suggestions. Problems were investigated so that effective solutions could be developed. Leaders ensured that staff had the knowledge, resources and skills needed to carry out processes in a reliable fashion, at all times. Care, compassion and respect towards our staff was clearly exhibited by the senior teams, by acknowledging their expertize and accepting inputs for solutions.

As an initial step in pandemic planning, our Quality Teams identified processes in which high reliability was critical. These included resuscitations and intubations, donning and doffing of PPE, and ensuring staff safety by prevention of contamination and patients' strolls through the hospital. Strategies were put in place to reduce the likelihood of error in high-risk processes (e.g., standardized workflows, checklists, direct observation of PPE donning/doffing, and Code Green announcements to name few).

For simpler and patient-friendly processes, multiple technology-enabled process automations were implemented, e.g., virtual-consultations, paperless registrations, online screening, thermal screens at the hospital entrances, bedside admission and discharge billing, digital and fixed doctors' rounds. Technology that digitizes processes at the point of care also helped reduce waiting times, paperwork and administrative tasks. Empowering our healthcare providers with the right tools helped in a seamless and positive patient experience.

Figure 5. Process-related Interventions

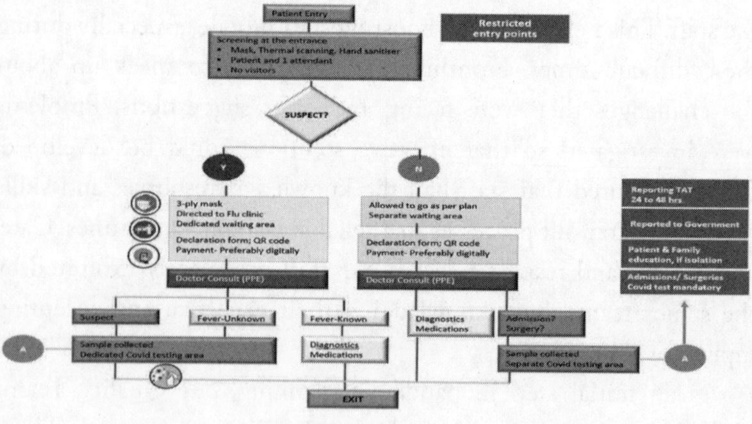

Modified process flow at entrances & exits

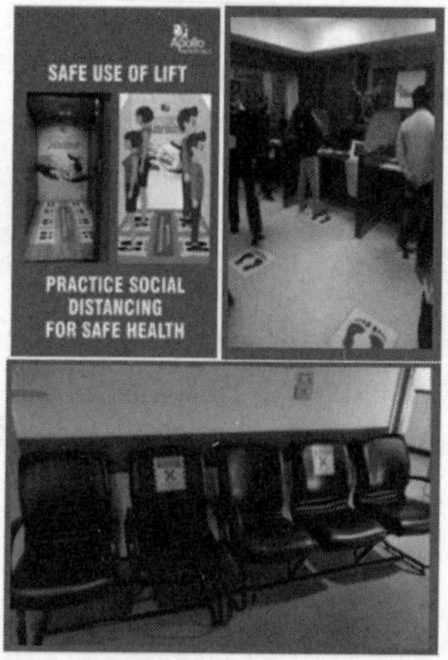
SAFE USE OF LIFT
PRACTICE SOCIAL DISTANCING FOR SAFE HEALTH

Courtesy: Apollo Hospitals

Through a 24x7 application with chatbot, users could get quick access to their health-information, driven by a self-learning AI-engine. It offered virtual consultation, online pharmacy and medical tests at home.

Online Screening: Alarmed by the number of people tested positive during manual screening, we also developed an in-house online self-screening for COVID-19. For scheduled appointments/admissions, an online screening link was pushed to patient's mobile for self-screening based on predefined criteria. Walk-in patients scanned a QR code at the entrance for screening. If any one of the screening criteria was marked positive, the patient was categorized as Grade-1, and was directed to the Fever Clinic.

Paperless Registration: For a 'touchless experience', as we have experienced while flying, we also installed kiosks/tabs in multiple locations for patients to self-register with current compliance of 87 per cent.

Clean-Seal: To boost patient confidence, our patient rooms were sealed after cleaning. The 'seal' was an indication that no one had entered the room before.

Bedside Admission/Billing: Waiting for admission paperwork or a bed could be emotionally draining and physically challenging for a patient. To eliminate the waiting time as well as crowding in the waiting area, we initiated bedside admission/billing processes. This drastically reduced our waiting time, helped move the patient and family comfortably out of public areas, and enabled initiation of care as soon as the patient arrived. Updates regarding bills were digitized and settled at the bedside. Fixed doctor rounds ensured that families got to meet to have an update on the patient's condition. Digital updates and calls were also done for families of COVID-19 patients. A digital application was launched to make it easier for the family members to ask questions and updates.

Prism: An online portal that provides access to patient's lab reports, discharge summaries and other clinical documents directly from the hospital—anywhere, anytime. The same could also be viewed on Apollo's 24/7 application.

E-education: E-brochures used to educate patients and their families were also uploaded on Prism. A robust communication team was created to give patient information to their families. This included using all available channels such as a telephone hotline, the hospital's website, social media and text messaging. The aim was to be transparent about the patient's condition and care plan.

Constant Monitoring: Patients could be monitored in home isolation based on the guidelines from the Indian Council of Medical Research/Ministry of Health and Family Welfare, for asymptomatic, post-discharged patients and COVID-19 positive/ suspected patients.

Follow-up Calls: Patient's primary doctor did a virtual follow-up call with the patient a week after discharge to get an update on their clinical condition.

Medical teams regularly observed simulations and patient care involving new processes. Infection Control Nurses and Link Nurses checked for sustainability of correct donning and doffing of PPEs. Multiple videos were created and circulated among the staff to ensure compliance to correct PPE donning and doffing processes, patient screening, physical distancing, cleaning and disinfection protocols. Cumulatively, more than 10,000 hours of training was conducted across all our locations continuously.

Staff were empowered to report challenges and deviations from the hospital protocols and policies, errors, near misses, and hazards through an online Apollo Incident Reporting System (AIRs), and these were reviewed by the respective process owners within 24–48 hours. Staff was also encouraged to provide suggestions for improvement. All incidents reported in COVID-19 areas were thoroughly analysed and discussed. The reporting had increased up to 38 per cent with zero adverse and sentinel events.

Fire Safety Drills and staff training were conducted in COVID-19 ICUs and wards for emergency response in all thirty-eight locations covering more than 3,000 frontline staff.

Commitment to Resilience

HROs are resilient systems: They have potential to immediately recover from setbacks or other challenging situations. They are able to do so through continuous training and re-training. Taking a cue from the HRO model, our frontline staff was trained through simulated systems and other innovative techniques. The aim was to develop strategies, techniques and systems that could prevent us from any catastrophe and system-wide failures.

Figure 6. Staffing and Training

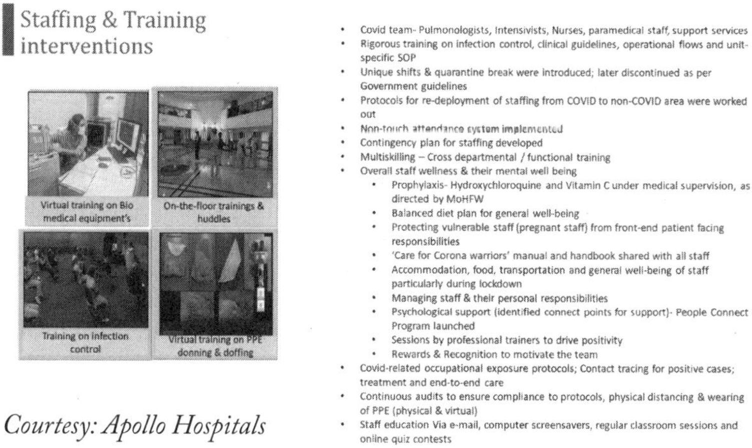

Courtesy: Apollo Hospitals

Process changes and information was shared using electronic platforms daily during morning huddles. The huddle team discussed the challenges, opportunities and concerns for the day ahead. The discussions at the ward level were reported to hospital leadership, including the unit head, medical director, nursing director and quality head during the leadership rounds.

Daily Quality Toolbox talks were conducted (more than 300 talks per month) to brief the on-staff multiple times a day to enhance situational awareness and fully understand the crucial practices and processes. The intention of these strategies was to use principles of high reliability to improve the safety of patients as well as staff. As the COVID-19 protocols required containment of patient care areas, limited access and fire safety become a concern. To address this concern, regular fire safety drills were conducted in the areas in different shifts to cover all the staff.

Green Corridor was created to transport patients for investigations within the hospital. Code Green starting from area 1 to area 2 was announced during transfers (e.g., Code Green starting now from ER to Level 5). Once the desired activity was completed, normal activities were resumed after sanitizing the complete area.

Intubation boxes were created in-house for emergencies and ICUs to safeguard our doctors and nurses while intubating suspected or confirmed infectious patients.

COVID-19 had challenged the healthcare workforce in new ways. The pandemic had not only affected the patients, but had also taken a toll on frontline workers. A virus that is highly transmissible and virulent, lack of essential supplies like PPEs worldwide, long working hours, etc. had added to their stress. To ensure mental and physical health of our staff working in the COVID-19 areas, mental health support, coping strategies and tools, and various yoga sessions and workshops were organized.

Deference to Expertize

When confronted by a threat like COVID-19, it was crucial for us to have mechanisms in place to identify the individuals with the greatest expertize relevant to managing such situation. The most experienced clinicians, infection control specialists and floor nursing supervisors were included in the task force to develop the protocols, modify the processes as per COVID-19 guidelines, and handhold the ground teams. Frontline staff played a key role in implementing the strategies, giving feedback and contributing to improvements continuously across the system. Leadership at Apollo Hospitals continue to acknowledge the expertize of frontline staff, our COVID Warriors, in all forums to encourage and keep up the morale.

Managing and guiding patients, visitors and employees in this very difficult phase was also a challenge as the pandemic changed human behaviour completely. This resulted in an increased workload for healthcare workers. Crisis management and risk-mitigation strategies are critical during these times for sustaining good management, thought leadership and a large number of organizational workforces.

The HRO principles helped us in many stages—detection, testing, isolation and treatment, and was deemed successful overall. Key takeaways from our experience include organizational governance through effective communication, standardization of policies and protocols, upscaling and integrating digital health tools, effective staff communication and innovating systems to deliver hospital-level care in the community. We believe that the basic HRO principles we have adopted at our hospitals will assist many other healthcare organizations in managing the potential pandemic surges in the best possible way.

References:

1. *The Statistics Portal*, Statista, https://www.statista.com/aboutus/our-research-commitment
2. 'Reason J. Human error: models and management', *BMJ*, Vol. 320 (7237), pp. 768–70.
3. K.E. Weick and K.M. Sutcliffe, *Managing the Unexpected*, 2nd ed. San Francisco: Jossey-Bass (2007).
4. M. Gaw, F. Rosinia, T. Diller, 'Quality and the health system: becoming a high reliability organization', *Anesthesiol Clin* (2018), Vol. 36 No. 2, pp. 217–226.
5. John Shook, 'How to Go to the Gemba: Go See, Ask Why, Show Respect', Lean Enterprise Institute, 21 June 2011, https://www.lean.org/shook/displayobject.cfm?o=1843.
6. G. Jacobson, '5 Principles of a High Reliability Organization (HRO)', 12 May 2022, https://blog.kainexus.com/improvement-disciplines/hro/5-principles
7. M.R. Chassin and J. M. Loeb, 'High-Reliability Health Care: Getting There from Here', *Milbank Quarterly* (2013), Vol. 91, No. 3, pp. 459–490.
8. 'COVID-19: Operational Crisis Management in Hospitals from a Leadership Perspective', International Hospital Federation, 30 September 2020, https://ihf-fih.org/news-insights/operational-crisis-management-in-hospitals-from-a-leadership-perspective/
9. Agency for Healthcare Research and Quality (AHRQ), https://www.ahrq.gov/
10. John R. Griffith, 'Understanding High-Reliability Organizations: Are Baldrige Recipients Models?', *Journal of Healthcare Management* (Jan–Feb, 2015), Vol. 60, No. 1, pp. 44–61, https://pubmed.ncbi.nlm.nih.gov/26529993/

11. Ellen Lanser May, 'The power of zero: steps toward high reliability healthcare', HealthExec (March–April, 2013), Vol. 28, No. 2, pp. 16–8, 20, 22, https://pubmed.ncbi.nlm.nih.gov/23556381/
12. S. Dekker, *Patient Safety: A Human Factors Approach* (CRC Press, 2011).
13. P. Pronovost, et al., 'Creating High Reliability in Health Care Organizations', Health Service Research (August, 2006), Vol. 41, No. 4, pp. 1599–1617, https://pubmed.ncbi.nlm.nih.gov/16898981/
14. J. Edwards, et al., 'Lessons Learned at a COVID-19 designated hospital', *American Journal of Surgery* (January 2021), Vol. 221, No. 1, pp. 62–64.
15. M. M. Shabot, 'Memorial Hermann: High Reliability from Board to Bedside', *Joint Commission Journal on Quality and Patient Safety* (2013), Vol. 39, No. 6, pp. 253–257, https://patientsafetymovement.org/speaker/m-michael-shabot-md-facs-fccm-facmi/
16. 'Supply Chain Disaster Preparedness Manual, Center for Preparedness and Response', National Center for Environmental Health, 22 September 2020, https://www.cdc.gov/cpr/readiness/healthcare/SupplyChainDisasterPreparednessManual.htm
17. 'The SAFER Matrix: A New Scoring Methodology', Joint Commission Perspective (May 2016), Vol. 36, No. 5, https://pubmed.ncbi.nlm.nih.gov/27263314/
18. Thomas Nolan, et al., 'Improving the Reliability of Health Care', IHI, https://www.ihi.org/education/IHIOpenSchool/Courses/Documents/CourseraDocuments/08_ReliabilityWhitePaper2004revJune06.pdf
19. C. Kemper and D. Boyle, 'High reliability in healthcare', *Nursing Management* (April 2009), Vol. 40, No. 4.
20. Karl E. Weick, Kathleen M. Sutcliffe, '*Managing the Unexpected: Resilient Performance in an Age of Uncertainty*', (Wiley, 2011), https://books.google.com/books/about/Managing_the_Unexpected.html?id=GU55MJOp1OcC

13

The Right Culture Drives Safety

Developing a safety culture is one of the core components in quality and patient safety in acute care settings. The leading accreditation bodies have also emphasized safety culture measurement and improvement in leadership standards.

An effective safety culture can be described as the corporate atmosphere in which safety and health is understood to be and accepted as an important core value. The safety culture is influenced by actual or perceived management's actions, expectations, the work environment and leader-member exchange.

'Safety work is today recognized as an economic necessity. It is the study of the right way to do things.'

—Robert W. Campbell

Introduction

SAFETY CULTURE IS a commitment to combining attitudes and behaviours towards the well-being of the patients conveyed while entering a health facility.

Joint Commission International defines the safety culture of an organization as 'the product of individual and group beliefs, values, attitudes, perceptions, competencies and patterns of behaviour that determine the organization's commitment to quality and patient safety.' It lists the following traits of an organization practising a safety culture:

- Management and staff promote the utmost levels of transparency, accountability and mutual respect.
- Safety is the topmost priority for everyone.
- Behaviours hampering a safety culture are impermissible.
- Staff detects that systems might fail and are, therefore, cautious of identifying hazardous conditions and close calls before any damage is done.

- Staff reports errors as they are aware that the information can be utilized for addressing the existing flaws in the system and contribute efficiently to patient safety events.
- Staff promotes a learning atmosphere and continuously improves by adopting new learnings from patient safety events.

Developing a culture of safety is one of the core components in quality and patient safety in acute care settings. Accreditation bodies have also emphasized safety culture measurement and improvement in leadership standards.

Measuring Safety Culture

Assess the safety culture of the organization, preferably every year, to track changes and improvements over time.

Organizations face the risk of the following adverse events when they do not prioritize a safety culture:

- Unsafe events not reported or underreported
- Higher workforce attrition and burnout
- Lack of improvement
- Higher rate of harm
- Increasing costs

According to a 2016 study by Health Catalyst, teamwork and enhanced safety culture can largely uplift health systems to minimizing any sort of harm to patients.

The Safety Culture Ladder

The Safety Culture Ladder measures relevant elements to show whether a health system is ailing (very low) or doing well (very high) with its safety culture.

Pathological: People rarely or don't care about safety and are only driven by regulatory compliance and not getting caught.

Reactive: Leaders take safety seriously only when things have gone wrong. Managers and supervisors feel upset about how the workforce won't do what they are told.

Calculative: More focus is given to systems and numbers. Substantial data is collected and analysed periodically. Multiple audits are undertaken, and people begin to feel they know 'how it works'. However, the efficacy of the collected data is not always established.

Proactive: Anticipating, taking action and being in control even in unfamiliar situations. The workforce ensures that actions are taken rather than waiting for things to happen on their own.

Generative: Organizations set extreme standards and challenge themselves to surpass them. They use lessons from previous failures to improve the system rather blaming the system or staff. Management is well aware of what is really is going on, because the employees share it with them. People strive to be completely informed as it prepares them for the crisis.

Culture change takes time to be embedded within the pulse of an organization.

The safety culture survey depicting that employees feel unsafe at work is a primary factor indicating that immediate action needs to be taken to mitigate possible risks likely to hamper the work environment predominantly.

Another important motive to conduct a safety culture survey is to bridge the gap between perception and reality in the organization. What do your employees really think about the work environment? Are you on the same page when it comes to managing risks?

Survey Tool

Several tools are available for measuring safety culture. However, the AHRQ Surveys on Patient Safety Culture™ (SOPS®) is one widely accepted tool used to assess the safety culture in healthcare.

It assesses the extent to which the organizational culture promotes safe practices for the well-being of patients.

Across facilities, a standard set of core items along with comparable survey content are included in all the SOPS.

Assessed by the AHRQ SOPS surveys, the areas of patient safety culture include:

- Communication of error
- Communication openness
- Organizational learning
- Continuous improvement
- Overall rating on patient safety
- How the staff, supervisors and organization as a whole respond to any error
- Staffing
- Supervisor and management support for patient safety
- Teamwork
- Work pressure management

AHRQ also has safety culture survey tools available for ambulatory care and for nursing homes.

Table 1. Examples of Items in Hospital's Safety Culture Survey

Background	What is your primary work area or unit? Since how long have you been employed in this hospital? Since how long have you worked in the current unit? Typically, how many hours per week do you work? What is your staff position in this hospital? Do you typically have direct contact with patients? How long have you worked in your profession?
Frequency of event reporting	When a mistake has been made, but is detected and improvised before affecting the patient, how frequently is this reported? When a mistake is made, however, it is not harmful for the patient, how often is this reported? When a mistake is likely to harm the patient, but does not, how often is this reported?
Rating overall perceptions of safety	Patient safety is never put at stake to perform more tasks. Our procedures and systems are good enough at averting risks. Just by chance, more serious errors don't take place here. We have patient safety problems in this unit.
Patient safety grade	Give your work area an overall grade on patient safety
Number of events reported	In the past year, how many event reports have you filled out and submitted?

Supervisor / manager expectations and actions	My supervisor/manager motivates by giving a positive feedback when he/she notices that a job done is done according to the guidelines. My supervisor/manager considers staff suggestions for enhancing overall patient safety. Under immense pressure, my supervisor/manager expects us to work faster, even if it means taking shortcuts. My supervisor/manager doesn't pay attention towards patient safety problems happening repeatedly.
Organi-zational learning	We are actively doing things to improve safety. Mistakes have led to positive changes here. After we make changes to improve patient safety, we evaluate their effectiveness.
Teamwork within units	People support one another in this unit. When a number of tasks need to be performed, we work together as a team to perform the tasks. In this unit, people treat each other with respect. When a particular unit is highly occupied, others help.
Commu-nication openness	Staff will freely speak up if they witness an element that is likely to affect patient care. Staff feels free to raise questions relating to the decisions or actions of seniors. Staff is afraid to raise their voice when something is not right.
Feedback and commu-nication about error	We are given feedback about changes put into place based on event reports. We are informed about errors that happen. We discuss ways to prevent errors from happening.

Non-punitive response to error	Staff feels like their mistakes are held against them. When an event is reported, it is experienced that instead of the issue, the person is being written up. Staff is worried that their mistakes/errors are kept in their personal file.
Staffing	We have enough staff to handle the workload. Staff in this unit works longer hours than is best for patient care. We use more agency/temporary staff than is best for patient care. We work in 'crisis mode' trying to do too much, too quickly.
Hospital management support	Management offers a work climate promoting patient's well-being. Their actions depict that patient safety is the utmost priority and they seem highly interested about safety of patients only after an adverse event takes place.
Teamwork across hospital units	There is good cooperation among hospital units that need to work together. These units work well together in order to offer best-in-class care to patients. These units do not coordinate well with each other. It is often inconvenient to work with staff of other hospital units.
Hospital hand-offs and transitions	Things 'fall between the cracks' when transferring patients from one unit to another. Pivotal details of patient care information are misplaced during shift changes. Problems often occur while exchanging information across hospital units and change in shifts become challenging for patients.

Second Victim	Have you heard the term second victim used to describe health care team members who have been emotionally traumatized by an unanticipated clinical event/outcome? In the past 12 months, were there any clinical events that caused personal problems such as anxiety, depression or concern about your ability to perform your job? Did you receive support from anyone at your unit when you had the second victim experience? Please describe your recommendations for supportive strategies if you or another healthcare peer/colleague was involved in a traumatic or unexpected clinical event.

Source: Adopted from AHRQ Patient Safety Culture tool.

Roll-Out Process

The process of conducting the safety culture survey takes sessions approximately four to six weeks.

Pre-survey notification is shared with employees about the upcoming survey in our monthly newsletter with details of how to ensure that confidentiality and anonymity of survey are maintained. Maintaining anonymity is important as people are not interested to participate in the survey if there is a doubt that their identity can be revealed. At Apollo Hospitals, we conduct the online survey every June. The survey link is shared through email and mobile to reach out to each and every staff in all departments.

Online tools normally provide built-in analytics. All the data is exported to excel spreadsheets for further analysis and multilingual surveys are performed to rule out any sort of language barrier.

While planning for the Safety Culture Survey, it is also important to consider the length of the survey. The average time to complete the survey should not exceed 10–15 minutes. A minimum expected sample size should be predicated on the size of the organization, with representation from all department disciplines and management.

Sample Size

Table 2. Minimum Sample Sizes by Total Number of Providers and Staff

Number of Providers and Staff	Minimum Sample Size	Expected Number of Responses (Assuming a 50% Response Rate)
500 (or fewer)	500 – a census of all providers and staff	250 (or fewer)
501-699	500	250
700-1,299	600	300
1,300 3,999	700	350
4,000 or more	750	375

Source: AHRQ 2019 Hospital Survey on Patient Safety Culture, Version 2.0 User's Guide

Analysis of Survey Responses

The scores derived via survey using a Likert scale of 1 to 5 can be included in a spreadsheet for seamless analysis. A typical data analysis focuses towards scores based on the average or mean that references either attribute. Colour coding helps as a good visual guide for interpreting the observations that correspond with each survey section.

Table 3.

Mean Score	Interpretation
5	Very positive response
3.5-4.9	Room for improvement
1.0-3.4	Considerable room for improvement

Attribute-wise scoring with top concerns should be identified in the post-survey analysis.

Action Plan

Analysis of the data should be completed within a reasonable time, ideally within fifteen to twenty days of the survey. The action plan can usually be divided into two segments—short-term tactical interventions and long-term strategic initiatives.

The idea is to use the survey data to monitor what is performing up to the mark and what needs to be enhanced for improvement, and then prepare a blueprint for making the required advancements.

The National Business Aviation Association (NBAA) uses 'SMART' goals for safety culture data analysis and action plan. The action plan should be:

- **Specific**—clearly defined
- **Measurable**—so that performance can be monitored
- **Agreed**—with those responsible and accountable
- **Realistic**—achievable and practical
- **Timely**—set deadlines for milestones or achievement

Providing follow-up information to employees relating to the safety culture survey is an essential action item. The follow-up communication should be as transparent as possible, and clearly identify any deficiencies that need to be addressed.

Strategies to Promote a Safety Culture

The Apollo Safety Culture Model

Strategies to promote a safety culture include multifaceted interventions including system-level changes.

Listen to patient stories: Every board meeting can begin with a patient story, such as a near-miss or an adverse event. These patient stories help board members to focus on the people the organization serves and not just the financials.

Leadership walk rounds: At Apollo, we call it the 'Chairman's Round'. This strategy engages organizational leadership directly with frontline care providers. Senior leadership visit frontline patient care areas with the goal of observing and discussing current or potential threats to patient safety, as well as supporting frontline staff in addressing such threats. The purpose of this round is to show leadership commitment to safety, foster trust and provide support for frontline providers to proactively address threats to patient safety and challenges faced by the staff.

Encourage, recognize and reward incident Reporting: Make error reporting transparent, and use adverse events as opportunities for improvement instead of punishment. At Apollo Hospitals, we have an online Incident Reporting Module called Automated Incident Reporting System (AIRS). It is an anonymous incident-reporting module through which any staff or doctors can raise a safety incident related staff, patient process or facility.

The automated incident management focuses on ensuring that crucial events are timely analysed, addressed and efficiently resolved. Automation is a great process allowing incident management tools to seamlessly integrate with each other and promotes immediate communication across the organization. Safety events are reported by personnel involved in the events themselves. The benefits of voluntary incident-reporting systems include their relative acceptability and the involvement of frontline staff in identifying safety threats for the organization.

We simulate possible adverse events as part of the training. Training programmes that stress quality and service safety measures are conducted for members of all units annually. To promote a culture of safety, options are provided to raise incidents anonymously.

Thank You Cards/Rewards: Recognize staff who report safety issues or have good ideas for improvement. Recognize staff who report incidents.

Supporting Second Victims: The second victim can be any healthcare worker involved in an adverse patient event and experiencing feelings of failure.

The Buddy Support Programme was developed at Apollo Hospitals by patient safety, risk management and clinical department leaders. This programme provides guidance on how staff can support each other during an adverse event. Educational campaigns introduced the second victim concept.

Handover Communication: Hand-off processes in a high-risk and high-volume environment of patients with highly complex care needs create room for error, which could potentially lead to life-threatening situations. Barriers that can cause hand-off failure are a lack of standardized handover tool, lack of staff training, and lack of supervision.

To address these concerns, we have implemented standardized verbal and written hand-off protocols in our policy. We have developed required processes for teamwork, communication and hand-offs among the team using tools such as SBAR, read back, briefings and de-briefings.

A safety culture is not limited to the healthcare space. The concept is widely used in other high-risk industries, such as nuclear power and aviation, which use this concept to understand safety incidents to prevent future disasters.

In its sentinel event alert on the role of leadership in developing a safety culture, JCI references James Reason's concepts about safety culture in his 1997 book on human error, *Managing the Risks of Organizational Accidents*. The three key elements of a safety culture are the following:

- **Fair and just culture** is a workplace culture built on trust and transparency. It empowers clinical and non-clinical staff to report safety concerns and errors without fear, and it holds both staff and the hospital's systems accountable by responding to safety events with reasonable, learning-based consequences.
- **Reporting culture**. Although adverse events and near misses are common in healthcare, they are almost ubiquitously underreported. Barriers to reporting include fear among healthcare providers regarding repercussions and cultural factors. In organizations where reporting culture is encouraged, people have confidence to report safety concerns without fear of being punished.
- **Learning culture** that resonates with your employees. In a learning culture, leaders play the role of a mentor. They ensure new employees succeed in the organization by creating all-inclusive departmental employee orientation programmes.

Safety culture is the way patient safety is thought about, structured and implemented in an organization. It is an important step towards high reliability. Such an organization is recognized by staff who are dynamic, engaged and collaborative. Individuals treat each other and patients with dignity and respect in an organization promoting a strong safety culture.

For an organization to have a strong safety culture, it requires leadership commitment along with the engaged and empowered employees.

A Case Scenario

Which One Is Yours?

Mr A
45 years/Male
History of illness: Diabetes from the past 7 years

Visited the hospital outpatient department with the chief complaint of shortness of breath and exertion.

He was referred by his primary consultant for a cardiology consultation, at which a stress test was ordered. After the test, patient left for home as the reception staff informed the patient that the reports will be sent to the patient's address. The results of the stress test results were not communicated back to his primary care provider, and the referring cardiologist they were sent to was on leave for the next ten days.

One week later, Mr A presented to the emergency department with severe chest pain and was diagnosed with an acute myocardial infarction. Upon further review of his medical records, the emergency care team reviewed his past test results and learnt about the positive stress test report done one week ago.

Placement of stent to open his coronary artery was planned on the same day, followed by two weeks of cardiac rehabilitation.

How Would You Respond to This Event as an Organization?

Action Taken by Organization A

A Root Cause Analysis (RCA) was performed by the Quality Department staff to identify the reasons for the patient's critical test result not being communicated to either him or his treating consultant. Action steps from the RCA focus on re-educating the cardiac diagnostics department about the policy for communication of critical and abnormal test results within a specified period of time.

A warning letter was issued against the staff and was put in his personnel file. The action plans were only focused on the training aspect and did not include metrics for sustainability. The RCA and actionables were not discussed with the relevant team members and the leadership.

Action Taken by Organization B

An RCA was performed by a team comprising staff and leaders of respective areas to identify the reasons behind the patient's critical test result not being communicated to either him or his treating consultant.

The RCA team proposed actionables, which included designing a new process for communication of test results with an escalation matric. The escalation matric clearly defined the steps of escalating the issue when it is not immediately possible to communicate critical test results to the ordering provider and/or the patient.

Strong action plans for improvement and metrics for sustainability were presented to the organization's leadership team for review and approval. The unit head presented the case and action plan to the Quality Steering Committee. Sincere apology was offered to the patient and his family, and they were further informed about these breakdowns in communication, and how the incident might have contributed to his myocardial infarction.

After three months, the Quality Department Team followed up with the frontline care team involved in the event to evaluate the action plan and review improvement metrics. These results were presented at the next board meeting by the Hospital Leadership.

Debrief

In most organizations, the response to handling Mr A's situation is similar to Organization A than to Organization B. This example illustrates as to why healthcare must create and improve systems that are committed to zero harm to patients and our workforce.

References:

1. L.T. Kohn, J. M. Corrigan and M. S. Donaldson, 'To Err Is Human: Building a Safer Health System', *A Report of the Committee on Quality of Health Care in America, Institute of Medicine* (Washington DC: National Academy Press, 2000), https://www.scirp.org/reference/ReferencesPapers.aspx?ReferenceID=1372005
2. K. G. Shojania, B. W. Duncan, et al, 'Making healthcare safer: A critical analysis of patient safety practices', *Evidence Report Technology Assessment* (2001), https://pubmed.ncbi.nlm.nih.gov/11510252/
3. J. Braithwaite et al, 'Cultural and associated enablers of and barriers to, adverse incident reporting'.
4. S. Singer, et al, 'Relationship of Safety Climate and Safety Performance in Hospitals'.
5. J. Sorra, et al, 'Exploring Relationships Between Patient Safety Culture and Patients' Assessments of Hospital Care'.
6. 'Measuring the hospital practice environment: A Canadian context', Unbound Medicine, *Research in Nursing and Health* (August 2002), Vol. 25, No. 4, pp. 256–268, https://neuro.unboundmedicine.com/medline/citation/12124720/Measuring_the_hospital_practice_environment:_a_Canadian_context_
7. J. Sexton, 'The Safety Attitudes Questionnaire: psychometric properties, benchmarking data, and emerging research'.
8. Our Standards, Joint Commission, https://www.jointcommission.org/accreditation-and-certification/health-care-settings/hospital/learn/our-standards/
9. 'Hospital Survey on Patient Safety Culture: 2010 User Comparative Database Report', Rockville, MD, Agency for Healthcare Research

and Quality, 2010, https://www.jointcommission.org/standards/national-patient-safety-goals/

10. S. Singer, and T. Vogus, 'Safety climate research: taking stock and looking forward'.
11. J. Sorra, T. Famolaro, et al, 'Hospital Survey on Patient Safety Culture: 2012 User Comparative Database Report', 2012, AHRQ, https://psnet.ahrq.gov/issue/hospital-survey-patient-safety-culture-2010-user-comparative-database-report
12. 'The Essential Role of Leadership', 8 March 2017, https://psnet.ahrq.gov/issue/essential-role-leadership-developing-safety-culture
13. D. S. Brown, 'What Is Patient Safety Culture?', Agency for Healthcare Research and Quality, https://www.ahrq.gov/sops/about/patient-safety-culture.html

14

IT in Healthcare Quality: An Optimistic Outlook

So is the power of Information Technology (IT), that Quality teams at Apollo have moved from doing data capture to using IT to monitor processes through IT, proactively analyse trends, build AI models and hence through Clinical Decision Support Systems, we will see the right decisions in every instance. Technology has evolved significantly in the last few decades and continues to expand rapidly. Leveraging IT in healthcare has resulted in avoidance of non-value-adding activities, increased staff satisfaction and cost reduction.

Digitization is causing a quantum shift in the quality of healthcare services. The purpose of this chapter is to provide a foundation for understanding regarding the use of information technology in healthcare quality and patient safety. The quality management and hospital administration depend upon the data and information generated through process performance, gathered in numerous means and analysed through tools and techniques. The digital transformations hugely and positively impact the process capabilities, through constant monitoring and overseeing. Critical clinical and administrative decisions are now taken based on relevant and timely data.

'The great growling engine of change—technology.'

—Alvin Toffler

Introduction

IS HEALTHCARE INFORMATION Technology in modern times a useful development, or just the buzzword? Are data automation, big data, data analytics, the internet of things, etc., just fancy terms? Are they just there to create hype, or are they the need of the hour? We must understand how IT has transformed our lives with just a 'digital' approach anywhere and everywhere. It seems the digital way is the path to improving accessibility and making lives easier.

We have witnessed the ever-changing health technologies since the early stages of medicine. Increasing knowledge and diagnostics, preventive treatment and rehabilitation possibilities have significantly altered the landscape of healthcare systems across the globe. This has certainly led the health systems to evolve into complex entities with fast-changing roles and responsibilities—not only for patients but also for health professionals, payers and regulators. The digital transformation of health services—though complex and multifaceted—is considered a very important and powerful process, which has created a considerable impact on the present status of healthcare delivery systems, and is expected to have a further tangible impact on futuristic healthcare systems.

Technology has evolved significantly in the last few decades and continues to expand at a very rapid pace. This has made possible present-day life brand-new and impressive. Furthermore, it is expected that this will continue for the times to come. Healthcare is the field where technology has been proven most remarkable or profound in its impact. Healthcare information technology has certainly provided a better quality of life for patients, and has considerably improved patient safety.

From making possible hassle-free accurate communication to improving diagnostic and clinical safety, IT has contributed to a large extent in making patient-centred care error-free and consistent. With the advent of various digital applications and online decision support systems, technology is truly proving to be an enabler of better quality of patient care, and a safer and more patient-centric environment.

Healthcare has expeditiously transformed from acute care to predictive and preventive care in the last few years. These colossal changes have moved us away from curative drug-based healthcare to consulting/service-based healthcare, with an appropriate focus on lifestyle and adapting behaviour to the prevention of illness.

The ever-changing landscape of the healthcare industry has drastically changed the IT requirements of hospitals. Health information technologies have become crucial now in improving proactive and preventive patient care, safety, and the overall quality of our healthcare systems. Healthcare IT and its advanced decision support systems reduce human error, improve the coordination between providers, and make the world of healthcare better every day.

How Information Technology Helps

- Enhances the overall service quality and makes it more efficient in terms of accessibility and delivery.
- Integrated electronic health records facilitate faster clinical decisions, communication, and care planning. It also enables clinical research as data is made available in a systematic manner, which helps to understand the trends, patterns, occurrences and recurrences, incidents and prevalence, etc.
- Electronic patient records automatically and easily gather each patient's blood group, known allergies, and other demographic variables. Manual collection of such data is minimized to a great extent.
- Facilitates the remote diagnosis and medical therapy of patients. As a result, people living in remote areas can have access to online consultations from specialty doctors from bigger hospitals.
- Enables ready access and Customer Relationship Management (CRM), as this is a necessary function for any hospital.
- Machine learning and artificial intelligence concepts are hugely beneficial models for the early detection and curing some of complex diseases.
- Helps patients to move seamlessly across different geographical locations with a standard set of clinical information.
- Provides flexibility in procuring and billing.
- Supports an accounting framework, helping with entire billing, inventory management, store management, laboratory management, etc. IT helps in maximizing the returns on every penny spent.

Information Technology Use in Healthcare

- Healthcare digitalization, the use of computers and electronic health records, remote and home monitoring of patients, electronic medical devices, the application of computer-aided visualization, clinical decision support systems, etc., have significantly and positively affected aspects of healthcare systems in terms of structure, processes, culture, mindsets, behaviours and outcomes. It is expected to impact many more areas.
- Some elements of digital transformation represent a fundamental change in the mode and culture of healthcare delivery for organizations. Changes and innovations in health technologies have a profound impact on healthcare delivery processes, and impact health, healthcare and health systems at a large.
- As a part of the constant change process—relying more and more on technology every day—advances in artificial intelligence and information technology will only continue to improve how we receive clinical care.
- Use of IT improves accessibility to patient safety data in real-time, and safety dashboards allow the decision-makers (i.e., clinicians and managers) to identify safety and quality indicators and their trends over a period of time, and facilitate timely interventions and continuous monitoring and evaluation.
- The objectivity, transparency and accessibility of performance data on a real-time basis facilitated by the digital transformation supports clinical decision-making and timely interventions.

Limitations of IT

- As digital data and systems work on the 'junk in and junk out' principle, timely data entries are very crucial for effective information and process.
- Digital technology changes very fast, so creating a sync with the same is not easy.
- Digital technology works based on the masses—the more the better. So, if it changes, then it will be a huge capital investment.
- Maximum systems are cloud-based, so cybersecurity is crucial and expensive.
- The healthcare industry has a high attrition/staff changeover rate, which leads to errors and underutilization of complex features of healthcare digital technology.
- It is very difficult to identify errors in digital technology, so if this technology doesn't work uniformly, then it will be laborious to identify and correct errors.

Digital Apollo: A Pursuit of Healthcare Quality Excellence

At Apollo Hospitals, we have been on an unending journey of excellence since inception, in 1983. Among the corporate groups, Apollo Hospitals has always been at the forefront of quality and safe healthcare delivery in India.

With the ever-increasing expansion of its activities, and the need for monitoring and measuring the quality, patient safety, and clinical outcomes, Apollo Group invented a novel approach to go digital to sustain excellence. It is also essential to constantly oversee the procedures and processes across the group, considering frequent and global concerns over issues of patient safety, outcomes of clinical care, and litigations.

Digitization is causing a quantum shift in the quality of healthcare delivered at Apollo Hospitals. A firm believer in quality care and patient safety culture, Ms Sangita Reddy envisioned the digital transformation of the group through various IT innovations and digital applications.

Besides the indigenous hospital information system, Apollo Hospitals Group has forayed into digital quality systems by internally developing and successfully implementing numerous e-quality monitoring, analytical and safety culture promoting utilities at corporate as well as individual hospital levels for various important functions.

Figure 1. Digital Quality Systems at Apollo

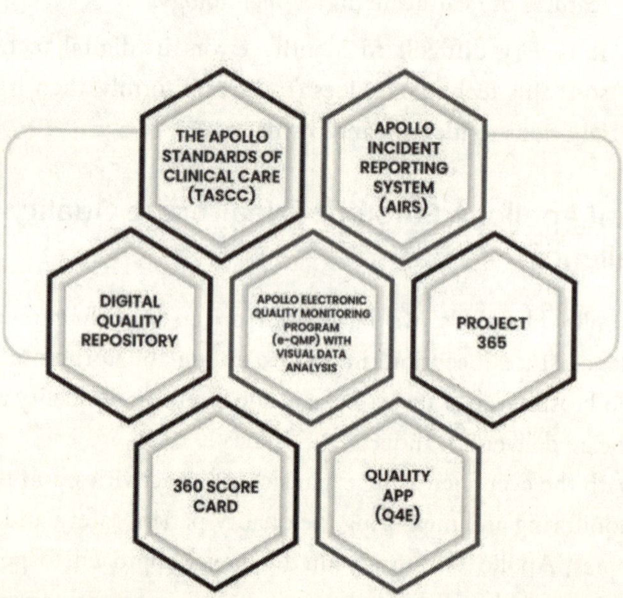

Courtesy: Apollo Hospitals

1. **The Apollo Standards of Clinical Care (TASCC):** An extensively planned digital programme that objectively monitors and evaluates special indicators, and the clinical and internal processes involved in patient care, helping in identifying opportunities for improvement. It seeks to improve patient care and outcomes through a systematic review of care against clearly defined criteria, and provide a mechanism through which action is taken to make and sustain those improvements.

Figure 2.

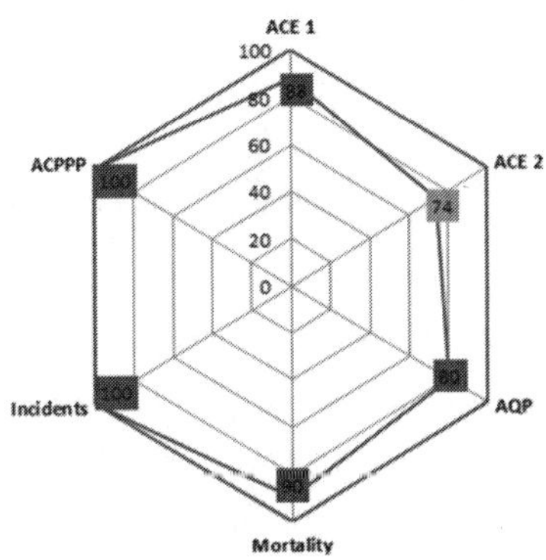

Courtesy: Apollo Hospitals

2. **Apollo Incident Reporting System (AIRS):** To establish clear systems for reporting information related to medical/healthcare errors, and to provide a confidential mechanism of identification, tracking, trending and follow-up of all incidences that pose an actual or potential safety risk to patients, families, visitors and staff.
3. **Apollo Electronic Quality Monitoring Program (e-QMP) with Visual Data Analysis:** To integrate all quality data in a single utility with appropriate backup and analytical capabilities.

4. **Digital Quality Repository:** One-stop online storage and making available all required resources for quality implementation and management, including best practices and innovations of individual hospitals.
5. **360^0 Score Card:** An annual on-site audit by experts on predefined standards and collating findings on a digital portal, thus arriving at a 360^0-performance score in each hospital. This helps us in comparing the performance of the hospitals over the years.
6. **Project 365:** It mandates each hospital of the Apollo Group to carry out departmental audits every month, which also includes compliance and adherence to these digital functions. Findings and scores are uploaded on a centralized digital portal, from where further analysis is carried out.
7. **Quality App:** Quality Application (as named Q4E: Quality for Excellence) has been designed and developed to ensure that each member of the Apollo Family can participate in and take advantage of this mobile-based quality application. Features of this application are very important and beneficial for all the Quality Professionals and for each staff. The Quality App is equipped with core healthcare quality functions and additional features such as:

    - Incident reporting and closure
    - Routine checklists
    - Real-time updates/reminders/notifications on completion of quality-related activities
    - Updates and reports on monthly activities, quality calendar activities
    - Galleries

- Training
- Surveys

Figure 3.

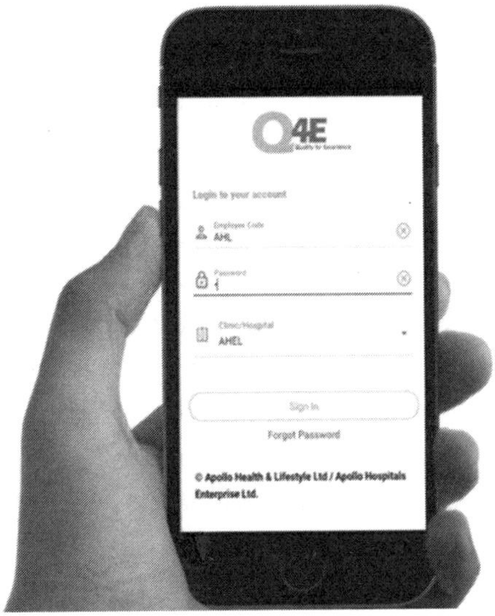

Courtesy: Apollo Hospitals

The Quality App can make audits and reports very easy to manage, and submission will be just a click away. The app can be used for multi-locations and for thousands of staff members together. One App will answer many activity-related questions. It captures data and presents it in real-time with the help of various reports and analysis.

It is very easy to share the data, reports and analysis by email and other communication tools.

Other Information Technology Tools for Healthcare

IT has helped in many digital initiatives and developed tools to make healthcare more efficient. A few examples are:

- HAI (Healthcare Associated Infections) Tracking Utility
- Single-use device tracking and follow-up utility
- Laundry materials usage data in hospitals
- RTLS (Real Time Location System) linked transport tracking mechanism
- Nursing services quality indicator analysis
- Healthcare-related training data collection and analysis
- Lighthouse—Clinical Intelligence dashboard using Apache Scoring

All these quality utilities were conceptualized, designed, tested, implemented, re-tested and upgraded in a gradually phased manner over the last year. A team consisting of senior management, corporate and unit level IT staff, quality staff, medical, nursing and operation leadership, etc. participated in the following steps of this project:

- Conceptualization and content writing
- Transcribing the requirements in IT parlance with specific interfaces and modules
- Coding and development of primary utility
- Running dummy utility under test environment
- Correction and trial run
- Piloting and staff training
- Roll-out for hospital/group-wide implementation
- Monitoring compliance and course correction

The variety of functions addressed by these innovations is very much essential and critical at times, to manage quality in the hospital. These functions are usually carried out manually (non-digitally) in other organizations. This takes a lot of effort, time, resources, etc., and leads to many fallacies, inaccuracies and failures in achieving the intended purpose.

To smoothen these processes and enhance accuracy and timeliness, Apollo Hospitals Group embarked on this unique digital journey to improve the overall quality and patient safety. After the development of these digital functionalities, process flows of each utility were developed and shared with each Quality Team member across the group. There were a couple of briefing sessions conducted through video conferencing. A structured and uniform training programme was chalked out and followed for individual hospital. Any changes/ upgradation in the digital platform were quickly communicated to all concerned.

Awareness and briefing of these digital functions were also made a part of the staff induction programme, and all new employees were trained at the time of joining, in order to develop and sustain their competency. Many changes upgrades were carried out in various functionalities, for better integration, retrieval and retention, data safety, etc. Where possible, automation and direct data fetching was done to further reduce the efforts spent on data collection and to eliminate inaccuracies. Analytics were introduced, through which customized reports could be generated, making decision-making faster and evidence based. Backup and data safety components were enhanced to ensure long-term term sustainability of the data for future reference.

The quality of quality management and hospital administration depend upon the data and information generated through process performance, collated by various means and analysed through tools and techniques. The digital transformations at Apollo Hospitals hugely and positively impacted the process capabilities, through constant monitoring and overseeing. Critical clinical and administrative decisions are now taken based on relevant and timely data. Besides, leveraging IT has also resulted in avoidance of non-value-adding activities, increased staff satisfaction, and cost reduction.

References:

1. 'Digital Healthcare Research', AHRQ, https://digital.ahrq.gov/
2. Health Information Technology (HIT), Agency for Healthcare Research and Quality, https://www.ahrq.gov/topics/health-information-technology-hit.html
3. Y. Alotaibi and F. Federico, 'The impact of health information technology on patient safety'.
4. 'Medical Device Interoperability', U.S. Food and Drug Administration, https://cacmap.fda.gov/medical-devices/digital-health-center-excellence/medical-device-interoperability
5. 'Patient Safety and Health Information Technology', ACOG, https://www.acog.org/clinical/clinical-guidance/committee-opinion/articles/2015/01/patient-safety-and-health-information-technology
6. Krishna Ganapathy, 'Healthcare IT in India: An Optimistic Outlook', https://www.asianhhm.com/information-technology/healthcareit-india
7. 'Healthcare in India: Digitization is the way forward', *The Financial Express*, 12 March 2021, https://www.financialexpress.com/opinion/healthcare-in-india-digitisation-is-the-way-forward/2210873/
8. Sreejith, 'The Application and Impact of Information Technology in Healthcare - Fingent Technology', https://www.fingent.com/blog/the-application-and-impact-of-information-technology-in-healthcare/
9. Simone Edelmann, 'Digitization: future of healthcare', Healthcare Transformers, 30 September 2019, https://healthcaretransformers.com/healthcare-business/digitization-future-of-healthcare/

10. 'Benefits of Health IT', Health IT, https://www.healthit.gov/topic/health-it-basics/benefits-health-it
11. Stephanie Watson, 'Telehealth: The advantages and disadvantages', Harvard Health Publishing, 12 October 2020, https://www.health.harvard.edu/staying-healthy/telehealth-the-advantages-and-disadvantages
12. M. Khammarnia, A. Kassani, and M. Eslahi, 'The Efficacy of Patients' Wristband Bar-code on Prevention of Medical Errors', 2015.
13. Patient Safety Movement, Patient Safety Movement Foundation, Global Non-profit focused on ZERO, https://patientsafetymovement.org/?gclid=EAIaIQobChMI4vP2yYKy-QIV1JNmAh0UqQ-_EAAYASAAEgLmNPD_BwE

Case Studies

Please note that all case studies have been developed for illustrative purposes only and do not bear resemblance to any person, living or dead.

Case Study 1

Medical Record Completion

A multidisciplinary team, a defined checklist, regular audits supported by interventions lead to a significant improvement in completion of medical records in a healthcare organization.

Introduction

MEDICAL RECORDS MANAGEMENT is one of the key functions in any healthcare setup. Physical medical records of patients who have been treated—in the Outpatient Department, Inpatient Department or Emergency Department of the hospital—are stored here. These records map out the patient journey, i.e., chief complaints, history, clinical findings, diagnostic test results, pre- and post-operative care, surgery notes, progress, medications, and most importantly, all the consents that were taken during the entire stay of the patient during treatment. These help healthcare providers to ensure that safe and appropriate care is provided to the patient.

Today, most of the hospitals/healthcare facilities in our country are facing challenges in the management of medical records. Additionally, completion of medical records is also a concern, as there are multiple stakeholders expected to make an entry.

The level of training and awareness varies among these stakeholders. Hence, for any healthcare organization, completeness, accuracy, correctness and legibility are always a concern. Though many organizations have adopted the 'digital' path, it will still take a few years to get there.

Problem Statement

Despite having a full-fledged medical record department, experienced clinical teams and brilliant operations team, incomplete documentation of medical records was the biggest concern for XYZ Hospital.

They had multiple litigations against them, and the overall patient satisfaction was a major issue. Insurance denial due to poor/incomplete documentation of records, improper discharge, and transfer summaries going out of the hospital to other organizations was adding to the problems. Hence, there was an urgent need to investigate the entire process and correct it at the earliest.

Immediate Intervention

A meeting was called with all the stakeholders to understand the status and challenges. The existing team, documents, forms and checklists were discussed in detail to understand the concerns.

Assessment of Problem and Analysis of Causes

A retrospective analysis of the medical records of patients was completed by the stakeholders to assess the gaps in the medical record documentation. The processes for open and closed medical record audits were also discussed. The parameters were reinvestigated as per the accreditation requirements. The team decided to call for a two-day workshop.

The invitees were all floor in-charge doctors, all floor in-charge nurses, dieticians, physiotherapists and medical social workers.

Agenda:

1. To review the existing process.
2. To evaluate the audit tools used for open and closed medical record audits.
3. To brainstorm among the team members for a long-term feasible solution.
4. To draft communication strategies with the team and leadership.

Strategy for the Change

A detailed fishbone analysis was charted to understand the reasons behind improper/incomplete documentation.

Figure 1. Fishbone Analysis

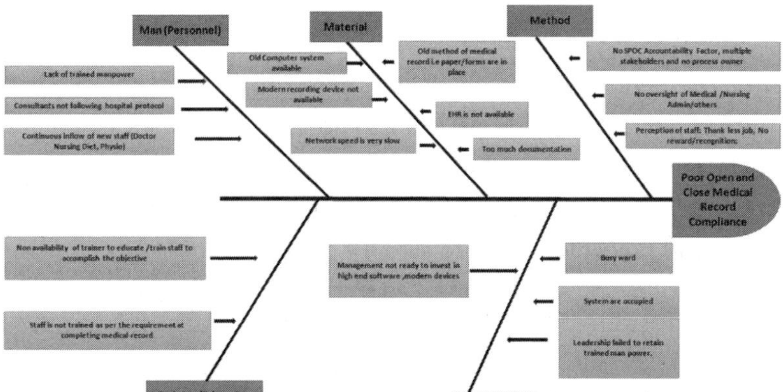

Pareto analysis was also conducted with the available data, which helped the team to understand the 20 per cent of the causes that had an 80 per cent impact on documentation compliance.

Figure 2. Category-wise Non-compliance in Medical Record Documentation

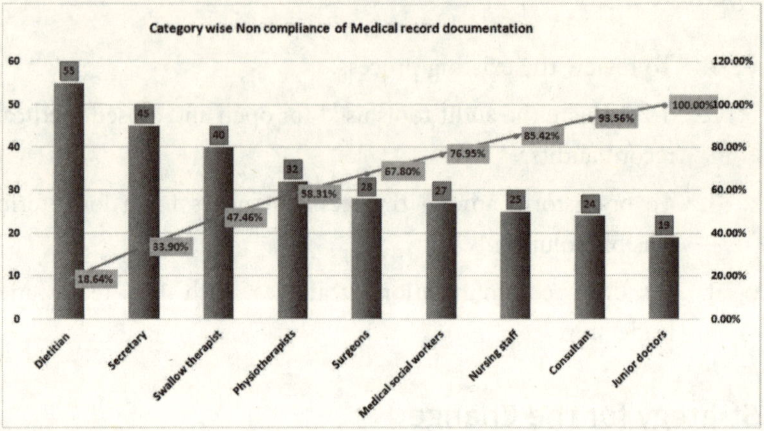

Solutions

Completing the records—which were deficient in a number of forms or content as per the established standard, was a basic exercise completed by the Medical Records department.

Initially, the Medical Records staff would review each case and note the deficiencies of physicians, nurses and other stakeholders. But later, to achieve 100 per cent compliance and better outcomes, we formed an interdisciplinary team, including a ward doctor, nurse, dietician, physiotherapist and a medical social worker. A weekly roster was prepared for the review.

The following steps were taken for this challenging task:

1. A roster of the identified team members was prepared.
2. A working space for the team was identified.
3. MRD team members shared the daily list of files for open and closed medical record audits.
4. The compiled report was discussed every week with the leadership and stakeholders.
5. Additional analysed data, including trends, was utilized.
6. The most compliant units were rewarded.

Medical Record Review Committee

For an overall approach using collaborative governance, a multidisciplinary team was constituted, which discussed the following agenda points at least once in a quarter:

1. Hospital statistics
2. MRD functions and quality indicators
3. Statutory compliances
4. Issues and challenges
5. Open and closed medical record audit reports
6. Compliance with the accreditation standards
7. Other issues

Interdisciplinary Team

Medical Record Review:

Two interdisciplinary teams were constituted. The teams were expected to complete open and closed medical record audits on a daily basis.

A) Open Record Audit Team

- Respective department head was responsible for ensuring that an audit was conducted by the doctor, nurse, dietician, physiotherapist and medical social worker for that area.
- Open record audit was conducted at the ward level.
- One in every fifth file was audited as a sample.
- Approved open audit tool was used.
- The sheets were thereafter collected back and analysed by the MRD Team.
- The findings and observations were discussed in the quarterly MRD Committee.

B) Closed Record Audit Team

- Medical Administration department developed a roster of doctors, nurses, dieticians, physiotherapists and medical social workers.
- Based on the same, the team assembled and conducted the audit.
- Closed record audit was conducted in the Medical Records department.
- 100 per cent of records based on discharge needs was audited.
- An approved closed audit tool was used.
- The sheets were collected back and analysed by the MRD team.
- The findings and observations were discussed in the quarterly MRD Committee.

Submission of the Report and Action Plan

- Medical records manager analysed the data collected in the open and closed record audits.
- Review findings, learning points, and suggestions for improvement were presented to the CEO/Committee by the Manager of the Medical Records department.
- Time-bound action plan was delegated to the respective medical and non-medical staff.
- A closure report was duly submitted to the medical head before the review meeting.

Analysis

Open Medical Record Audit Analysis

Figure 3. Overall Compliance Percentage of Open File Audit

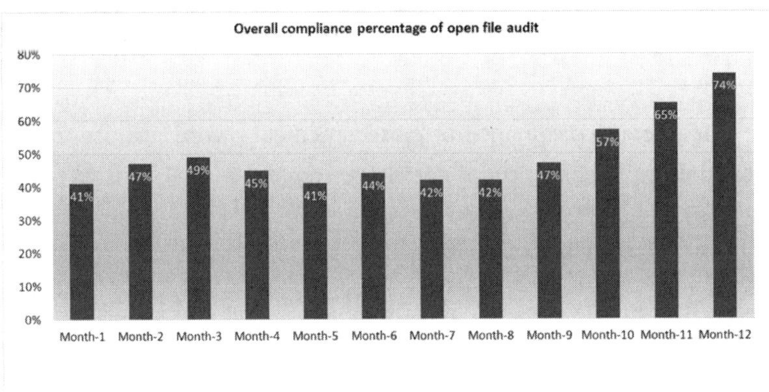

The overall compliance of open medical record audit improved from 43 per cent to 74 per cent as a result of a structured approach and regular follow ups.

Closed Medical Record Audit Analysis

Figure 4. Overall Compliance Percentage of Closed File Audit

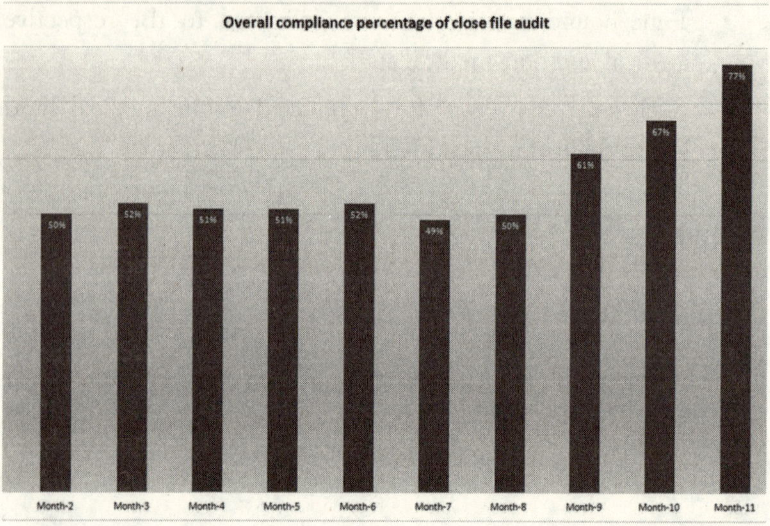

The overall compliance of closed medical record also improved after the implementation of corrective steps.

Sustenance Plan

It was decided that the same process of medical record review shall be continued in the future as well. All the respective staff must be trained on proper documentation. A weekly meeting was scheduled with the respective stakeholders and leadership to discuss the compliance.

Table 1. Department-Wise Data

PHYSICIAN DOCUMENTATION																		
WARD	SAMPLE SIZE	Source of history	Chief complaints	Medical history	Drug allergies	Vitals document ed	Pain assessmet iscore & location)	Infection risk assessmen t	Physical / Systemic Examinatio n	Diagnosis (Sign, Date & Time)	document ation review	Plan of care & measurabl e goals	Expected outcome at discharge	Medicatio n reconciliati on	Cosultant Sign, Date & Time	Completio n Rate	Previous Week - 14.12.18	Previous Week - 07.12.18
ACCU	5	100	100	100	100	100	100	100	100	100	100	100	100	100	100	100	96	100
CCT	4	100	100	100	100	100	100	100	100	100	100	100	100	100	100	100	100	67
CHEMOTHERAPY	7	100	100	100	100	100	100	100	100	100	86	100	100	100	100	99	98	100
CICU	9	100	100	100	100	100	100	100	100	100	67	89	100	100	100	97	79	88
CSICU	4	100	100	100	100	100	100	100	100	100	100	100	100	100	100	100	100	96
CT POST	5	100	100	100	100	100	100	100	100	100	100	100	100	100	100	100	100	100
FGW/MGW	19	100	100	100	100	100	100	100	100	100	79	95	100	95	95	97	93	92
FIRST FLOOR	5	100	100	100	100	100	100	100	100	100	60	100	100	100	80	96	74	94
INTER SECOND	12	100	100	100	100	100	100	100	100	100	100	75	100	92	100	98	88	88
INTER THIRD	18	100	100	100	100	100	100	100	100	100	39	94	94	94	94	94	85	93
MICU 1	5	100	100	100	100	100	100	100	100	100	80	80	100	100	100	97	96	98
MICU 2	7	100	100	100	100	100	100	100	100	100	86	100	100	100	100	99	94	93
NICU 1	4	100	100	100	100	100	100	100	100	100	75	100	100	100	100	98	100	100
NICU 2	3	100	100	100	100	100	100	100	100	100	33	100	100	100	100	95	100	98
ONCOLOGY	5	100	100	100	100	100	100	100	100	100	80	80	100	100	100	97	96	96
PAEDIATRIC	4	100	100	100	100	100	100	100	100	100	50	100	100	100	100	96	64	91
REGENCY -2	20	100	100	100	100	100	100	100	100	100	85	100	100	100	100	99	92	97
SECOND FLOOR	25	100	100	100	100	100	100	100	100	100	72	92	100	92	100	97	83	76
SICU	10	100	100	100	100	100	100	100	100	100	90	90	100	100	100	99	100	100
THIRD FLOOR	31	100	100	100	100	100	100	100	100	100	74	100	100	100	100	98	71	80
TRACHEOSTOMY																		
Completion Rate		100	100	100	100	100	100	100	100	100	78	95	100	99	98	98	90	92

Department-wise data was analysed and presented in this meeting. The low-scoring areas/sections were dealt with in detail. Weekly comparison of data was also completed to identify opportunities for improvement.

Conclusion

A dedicated task force, a well-defined checklist and regular follow ups on audit findings helped improve the compliance as well as accuracy and completeness of documentation.

References:

1. Our Standards, Joint Commission, https://www.jointcommission.org/accreditation-and-certification/health-care-settings/hospital/learn/our-standards/
2. Medical Records Maintenance, AIHMS Blog, 6 March 2021, https://aihms.in/blog/medical-records-maintenance/
3. P. Esposito and A. Dal Canton (2014), 'Clinical audit, a valuable tool to improve quality of care: General methodology and applications in nephrology', *World Journal of Nephrology*, Vol. 3, No. 4, pp. 249–255, https://doi.org/10.5527/wjn.v3.i4.249
4. R. G. Hughes, 'Tools and Strategies for Quality Improvement and Patient Safety', *Patient Safety and Quality: An Evidence-Based Handbook for Nurses* (Rockville, MD: Agency for Healthcare Research and Quality), https://www.ncbi.nlm.nih.gov/books/NBK2682/

Case Study 2

Patient Falls

'Please Call, Don't Fall.' Reducing the risk of harm related to patient falls.

Introduction

PATIENT FALLS IN any hospital is a major patient safety concern for the hospital systems and the Quality Teams. The addressal of this issue is essential to demonstrate the organization's competency in risk reduction, health promotion and implementation of evidence-based practices.

Fall has a negative impact on patient outcomes and sometimes could possibly lead to adverse/sentinel events. Most hospitals follow evidence-based assessment scales to evaluate the patients for fall risk factors, based on which they identify patients who are vulnerable and at a higher risk of fall. The accreditation bodies also consider patient falls as a major patient safety concern, and they are considered as one of the National/International Patient Safety Goals (IPSGs).

The clinical condition of the patient, i.e., acute or chronic illness, post-surgery status, bed-bound status, medications, treatments and placement of various tubes and catheters, increases the vulnerability to fall.

Most patient falls neither cause major injuries not require any major intervention; however, there is always a high risk of serious injuries post fall.

Patient falls are always disturbing and create fear among patients, family members and care-providers. At an individual level, patient falls may result in a fear of falling again, leading to reduced mobility and loss of confidence, adversely affecting recovery and increasing the length of stay in the hospital.

While not all patient falls are preventable, most of them are. Falls could be prevented by assessing risks and implementing interventions to reduce these risks. It is also vital to encourage a culture of vigilant safety among patients through continuous education and feedback. While the staff should participate in continuous education and learning from adverse events, preventing falls by guiding, educating, handling, and managing patients and their needs in a hospital is everyone's responsibility.

Undoubtedly, mobility is an essential feature of recovery from illness; sometimes, it indicates wellness of the patient, and in other instances, it is a symbol of recovery.

While reviewing incidents, it was observed that patients often suffered falls because they refused assistance from the care-providers, stating that they are fine, but later felt dizzy and fell down. Despite extensive and repeat patient education, it has been observed that patients continue to move out of bed for using washrooms, without calling/informing anybody for assistance. It has also been observed that patients don't accept any assistance inside the washrooms.

Best Practices

At the time of admission, every patient is assessed thoroughly by a nurse, and a modified fall risk assessment tool named AFRAT (Apollo Fall Risk Assessment Tool) is used to evaluate the risk of patient fall (though adapted from the Morse Scale, credit for improvising and adapting this scale goes to the nursing team at Apollo Hospitals Group).

The AFRAT score is calculated as per the clinical and physical condition of the patient. Patients who score >45 are considered vulnerable and at a high risk of fall. Additionally, if any patient belongs to a defined vulnerability criterion, they are also considered to be at a high risk for fall.

For prompt identification of such patients, a different colour band (yellow/blue/red) is tied on their wrist along with the usual ID band. A SAFETY FIRST sticker is placed at the head end of the patient's bed.

All healthcare providers stay vigilant in the inpatient units at all times. Patient and family education is provided by the doctors, nurses and physiotherapists (if required). There are few areas in the hospital that are pre-identified 'Vulnerable Patient Zones', such as ICU or the OT; patients admitted in those areas are considered vulnerable, and hence, prone to falls.

There is a protocol of conducting 'Post Fall Huddle', wherein representatives from Nursing Leadership, Physiotherapy, Clinical Care Coordinator Team, Engineering, Housekeeping and Quality Team meet the patient and assigned nursing staff to discuss the details of the incident using tools such as 5-Why analysis. The objective of the Post Fall Huddle Team is to identify the contributing factors of patient fall, and strengthen or develop such an environment across the organization which does not promote recurrence of such incidence.

Immediately after a fall incident occurs, the staff nurse stabilizes the patient, checks their vital signs, and conducts assessment for injury. Thereafter, the nurse calls the primary consultant and physicians from Orthopaedics, Neurology and Medicine departments. These physicians assess the patient thoroughly and order diagnostic investigations, if required. The nurse reassesses the patient using AFRAT to identify if there is an increased risk of fall based on the scoring.

Data Analysis

A sample dataset for one of the units (presented here) indicates that the majority of the falls were not true accidents. They were not inevitable consequences of ageing. Sometimes, they were the results of multiple intrinsic factors (cultural beliefs and behavioural issues) and extrinsic factors (environmental influences, medication and IV tubes, etc.), which further increased the risk of fall. Unfamiliar hospital environment coupled with acute physical and/or mental factors, too, amplify the risk of falls among patients.

Fall incident data of the study period was analysed based on age, timing of fall incident, ward/unit, location or site, medicines administered to the patient and their respective side effects. Higher fall rates were observed among male patients. The analysed data also indicated that in maximum cases, the patient got out of the bed and did not call any staff for assistance despite the hospital providing education as well as assistive tools like call bells.

The general remark has always been, 'I felt fine, and I can walk. I always go alone.'

Ward-wise analysis of data indicated that half of the fall incidents happened among the patients over the age of 60, and maximum fall incidents happened during late nights, midnight or early in the morning, when the patient had an urgency to pass urine.

Thus, patients are more likely to have a fall either while going to or coming from the washroom. Loss of balance and feeling of giddiness while coming/going to the washroom was the top reason of most of the fall incidents.

Figure 1. Fishbone Analysis

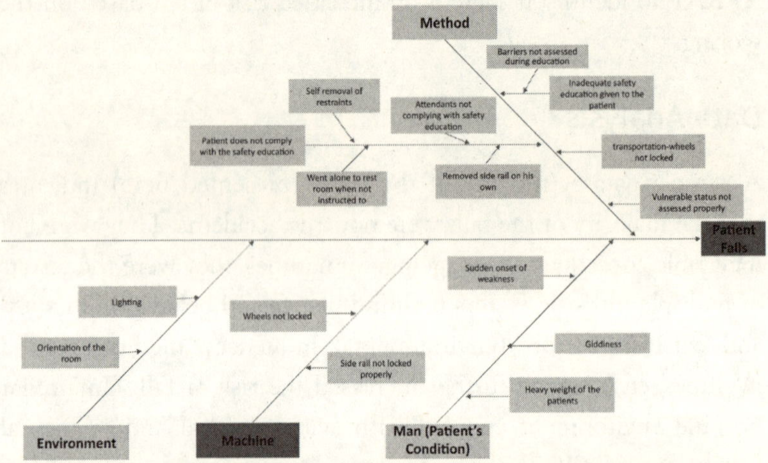

Interventions

The analysed data was discussed with the Senior Leadership and various modifications in the existing processes were undertaken to strengthen the patient fall prevention protocols.

The following interventions were taken into consideration to reduce fall incidences:

Strengthened 'Safety First Programme': Regular and vigorous training imparted to all the care-providers.

Figure 2. 'Safety First Programme' Training

Training Session- Return Demonstration SAMPLE

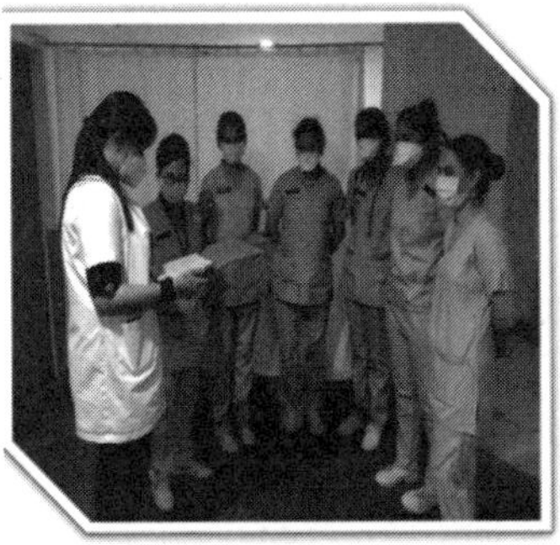

Reinforcement training on safe mobilization of post operative patients.

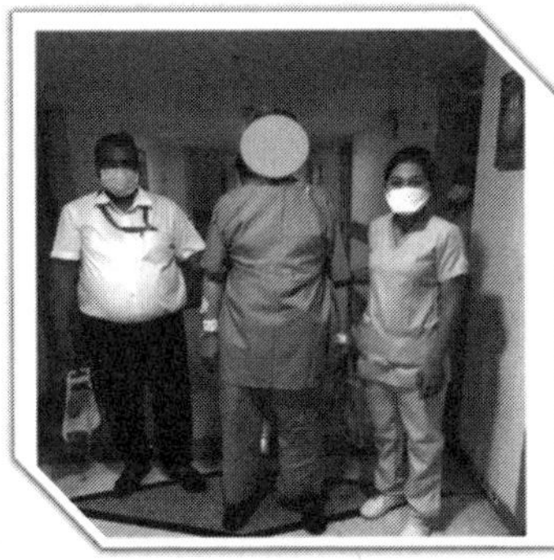

Demonstration on effective assistance

Hands On Training for Fall Prevention

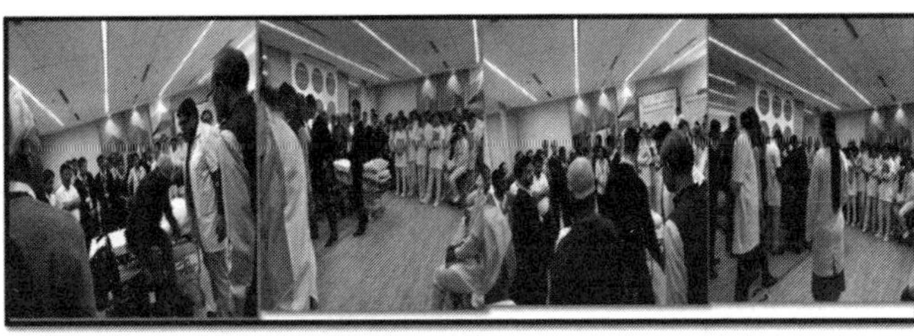

Theme - "Engaging all for prevention of fall".

Conducted by physiotherapy department on 19.02.2020.

Safe transfer of patients and ergonomics was demonstrated.

Attended by nursing as well as house keeping staff.

Courtesy: Apollo Hospitals

Periodic Audits Conducted to Ensure Correct AFRAT Scoring: Nurses were trained and periodic audits were undertaken to check the accuracy of scores calculated. *More accurate the score, better the identification of patients at a high risk of fall.*

Figure 3. Compliance Monitoring of AFRAT

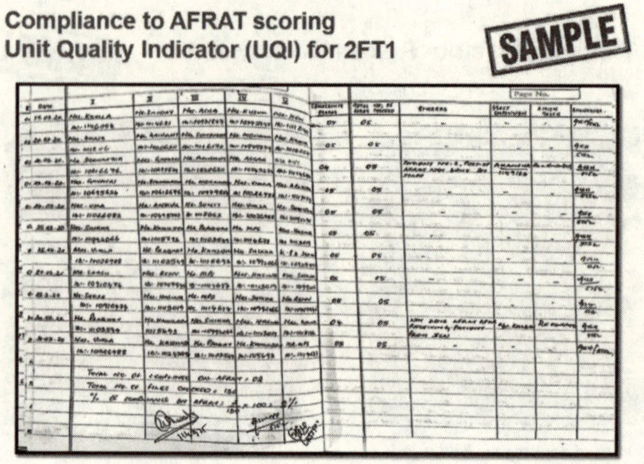

Don't Fall, Please Call: Bilingual patient and family education forms were incorporated for patient care to remove the language barrier.

Figure 4. Bilingual Patient and Family Education Form

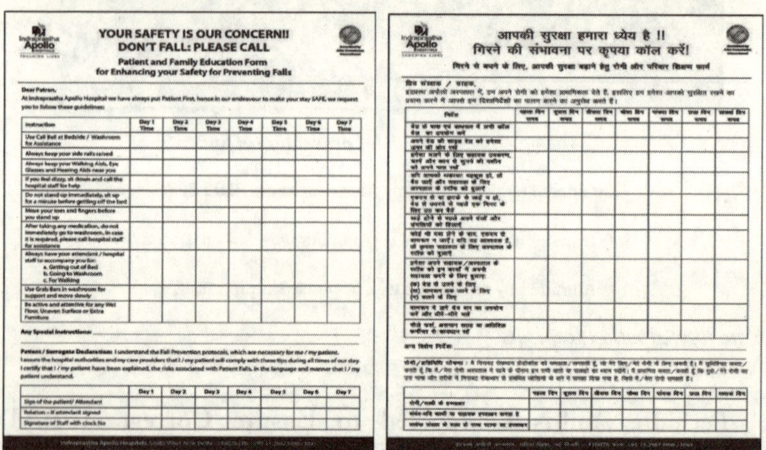

YOUR SAFETY IS OUR CONCERN!!
DON'T FALL: PLEASE CALL
Patient and Family Education Form for Enhancing your Safety for Preventing Falls

Dear Patron,
At Indraprastha Apollo Hospital we have always put Patient First, hence in our endeavour to make your stay SAFE, we request you to follow these guidelines:

Instruction	Day 1 Time	Day 2 Time	Day 3 Time	Day 4 Time	Day 5 Time	Day 6 Time	Day 7 Time
Use Call Bell at Bedside / Washroom for Assistance							
Always keep your side rails raised							
Always keep your Walking Aids, Eye Glasses and Hearing Aids near you							
If you feel dizzy, sit down and call the hospital staff for help							
Do not stand up immediately, sit up for a minute before getting off the bed							
Move your toes and fingers before you stand up							
After taking any medication, do not immediately go to washroom, in case it is required, please call hospital staff for assistance							
Always have your attendant / hospital staff to accompany you for: a. Getting out of Bed b. Going to Washroom c. For Walking							
Use Grab Bars in washroom for support and move slowly							
Be active and attentive for any Wet Floor, Uneven Surface or Extra Furniture							

Any Special Instructions:

Patient / Surrogate Declaration: I understand the Fall Prevention protocols, which are necessary for me / my patient. I assure the hospital authorities and my care providers that I / my patient will comply with these tips during all times of our stay. I certify that I / my patient have been explained, the risks associated with Patient Falls, in the language and manner that I / my patient understand.

	Day 1	Day 2	Day 3	Day 4	Day 5	Day 6	Day 7
Sign of the patient/ Attendant							
Relation – If attendant signed							
Signature of Staff with clock No							

आपकी सुरक्षा हमारा ध्येय है !!
गिरने की संभावना पर कृपया कॉल करें!

Courtesy: Apollo Hospitals

Night-time PFE (Patient Family Education): In some cases, it was observed that there was a different attendant/family member with the patient every day. Hence, the education provided to the attendant at the time of admission was not effective in preventing falls as this attendant/family may not have remembered the instructions well or may not have passed on the information to the next attendant accompanying his patient. Therefore, a mandatory bedtime or night-time PFE was initiated. This ensured that every patient and accompanying attendant, if any, gets educated on all Dos and Don'ts each night before bedtime.

Figure 5. Night-time Patient and Family Education

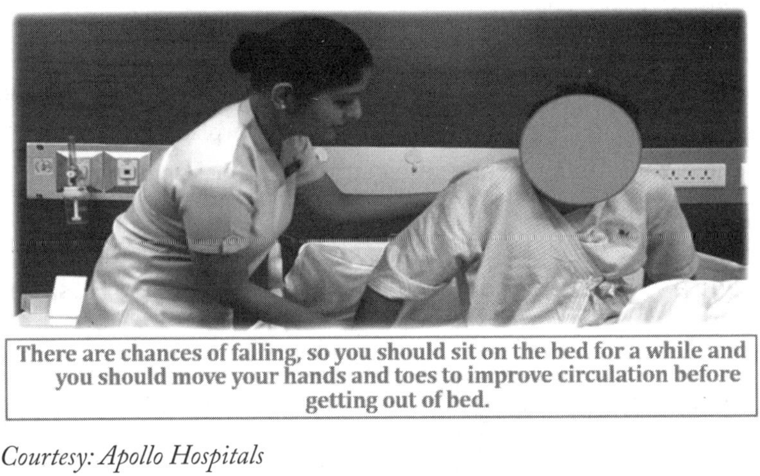

Courtesy: Apollo Hospitals

The education material was improvised with a focus on the falls due to orthostatic hypotension.

Figure 6. Patient Education Materials

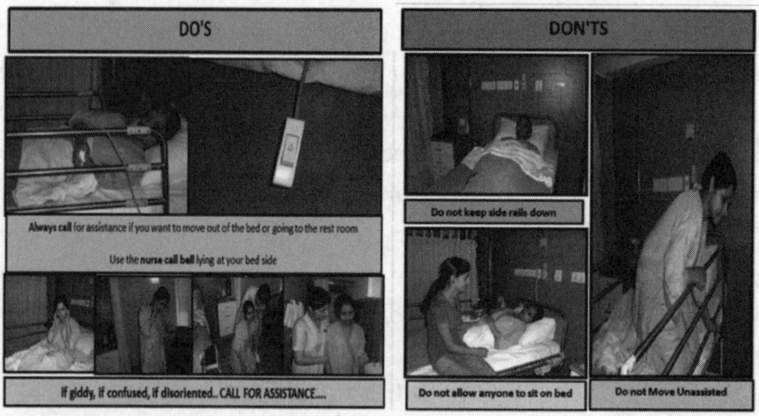

Courtesy: Apollo Hospitals

Modified Posters for Vulnerable Patient Zone and Fall Prevention Strategies: Bilingual posters were placed in vulnerable patient zones and patient waiting areas to emphasize the *Don't Fall, Please Call* initiative.

Figure 7. Identification of Vulnerable Zones in the Hospital

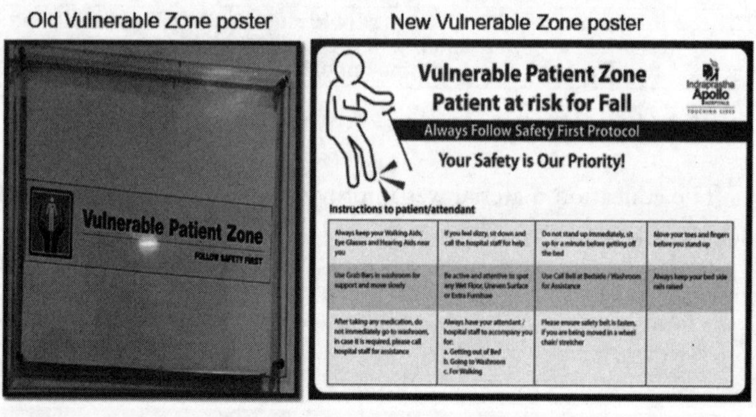

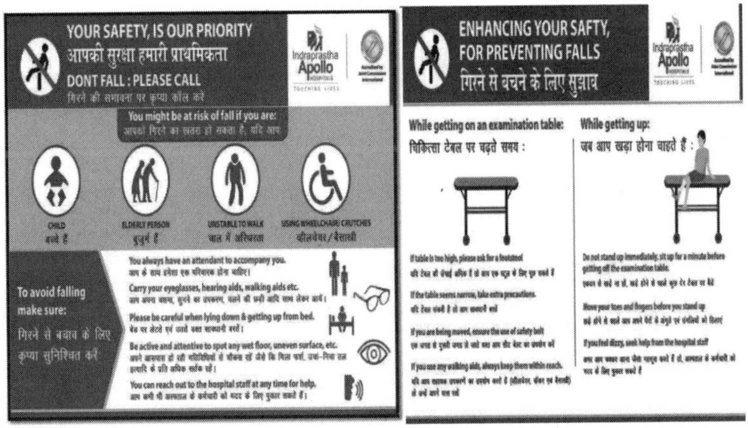

Courtesy: Apollo Hospitals

Your Safety is Our Priority: Since maximum patient falls happened either in the room or the washroom, patients were specifically educated to not move from the bed alone, along with various other measures for fall prevention. Posters were also placed inside the restroom, on doors, to catch the attention of the patient and disseminate fall-prevention education.

Figure 8. Display of Patient Education on Falls Prevention and Assistance in the Washrooms

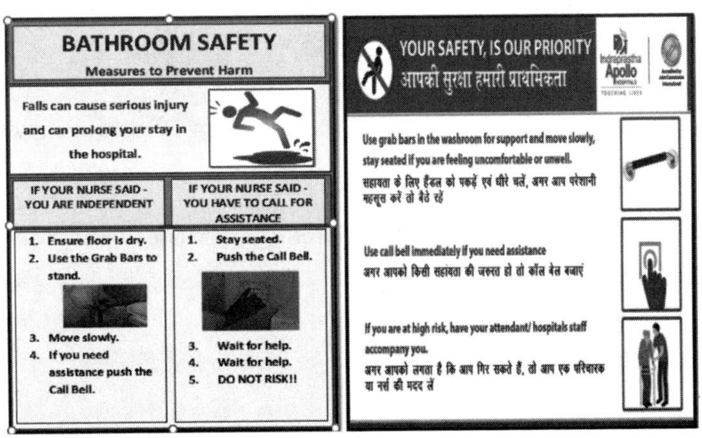
BATHROOM SAFETY
Measures to Prevent Harm
Falls can cause serious injury and can prolong your stay in the hospital.
IF YOUR NURSE SAID - YOU ARE INDEPENDENT
1. Ensure floor is dry.
2. Use the Grab Bars to stand.
3. Move slowly.
4. If you need assistance push the Call Bell.
IF YOUR NURSE SAID - YOU HAVE TO CALL FOR ASSISTANCE
1. Stay seated.
2. Push the Call Bell.
3. Wait for help.
4. Wait for help.
5. DO NOT RISK!!
YOUR SAFETY, IS OUR PRIORITY
आपकी सुरक्षा हमारी प्राथमिकता
Use grab bars in the washroom for support and move slowly, stay seated if you are feeling uncomfortable or unwell.
Use call bell immediately if you need assistance
If you are at high risk, have your attendant/ hospitals staff accompany you.

Courtesy: Apollo Hospitals

Extension boards were attached to the beds of the patients to prevent falls in vulnerable patients. These boards prevent the patient from falling/coming out of the bed from the gap between the side rails and foot end.

Figure 9. Additional Extension Boards to Cover the Gap

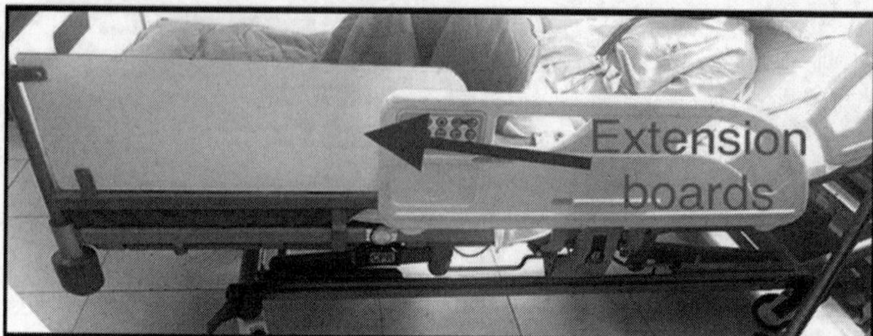

Campaign on Fall Prevention: A campaign was organized to create awareness among the nursing staff to be more cautious while handling inpatients.

Figure 10. Campaign on Fall Prevention

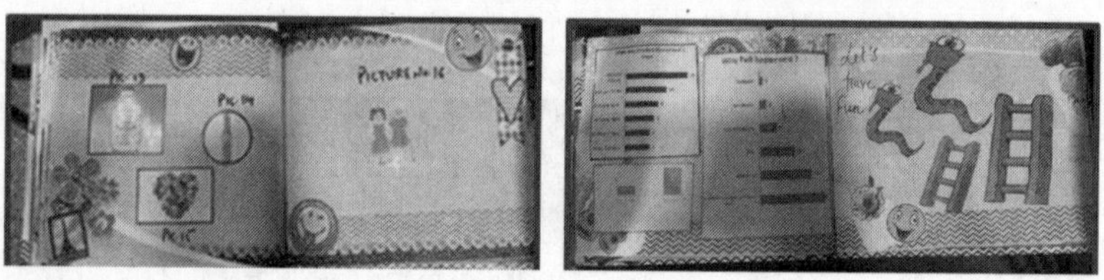

Courtesy: Apollo Hospitals

1. Fall incidents of each ward/unit was discussed with the staff.
2. Random audits were undertaken to check compliance with fall prevention measures.

3. Assessment was undertaken to gauge awareness levels among patients and families regarding fall prevention measures.
4. Brainstorming activities were conducted, wherein a scrapbook was created and 'fall culprit drugs' and other causative factors' pictures were added. Staff was asked to identify and give answers.
5. Nurses took a resolution to adhere to fall prevention protocols and focus on patient education in their respective areas.

Figure 11. Resolution to Prevent Falls

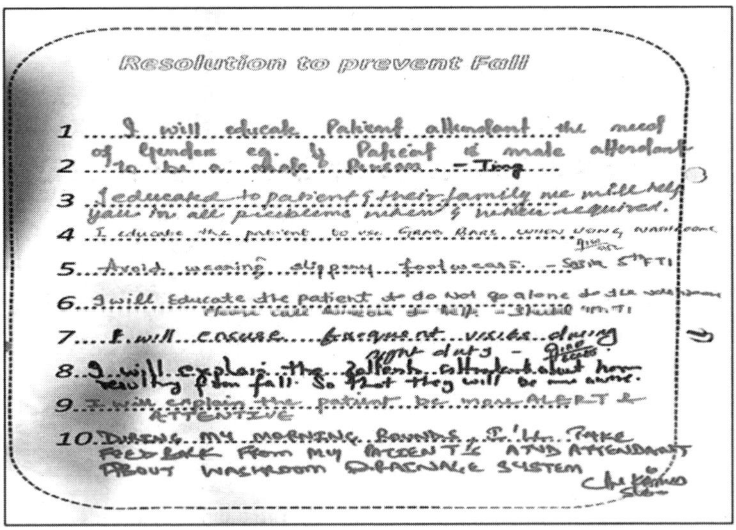
Resolution to prevent Fall

1 I will educate Patient attendant the need of [illegible] eg. if Patient is male attendant
2 to be a [illegible] person
3 I educate to patient & their family we will help you in all problems when & where required.
4 I educate the patient to use [illegible] when using washroom
5 Avoid wearing slippery footwears.
6 I will educate the patient to do not go alone to the washroom [illegible]
7 I will ensure frequent visits during [illegible]
8 I will explain the patient attendant about how [illegible] from fall. So that they will be aware.
9 I will explain the patient be more ALERT & ATTENTIVE
10 During my morning rounds, I'll take feedback from my patients and attendants about washroom drainage system

Courtesy: Apollo Hospitals

Revised AFRAT: Based on analysis, the drugs that posed a high risk of falls—culprit drugs—were incorporated in the AFRAT form. The addition of culprit drugs in the form has helped accurately identify patients who are at a high risk of fall.

Figure 12: Revised AFRAT Form

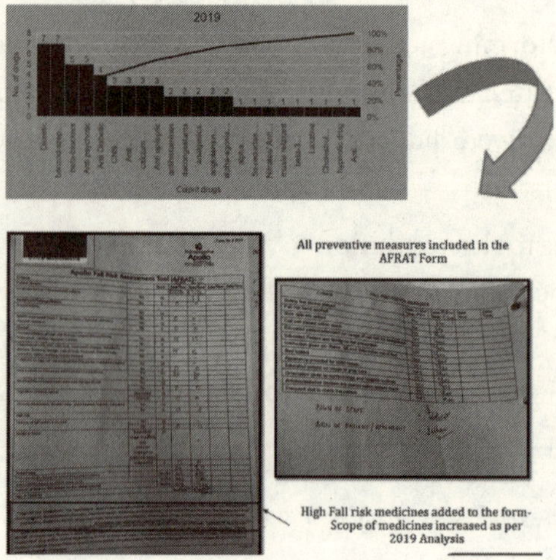

Courtesy: Apollo Hospitals

Introduced a Code White Team: The Code White Team acted as a rapid response team in case of any incidence of fall. A team of designated doctors was alerted about the incident through the addressal system, reducing the response time for initiating definitive treatment.

Results

Significant reduction in the number of falls was observed in Year 2, compared to Year 1. However, while reduction in the number of falls was noted among vulnerable patients, there was a rise in fall incidents among non-vulnerable patients.

Figure 13. Reduction in Patient Falls Post Interventions in Year 2

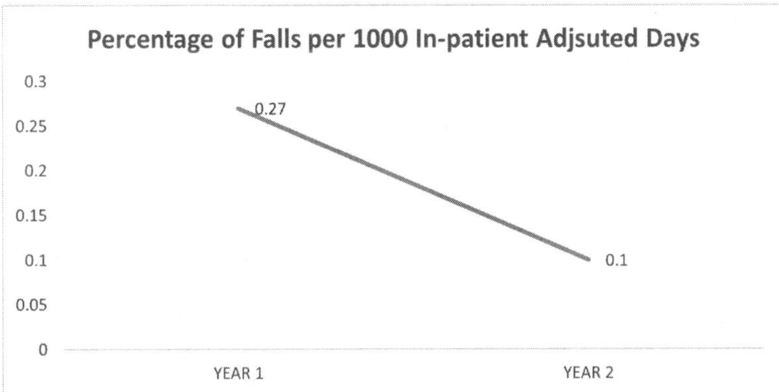

As a result of our Night-time PFE initiative, decline in the number of fall incidents could be seen in the Year 2.

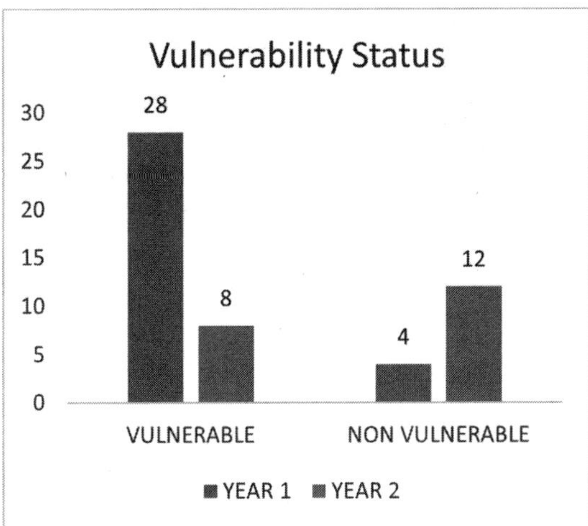

Courtesy: Apollo Hospitals

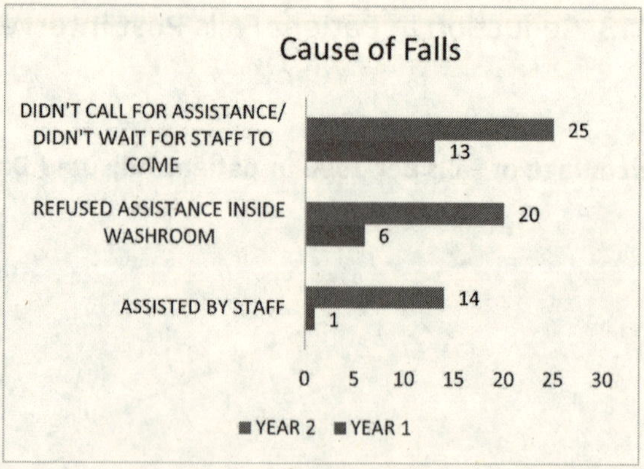
Cause of Falls
DIDN'T CALL FOR ASSISTANCE/ DIDN'T WAIT FOR STAFF TO COME
REFUSED ASSISTANCE INSIDE WASHROOM
ASSISTED BY STAFF
25
13
20
6
14
1
0 5 10 15 20 25 30
YEAR 2
YEAR 1

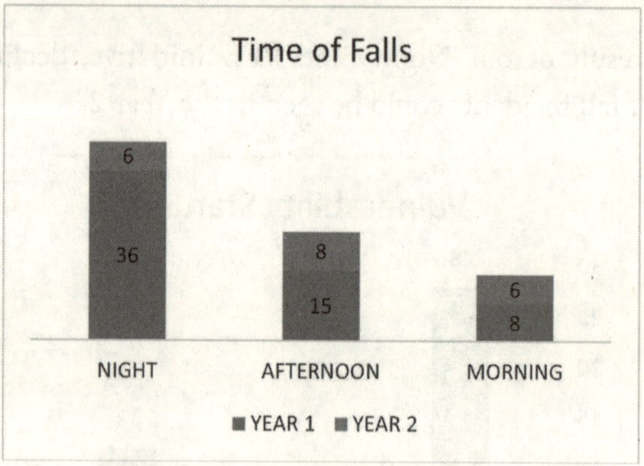
Time of Falls
6
36
8
15
6
8
NIGHT
AFTERNOON
MORNING
YEAR 1
YEAR 2

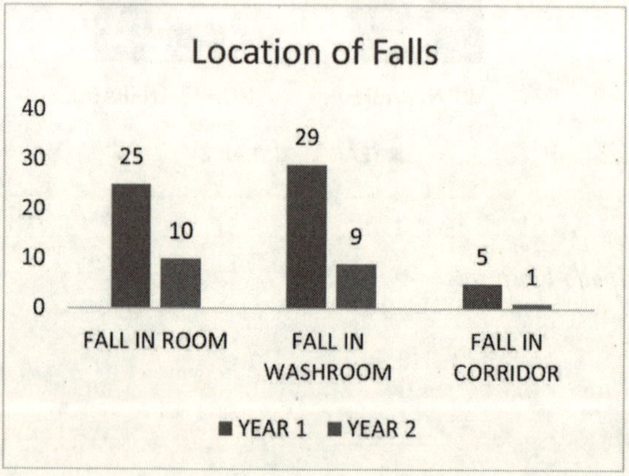
Location of Falls
40
30
20
10
0
25
10
29
9
5
1
FALL IN ROOM
FALL IN WASHROOM
FALL IN CORRIDOR
YEAR 1
YEAR 2

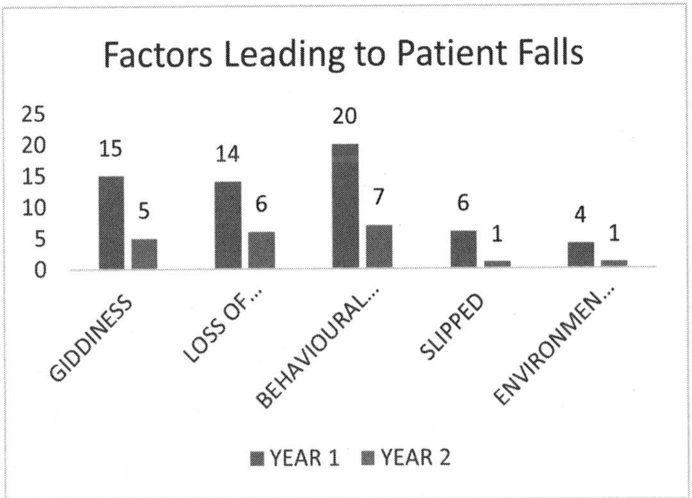

Courtesy: Apollo Hospitals

Reinforcement of nurses to emphasize patient and family education and placement of vibrant posters in different areas for educating patients to follow fall prevention strategies has reduced the overall fall numbers in all areas—including patient rooms, washroom and other locations.

Moreover, with focused interventions such as the revised AFRAT form that identifies culprit drugs, falls due to giddiness, loss of balance and behavioural issues have been on a steady decline.

Lesson Learnt

Because healthcare delivery has become complex in the current scenario, every hospital must institutionalize the approach of risk assessment for patient safety. Though traditionally, the basic protocols of detailed clinical and nursing assessments, patient rounding, patient and family education and care planning must be followed, we also need to be proactive when it comes to risk management. Hence, we need to conduct patient falls risk assessment at various stages.

This is still a new concept in the healthcare system, though it has existed in other industries for a long time. All healthcare accreditation standards are now emphasizing proactive risk assessment and mitigation in all hospitals, and they encourage the use of quality/safety tools such as Failure Mode Effect Analysis (FMEA), Hazard Vulnerability Analysis (HVA) and Risk Registers.

During the various phases of analysing patient fall data, we realized that in addition to all basic protocols being in place, there is a strong need for out-of-the-box thinking and formulating solutions specific to the needs of patients and families. The healthcare providers should create an atmosphere that facilitates the theme of PATIENTS AS PARTNERS in their care process. Visual reminders on patient safety through bilingual posters and patient fall education forms have also helped us in reducing the fall events. There are many aspects that need attention, such as type of medications, bed design, floor, and positioning of call bells in creating a safe environment for patients.

Conclusion

Falls are the most commonly reported patient safety incidents in acute hospital settings. There are multiple risk factors for falling in a hospital, but no single methodology can be described as the best to eliminate fall risk. Hence, a collaborative and multipronged approach needs to be undertaken by healthcare providers.

Identifying risks in a proactive manner and providing effective interventions wherever possible can reduce falls by 20–30 per cent. Building safety consciousness among all healthcare providers—doctors, nurses, physiotherapists, pharmacists, housekeeping, engineering and regular training—is one of the key factors.

References:

1. 'Falls Risk Assessment Tool (FRAT): An Overview to Assist Understanding and Conduction', Physiopedia, https://www.physiopedia.com/Falls_Risk_Assessment_Tool_(FRAT):_An_Overview_to_Assist_Understanding_and_Conduction
2. R. Morris and S. O'Riordan, 'Prevention of falls in hospital', *Clinical Medicine*, Vol. 17, No. 4, pp. 360–362, https://doi.org/10.7861/clinmedicine.17-4-360.
3. H. Heng, D. Jazayeri, et al., 'Hospital falls prevention with patient education: A scoping review', *BMC Geriatrics*, Vol. 20, No. 1, https://doi.org/10.1186/s12877-020-01515-w
4. D. Avanecean, et al., 'Effectiveness of patient-centered interventions on falls in the acute care setting compared to usual care: a systematic review', *JBI database of systematic reviews and implementation reports* (2017), Vol. 15 No. 12, pp. 3006–3048. https://doi.org/10.11124/JBISRIR-2016-003331
5. M. Luzia, et al., 'Incidence of falls and preventive actions in a University Hospital', *Incidência de quedas e ações preventivas em um Hospital Universitário, Revista da Escola de Enfermagem da USP* 52, e03308, https://doi.org/10.1590/s1980-220x2017024203308
6. T. Dunne, et al., 'Falls in hospital increase length of stay regardless of degree of harm', *Journal of Evaluation in Clinical Practice* (2014), Vol. 20, No. 4, pp. 396–400, https://doi.org/10.1111/jep.12144
7. D. Evans, B. Hodgkinson, et al., 'Falls in acute hospitals: a systematic review', *Joanna Briggs Institute for Evidence Based Nursing and Midwifery, Systematic Review* (1998), Vol. 1.

Case Study 3

Surgical Safety

An initiative to reduce the incorrect count of material/ equipment, leading to safe surgery.

Introduction

HEALTHCARE HAS ALWAYS been a complex environment and adverse events are a reality. This becomes even more crucial when surgical patients are involved. The World Health Organization (WHO) Safe Surgery campaign aimed to implement safe surgical procedures and patient safety best practices to reduce the incidence of adverse events, both in the operating room and in the patient care areas.

For decades, the main focus of safe surgery was on technical procedures. More recently, promoting an organizational culture of safety and improving teamwork and interpersonal communication have been found to play a significant role in preventing harm in surgical care settings.

Many studies (Leape et al., 1991; Vicent, Neale, & Woloshynowych, 2001; WHO, 2002; Wilson et al., 1995) indicate that the incidence of adverse events range from 3.8 per cent to 16 per cent, of which 48 per cent are linked to surgery. The implications of these events directly reflect on the patient's increased length of hospital stay, temporary or permanent disability, or even patient deaths. In addition, they are associated with a considerable amount of increased costs, which ultimately, the patients have to pay for. The concern is even greater when it's evident that about half of these events were preventable.

It's also noted that given the increasingly complicated modern healthcare atmosphere and patient population, reduction of medical errors is becoming a highly significant job. While the incidence and outcomes of specific types of surgical errors are relatively well described, the knowledge of why these errors occur need a thorough examination. Retention of surgical foreign bodies such as sponges, instruments, needles, etc., are the most well-known examples of serious surgical errors in healthcare. Retained surgical foreign bodies may cause harm to the patient and can result in serious professional and medicolegal consequences, impacting surgical practice. Thus, special emphasis needs to be laid on problem identification, preventive strategies, and system-based education and improvement. Hence, even WHO advocates that the surgical count process should be performed in any surgery.

Unintentional retention of foreign body is the cause of 70 per cent of re-interventions, with a morbidity of 80 per cent and mortality of 35 per cent. The most common foreign bodies are sponges or gauze. Perioperative counting of equipment and materials is the most common method of screening for retained surgical item, while a diagnosis can later be confirmed by the imaging study and clinical appearance.

The diagnosis of retention of surgical items is extremely important, and safe surgical practices including the sign-out process should be encouraged to identify such incidences.

Retained Surgical Foreign Bodies: Preventive Measures

The best approach to prevent retained surgical foreign bodies is to prevent their occurrence, which avoids all its deleterious consequences, including the need for unnecessary invasive procedures and associated medico-legal consequences.

The most essential preventive measure is to precisely count all the pieces of surgical gauze and surgical instruments used during a surgery. If a sponge or an instrument count at the end of the procedure is not matching with those performed at the beginning of the procedure, or if there is any suspicion among the operative team members that retained surgical foreign bodies may have been left behind, then the team should do a 're-count' of sponge, instruments, etc. This could be followed either by radiography (to confirm absence of intracorporeal-retained surgical foreign bodies) and/or surgical re-exploration.

Case Study

A forty-two-year-old patient was admitted to the hospital for left cervical lymph node selective nodal excision under general anaesthesia. As part of the hospital process, Pre-Anaesthesia Check (PAC) was completed by the anaesthetist on set criteria. The patient was wheeled into the operation theatre (OT) for the procedure of cervical lymph node selective excision.

The WHO surgical safety checklist was followed, and as per the checklist, sign-in was completed.

The patient was identified correctly, checked for difficulty in airway/aspiration/dentures, assessed for possibility of hypothermia,

Figure 1. WHO Safe Surgery Checklist

Patient Name:
UHID:

SAFE SURGERY CHECKLIST

Date:

SIGN IN

A. IN PREOP AREA BEFORE SHIFTING PATIENT TO OPERATING ROOM (O.T.)

B. IN PREOP AREA/ IN OPERATING ROOM BEFORE INDUCTION OF ANAESTHESIA

A. IN PREOP AREA BEFORE SHIFTING PATIENT TO O.T., REVIEW WITH PATIENT & CHECK CASE FILE

1. Patient identification(Name, Age, IPID, ID Band)
2. Surgical procedure to be performed
3. Site/Side of surgical procedure with marking
4. Consent Forms (Surgery, Anesthesia) complete & signed
5. Known allergies
6. Airway assessed for difficulty
7. In case of difficult airway whether equipment / assistance available

Yes No NA

Anesthetist Sign......................................

8. Special equipment for surgeries after discussing with the surgeon.

Nurses Sign......................................

OT Technician to transfer the patient to O.T. only after part A is completed and signed by Anaesthetist

B) IN PREOP AREA/ IN O.T. BEFORE INDUCTION ANESTHESIA REVIEW :

9. Is Patient identification reconfirmed ? Yes No
10. Any Anesthesia equipment issues or concerns Yes No
11. Anesthesia safety check has been completed Yes No
12. Risk of blood loss > 500 ml/ 7ml/kg in children Yes No
13. Blood products arranged NA Yes
14. Have all ornaments been removed from patient body Yes No

16. Beta blocker medication given Yes No NA

Time patient wheeled In O.T. :..............................

Anesthetist. ....(After Time Out)

(Surgeon)

TIME OUT (Operation Theater)

C. BEFORE SKIN INCISION (SAFETY PAUSE)

1. Does everyone know each other?

Yes No (If No, introduce-name, role)

SURGEON REVIEWS WITH THE TEAM :

2. What is the Patient's name ?
3. What is the UHID No :
4. Name of the procedure planned, operating plan

....

5. Is the correct site prepared and draped?

Yes No

6. Expected duration of the surgery......................
7. Discuss if there is anything unique or non - routine about this surgery?

Routine Non routine / Any issues

....

....

8. Implants or special equipment required

NA Yes

9. Is essential imaging displayed?

Yes Not applicable

ANAESTHETIST REVIEWS WITH THE TEAM :

10. Antibiotic Prophylaxis given within last 15-60 minutes (90-120 for Vanco, Metro, etc)?

Yes No Not applicable

Name of Drug ....

Time of administration..............................

11. Is there anything unique or non-routine about anesthesia administration?

No

If Yes......................................

12. Normothermia attended to Yes No

NURSING TEAM REVIEWS

13. Has sterility been confirmed

Yes No

Incision Time :......................................

14. VTE prophylaxis ordered Yes No NA

Circulating Nurse / Person doing the Time Out

....

SIGN OUT (Operation Theater)

D. BEFORE PATIENT LEAVES OPERATING ROOM

NURSE REVIEWS WITH TEAM :

1. Instrument, sponge and needle counts are correct

Yes Not applicable

No

2. Name of the actual procedure performed

....

3. Specimen labeling
Read back specimen labeling including patient's name & UHID / IPID

SURGICAL TEAM DISCUSSES :

4. Any equipment problems that need to taken in Post Operative Patient Management

No

If Yes......................................

Discussion on wound classification Yes No

To all team members What are the key concerns for recovery and management of this patient

....

....

....

Time patient wheeled out :..............................

Circulating Nurse.....................................

(Anesthetist In-charge) (After Sign Out)

This Checklist is only a Quality Improvement Tool. To be included in patient file.

Courtesy: Apollo Hospitals

and preoperative medications were given. All concerned anaesthesia equipment and medications checks were completed.

Timeout was then conducted and documented by the team members by introducing themselves with their names and roles. Patient was identified by two identifiers, correct procedure, site, side, position, and consents were checked as well. Required equipment and implants were checked for their availability, along with essential imaging. The timeout process stringently followed the format of the WHO Surgical Safety Checklist. On completion of the timeout procedure, surgery commenced.

On completion of the surgery and after closure of the surgical site, dressing was completed. Patient was stable at the end of the surgery.

Post-surgery, sign-out was conducted and documented. Circulating nurse, along with the surgical team, confirmed:

- the name of procedure performed (left cervical lymph node selective excision),
- quantity and labelling of all specimens to be sent to lab (Level 1A lymph node left; Level 1B lymph node left; tissue over the left carotid sheath; Level 2 to Level 5 with skin over the left side of neck; revised margin from left buccal mucosa lesion; frozen section).

No equipment or instrument failure was noted. Sponge and needle count was then checked, and surprisingly, it did not match with the numbers counted at the beginning of the procedure. Two gauze pieces were missing.

Immediately, re-count was performed, followed by radiography examination through C-ARM machine (to confirm absence of intracorporeal-retained surgical foreign bodies). Unfortunately, there was no gauze piece found in the surgical opening. The whole incident was reported for further investigation.

Analysis

Investigation of such a serious incident revealed that all the prerequisite consumables were arranged and counted before the surgery. As a part of safe surgery check, sign-in and timeout were done appropriately, with all stakeholders participating in the process as per the protocol.

Incidentally, during the surgery, the primary surgeon requested for two more packets of gauze pieces. While handing over the gauze piece to the surgeon, the circulatory nurse missed counting the gauze pieces before giving it to the surgeon. Even the surgeon did not check how many he ended up using during the procedure.

Thus, incorrect counts as well as count discrepancies led to the unintentional retention of a surgical item after surgery.

Further Study and Results

It was further analysed that while the surgery was ongoing, the assigned circulatory nurse went out of the OT due to some emergency and another circulatory nurse came into the room to assist with that surgery.

When the surgeon asked for additional gauze pieces, the new circulatory nurse gave it to the surgeon, but unfortunately, since there was no communication or handover between the two circulatory nurses, the exact number of gauze pieces being used for the patient were not recorded.

During the sign-out process, it was observed that two gauze pieces were missing. The wound was examined with the help of C-ARM machine, but the missing gauze piece could not be found. All the surrounding areas were checked. Finally, as a final check, a few of the unused gauze piece packets were opened to check how many gauze pieces were there in each packet. Luckily, instead of five gauze pieces in each packet, there were four in each packet. Hence, it was concluded that the total gauze pieces were the same that were issued and used.

When the surgeon requested for extra gauze pieces during the procedure, the circulating and scrub nurse didn't count them before handing them over to the surgeon. Even the surgeon did not check how many he used in the procedure. Moreover, there was no handover communication between the two circulatory nurses who were replaced during the surgery.

It was also noted that there was a wide variation in the type of worksheets used to tally intraoperative counts (e.g., whiteboard, count sheet, sheet of unmarked paper). These disparities contributed to an incorrect count and count discrepancies associated with documentation errors. Incorrect counts also added time to the procedures, resulting in additional radiation exposure to patients.

The findings revealed a need to standardize the count process. After it was determined that nurses were documenting counts in various ways, the count practice expectations and updates were reinforced during several educational in-service programmes, staff meetings and electronic communication. The nurse supervisors enforced the established protocol of having two nursing team members 'count'—audibly and visibly. Education included the sequence of counting from the surgical field back to the back table, and then to the sponge receptacle.

The nurses also updated the instrument count sheets to create a seamless workflow during counting without any disturbance. Furthermore, the instrument count slip and the string of instruments were set in the same order for comfort of counting.

The goal was to reduce the number of reported incorrect counts and count discrepancies, thereby reducing patient exposure to radiographs, decreased time and expense, and lower risk of unintentional retention.

Interventions

The trends in improper counts were examined further in detail. Nursing administrator along with the Quality Department head implemented a root cause analysis (RCA) to gather pertinent information on instances of improper counts.

The quality team monitored all procedures in which an incorrect count happened. The team then discussed the findings with the perioperative team members who were involved, and strengthened the counts policy and practices as needed.

RCA specified that the majority of incorrect counts involved gauze pieces. Through detailed RCA, the following trends were also diagnosed that contributed to incorrect counts of gauze pieces:

- Surgical procedures that continued for more than eight hours
- Numerous staff movement and turnover during a procedure
- Documentation inconsistencies or lack of oversights of items added in between the surgery
- Communication failure among team members during the surgery
- A lack of standardized practices due to inconsistency and clarification of count policy

Way Forward

Recognizing the significance of this initiative, a small task force developed a methodical approach that included:

- reviewing reported wrong counts and count discrepancies
- working together with the radiology department
- reviewing the existing count policy
- standardizing practices across all team members
- using a team approach to the count process
- conducting observational audits on regular intervals

To overcome the process variation in incorrect counts and count discrepancies during a surgery, the hospital identified perioperative nursing metric priorities that were directly related to improved patient care and outcomes in the perioperative programmes.

Staff members agreed that a quality improvement initiative to reduce the number of incorrect counts and count discrepancies and prevent retention of surgical items was a top priority. Nursing supervisor made perioperative nursing staff members aware of the new initiative to reduce incorrect counts through staff meetings and e-mails.

Enthusiastic verbal and written feedback were received from the nursing staff members, who supported this endeavour. This enthusiasm ultimately contributed to the success of the initiative.

Efforts were made to standardize the number of gauze pieces packaging in CSSD, and from then on, a protocol was developed to ensure there were five gauze pieces in each packet. Random audits were done to check on the standardization of those numbers as well.

The hospital thus adopted a team approach to the count process, based on recommendations from the nursing supervisor, quality team, doctors and the nursing staff in the prevention of retention of surgical items.

Lessons Learnt and Recommendations

Implementing the policy through a methodical multidisciplinary team, supported by continuous handholding and monitoring, that meets recommended practices and the needs of the institution appears to be a logical way to reduce the number of retention of surgical items and count discrepancies.

It is recommended that surgeons take an active role and 'stop to counting the gauze'. This includes performing a precise wound exploration in every procedure, actively looking for sponges and gauze pieces, and announcing that all sponges are removed.

All sponges and gauze pieces used for the surgery must be kept in the holder at the end of each procedure for the whole team to check and verify during the final count. This process provides the surgeon and nurse with evidence that all the sponges and gauze pieces have been removed before wound closure. Perioperative team members should conduct a 'wound closure timeout too as a best practice'.

During this process, all the team members—which includes the surgeon and nurses—are expected to avoid disturbances or distractions and focus on wound closure time-out. Any break of staff members during the count process should not be allowed. The surgeon is responsible for checking the wound for any unintentionally retained items. The nursing team then completes the closing count by loudly and visibly conducting surgical counts. The nursing team is accountable for announcing the closing count status to the team. After the wound closure timeout is achieved, the team can proceed to conducting the remaining part of the sign-out process as described in the WHO safe surgery checklist.

Conclusion

The accurate application of the surgical count process by the perioperative team may lead to preventing retained surgical items during surgery, thereby securing the safety of surgical patients to a greater extent. Nurses can use this review to support in decision-making, focused on preparing, updating and implementing a dependable system for the surgical count process based on recent evidence-based guidelines. The perioperative nurse plays a pivotal role in the implementation of this practice in healthcare service delivery.

The system is designed to have safety checklists, standardize and streamline standardized process flows, integrate computerization, and provide a final restriction to prevent wrong counting.

References:

1. J. Devine, N. Chutkan, 'Avoiding wrong site surgery: a systematic review', *Spine* 35 (2010), S28–36, doi: 10.1097/BRS.0b013e3181d833ac 2.
2. M. A. James, J. G. Seiler, 'The occurrence of wrong-site surgery self-reported by candidates for certification by the American Board of Orthopaedic Surgery', *J Bone Joint Surg Am* (2012), Vol. 94 (Suppl. 1), doi: 10.2106/JBJS.K. 00524.
3. S. Hempel, et al., 'Wrong-Site Surgery, Retained Surgical Items, and Surgical Fires'.
4. Pennsylvania Patient Safety Authority, 'Beyond the count: preventing retention of foreign objects', *Patient Safety Advisory* (2019), Vol. 6, No. 2, pp. 39–45, http://patientsafety.pa.gov/ADVISORIES/Pages/200906_39.aspx
5. C. Greenberg, et al., 'The Frequency and Significance of Discrepancies in the Surgical Count'.
6. *Sentinel Event*, Joint Commission, https://www.jointcommission.org/resources/patient-safety-topics/sentinel-event/
7. A. Rowlands, 'Incorrect Surgical Counts: A Qualitative Analysis'.
8. A. Gawande, 'Risk Factors for Retained Instruments and Sponges after Surgery'.
9. S.P. Stawicki, D.C Evans, J. Cipolla, M.J. Seamon, 'Retained Surgical Foreign Bodies: A Comprehensive Review of Risks and Preventive Strategies', https://journals.sagepub.com/doi/pdf/10.1177/145749690909800103
10. 'Why safe surgery is important', WHO *Safe surgery*, https://www.who.int/teams/integrated-health-services/patient-safety/research/safe-surgery

11. 'Impact of the COVID-19 pandemic on delays in surgical procedures in Germany: a multi-center analysis of an administrative registry of 176, 7', *Patient Safety in Surgery*, BioMed Central, https://pssjournal.biomedcentral.com/

12. Liam Donaldson, Pauline Philip, WHO Guidelines for Safe Surgery, http://apps.who.int/iris/bitstream/handle/10665/44185/9789241598552_eng.pdf; jsessionid= 5D2E1301E4EEBAEB584519ECB2F12C8F?sequence=1

Case Study 4
Medication Error Analysis

'Data are just summaries of thousands of stories—tell a few of those stories to help make the data meaningful.'

—Dan Heath

Introduction

MOST OF THE healthcare organizations today have a process to spot and report medication errors and near misses. The process includes defining a medication error and near misses, employing a standardized format for reporting, and educating staff on the process and the importance of reporting.

The reporting process is a crucial part of the organization's quality and patient safety programme. The programme focuses on preventing medication errors by analysing the sort of errors that occur in the organization, and eventually comparing it with other organizations. Process improvements and staff training are used to prevent these errors in the future.

Case Presented

A multispecialty hospital identified reporting of medication errors and near misses as an area for improvement based on a prioritization grid. They addressed the related issues by adopting a structured approach using multiple tools such as control charts, process maps and fish bone analysis.

- Drawing out the process
- Identifying measurables with appropriate definitions
- Plotting the data (after validation)
- Identifying opportunities for improvement

The Medication Process: Possible Errors

Figure 1: Medication Process with Error Spots

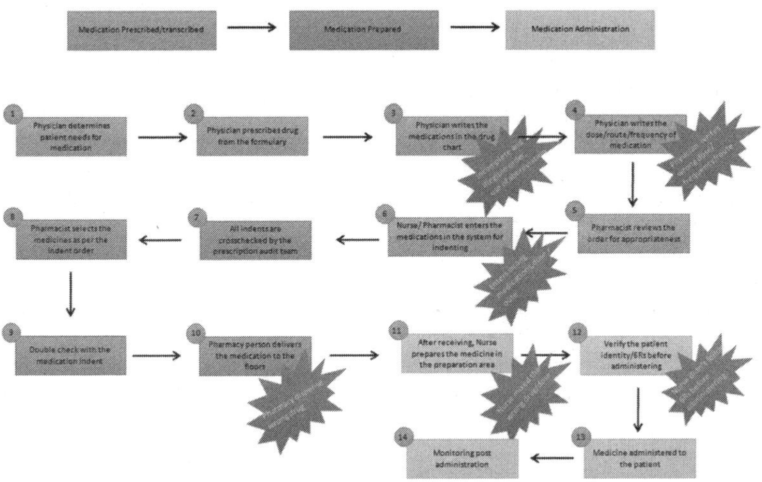

Courtesy: Apollo Hospitals

Table 1. Prioritization Grid

Criterion	Score 3	Score 2	Score 1	Score 0	SCORE
Patient needs/ expectations	Indicated by survey/ complaints	Possible high positive effect	Possible moderate effect	Minimal or no effect	3
Patient outcome	Important improvement	Some improvement	Little improvement	No improvement	3
Strategic plan	Strong relationship	Moderate	Minimal	None	3
Regulatory compliance	Required	N/A	N/A	Not required	0
Cost to implement	No cost/Budgeted item	One time, <5% of operating budget	5-10% of operating budget	Ongoing increase in costs	2
Impact on efficiency/budget	Reduction of 1 FTE or >10% reduction	Reduction of 0-1 FTE or 1-10% red.	No impact	Increase in staff or operating costs	0
Patient volume affected	100% of patients	50-75% of patients	25-50% of patients	0-25% of patients	3

Criterion	Score 3	Score 2	Score 1	Score 0	SCORE
Patient risk	May cause death	Permanent serious complications	Temporary serious complications	Temporary or no risk	3
Problem prone	Increased risk to staff or patients	Moderate risk	Low risk	No risk	3
				TOTAL	**20**

Score of >18 = Top priority
Score of 14–18 = Moderate priority
Score of 10–14 = Low priority
Score of <10 = Not a priority
Thus, medication errors are prioritized indicators for a healthcare organization

What Is a Medication Error

A medication error is defined as any preventable event that will cause or result in inappropriate medication use or patient harm, or which has the risk of being administered in a manner different from the prescribed norms while the medication is within the control of the healthcare professional or the patient.

Such events could also be associated with professional practice, healthcare products, procedures, and systems, including prescribing; order communication; product labelling, packaging, and nomenclature; compounding; dispensing; distribution; administration; education; monitoring; and use.

Problems can include adverse reactions and interactions with other medications as well as basic administrative errors such as patients being given the incorrect medication or wrong dosage. Therefore, such incidents are crucial and should be closely monitored.

Types of Errors

On the concept of whether the medication error has reached the patient or not, errors are classified as:

- Intercepted errors
- Actual errors

Both the type of errors are further divided into:

- Prescription error
- Transcription error
- Dispensing error
- Administration error

Except for administration errors, all errors are rectified by 'prescription auditing'. Prescription errors that are corrected and prevented by the Prescription Auditing Team are called 'intercepted errors'.

Prescription Error

- No route specified
- Order without an indication
- Drug indicated but the dose is inappropriate
- Order without a time interval
- Dose change order without discontinuation of a previous order
- Order illegible
- Order incomplete in specifying doses or frequency

Transcribing Error

- Order is not transcribed at all
- Order is transcribed incorrectly
- Allergy not documented on the medication administration record
- Allergy not documented on the order sheet

Dispensing Error

- Wrong drug or dilution dispensed
- Wrong preparation dispensed

Administration Error

- Scheduled dose is not documented as administered
- Drug administered without a physician's order
- Dose missed

NCC MERP Index for Categorizing Medication Errors

- **Category A:** Circumstances or events that can cause an error.
- **Category B:** An error occurred but the error did not reach the patient ('error of omission' does reach the patient).
- **Category C:** An error occurred that reached the patient but did not cause the patient harm.
- **Category D:** An error occurred that reached the patient and required monitoring to confirm that it resulted in no harm to the patient and/or required intervention to preclude harm.
- **Category E:** An error occurred that may have contributed to or resulted in temporary harm to the patient and required intervention.
- **Category F:** An error occurred that may have contributed to or resulted in temporary harm to the patient and required initial or prolonged hospitalization.
- **Category G:** An error occurred that may have contributed to or resulted in permanent patient harm.

- **Category H:** An error occurred that required intervention necessary to sustain life.
- **Category I:** An error occurred that may have contributed to or resulted in the patient's death.

Measure Type: Process Indicator

Improvement Noted As: Decrease in the errors

Numerator Definition (with exclusions if any): Total number of medication errors

Denominator Definition (with exclusions if any): Total number of discharges

Calculated as: Medication errors per 100 discharges

Data Collection Approach: Data is collected by the Prescription Audit Team and through incident reports, and sent to the Quality Systems department every month.

Sampling: Every medication prescribed, indented, issued and administered to a patient is recorded.

Reporting Cycle: Monthly

Responsible Department:

- Medical
- Pharmacy
- Nursing

Benchmark: ISMP (Institute for Safe Medication Practices) <2 per cent

Figure 2. Graphical Presentation

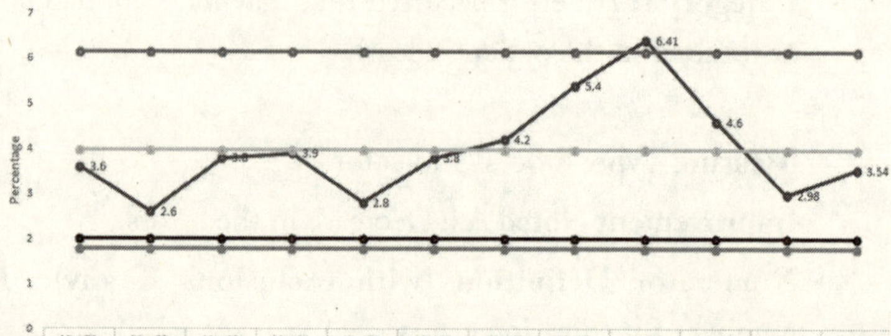

	Mon 01	Mon 02	Mon 03	Mon 04	Mon 05	Mon 06	Mon 07	Mon 08	Mon 09	Mon 10	Mon 11	Mon 12
Benchmark	2	2	2	2	2	2	2	2	2	2	2	2
Trend	3.6	2.6	3.8	3.9	2.8	3.8	4.2	5.4	6.41	4.6	2.98	3.54
Mean	3.97	3.97	3.97	3.97	3.97	3.97	3.97	3.97	3.97	3.97	3.97	3.97
UCL	6.15	6.15	6.15	6.15	6.15	6.15	6.15	6.15	6.15	6.15	6.15	6.15
LCL	1.79	1.79	1.79	1.79	1.79	1.79	1.79	1.79	1.79	1.79	1.79	1.79

Courtesy: Apollo Hospitals

Figure 3. Fishbone Analysis of Medication Errors

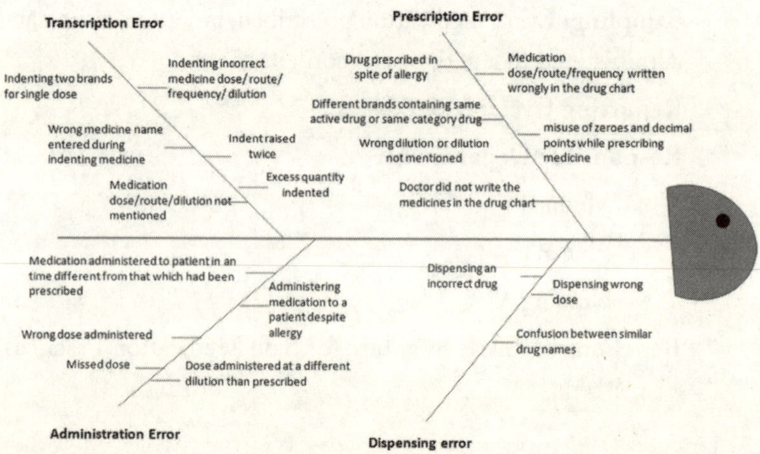

Courtesy: Apollo Hospitals

Table 2. Common Medication Errors in Type, Category, Subtype and Class as per the Analysis

ANALYSIS	MEDICATION ERROR	TRANSCRIPTION ERROR	DISPENSING ERROR	ADMINISTRATION ERROR
MOST COMMON TYPE	Prescription error	Wrong Drug Strength	Wrong Drug	Wrong Fixed-dose Combination
MOST COMMON SUBTYPE OR CLASS	Reconciliation Discrepancies	Wrong Drug Strength	Proton Pump inhibitors	Anti-Platelet Agents
MOST COMMON CLASS	Most common are Anti-Diabetics and Antihypertensives	Most common are Cardiovascular Drugs	Proton Pump inhibitors	Anti-Platelet Agents

Medication Error Analysis

Prescription Error

The sub-type of prescription errors was studied to grasp the vital areas of concern in managing medication errors. A Pareto Chart was plotted (see Graph 1) to show the relative importance of problems. An audit of all medication errors was conducted to see the categories (types) of errors and their frequency. The results were collected initially during a Tally Sheet, then the information was placed in descending order of frequency in a Pareto Chart Template in Excel.

Some prescription errors constitute the 80 per cent cut-off line—the 'vital few' types of medication error that ought to be addressed on priority, as they contribute most to the problem. These are:

- Reconciliation discrepancy in discharge
- Advised not added
- Dose not advised/wrong dose
- Therapeutic duplication
- Wrong/no frequency advised
- Relation with food not advised
- Route of administration

The types of medication errors that fall above the 80 per cent cut-off line are referred to as the 'trivial many', and are generally not seen as a high priority to deal with in comparison to the 'vital few' factors. However, several 'trivial many' factors could also be simple to deal with (low-hanging fruits), and thus it is also acted upon and may be acted upon earlier instead of later. Similarly, a category of drugs was also plotted to work out any vital group of medicines contributing to the medication errors.

Figure 4. Breakup analysis of Prescription Errors through Pareto chart

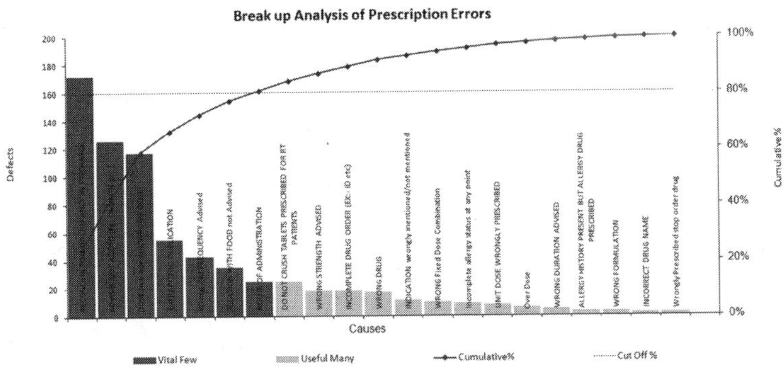

Courtesy: Apollo Hospitals

Table 3. Prescription Errors with Causes and Action Plan

Common Causes of Prescription Errors	Action Taken
Excessive workload and fatigue due to COVID-19 pandemic	• Regular handholding. Campaigns and fun activities on the floor on medication safety practices. • Interactive sessions with the doctors for writing complete medication orders.
Newly recruited doctors leading to high number of prescription errors	• Medication error briefing as part of induction trainings. • Intensive training programme for doctors by the Director Medical Services Office as well as the clinical pharmacologist. • Close monitoring of discharge summaries for medication oversight.

	• Emphasis on use of drug formulary. • Legibility analysis of prescriptions. The result shared with doctors. Emphasis on legible prescription writing. • Collaborative rounds initiated on the floors wherein random files are picked up from every floor by the team of doctors and pharmacists to check any medication errors. • Regular open file audit and tracers on floors.
Vital Causes	**Action Plan**
Reconciliation discrepancy in discharge	• Primary consultant to verify all the medications before finalizing the discharge summary.
Advise not added	• Primary consultant to verify all the medications before finalizing the discharge summary.
Dose not advised	• Prescriber to refer drug formulary and online drug info for the correct dose.
Therapeutic duplication	• Doctors are instructed to review current medications before prescribing new medications.
Wrong/no frequency advised	• Doctors instructed to ensure frequency is mentioned.
Relation with food not advised	• List of most common drug food interactions circulated.
Route of administration	• Doctors instructed to ensure route of administration is mentioned.

Transcription Error

Figure 5. Breakup analysis of Transcription Errors through Pareto Chart

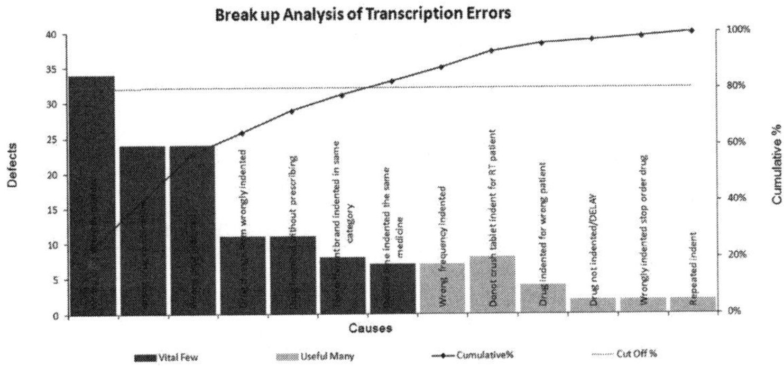

Courtesy: Apollo Hospitals

Table 4. Transcription Errors with Causes and Action Plan

Common Causes of Transcription Errors	Action Taken
Excessive workload and fatigue due to COVID-19 pandemic	• Regular interaction with floor staff by the hospital leadership for motivation. • Leadership walk rounds.
High staff turnover. New joinees in the system.	• Intensive training programme for floor pharmacists and nurses. • Medication error briefing as part of induction trainings. • Introduction of the concept of 'disturbance-free indenting' and 'lean-hours indenting'.

Environmental factors—noise level, interruption by patient/ attendants other staff while indenting/transcribing	• Medication safety week was organized for staff awareness on medication safety.
	• Focus on trainings related to medication indenting. • Slotted hours during night-time for medication returns to reduce day-time transactions. • Routine medications to be indented during early morning 'lean hours' for regular fills of the patients rather than raising single indent multiple times.

Vital Causes	Action Plan
Wrong drug strength indented	Staff instructed on referring drug formulary for specific strength.
Wrong drug combination	Staff trained on list of most common fixed dose combinations.
Wrong drug indented	Training given to indenting pharmacist on different class of drugs.
Drug dosage form wrongly indented	Staff counselled on correct drug formulation indenting.
Drug indented without prescribing	Indenting pharmacist to follow prescription orders written in the drug chart before indenting.
Two different brands indented in the same category	Staff to review the indent before finalizing.
Double time indented for the same medicine	Staff to follow 'up on' previous indents before raising a repeat order.

Administration Error

Figure 6. Breakup Analysis of Administration Errors through Pareto Chart

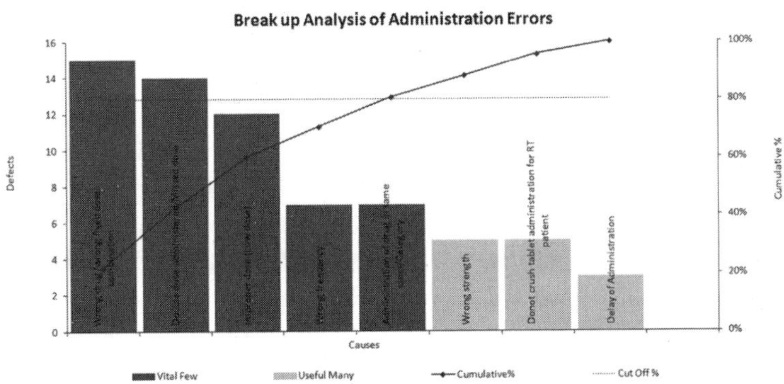

Courtesy: Apollo Hospitals

Table 5. Administration Errors with Causes and Action Plan

Common Causes of Administration Errors	Action Taken
Excessive workload and fatigue due to COVID-19 pandemic.	• Regular interaction with floor staff by the hospital leadership for motivation. • Leadership walk rounds.
High staff turnover. New joinees in the system (lack of knowledge, failure to follow policies, and poor documentation).	• Intensive training programme for nurses. • Intense training and monitoring of 7 Rights of Medication administration. • Spot checks by supervisors on nurses handover, medication administration protocol and documentation.

	• Increased focus of senior nursing team on reducing administration errors. • Improved patient and family involvement—through education —to speak up and ask questions. • Increased vigilance and pharmacist's interventions to ensure thorough reporting of administration errors.
Environmental factors—noise level, interruption by patient/attendants/other staff while indenting/transcribing	• Medication Safety Month organized for staff awareness on medication safety. • Focused on IPSG and safe medication administration. • 5S campaign.

Vital Causes	Action Plan
Wrong drug/wrong fixed dose combination	• Staff instructed on referring drug formulary for specific strength.
Double dose admin/stored/missed dose	• Staff instructed to document immediately after drug administration.
Improper dose (low dose)	• Staff instructed to check the right dose before administration.
Wrong frequency	• Staff instructed to plan due time for the next dose as per the prescription (refer standard administration timings).
Administration of drug in the same class/category	• Staff instructed to perform second level of check to identify same category drugs.

Dispensing Error

Figure 7. Breakup Analysis of Dispensing Errors through Pareto Chart

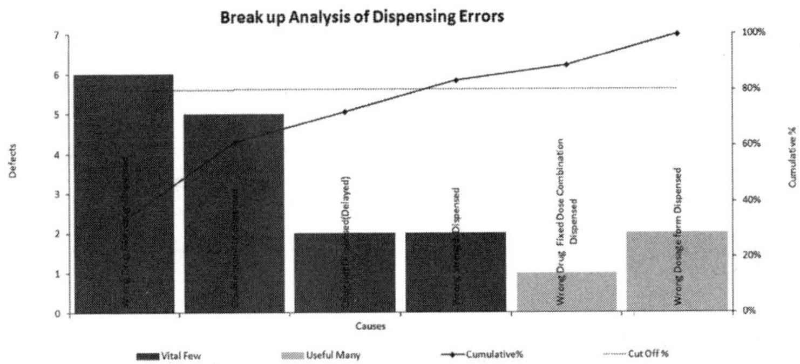

First 4 causes cover 83.33 per cent of total Dispensing Errors

Courtesy: Apollo Hospitals

Table 6. Dispensing Errors with Causes and Action Plan

Common Causes of Dispensing Errors	Action Taken
Excessive workload and fatigue due to COVID-19 pandemic.	• Staff shift allotment planned for better workforce utilization during peak hours.
High staff turnover. New joinees in the system (lack of knowledge, failure to follow policies, and poor documentation).	• New joinees given intensive training during induction about the policies, procedures and JCI accreditation.
Environmental factors—noise level, disorganized workspace	• 5S campaign

Vital Causes	Action Plan
Wrong drug/non-drug dispensed	• Dispensing pharmacist to verify before dispensing.
Double quantity dispensed	• Staff instructed to verify the picked medication quantity with the issued quantity in the indent copy before dispensing.
Drug not dispensed (delayed)	• SMS alert service initiated for indents exceeding TAT.
Wrong strength dispensed	• Medications of same generic with different strength stored separately.

Medication Error Action

1. Daily rounds by the Prescription Audit Team, Quality Team, Nursing Team to reduce prescription errors, administration errors, transcription errors and dispensing errors.
2. On-spot action on the detection of medication errors by educating on specific mistakes or counselling.
3. Continuous trainings for pharmacists.
4. Prescription error on detection—explanation, and on-the-spot education for doctors.
5. Drug administration error. Education provided wherever necessary.
6. Wrong indent. On-the-spot explanation provided to the pharmacist and nurses.
7. Dispensing error. On the spot education provided to the concerned.

8. Monthly analysis of various errors. Steps taken to minimize errors. Focused initiatives implemented.

Factors Contributing to Medication Errors

1. Illegible handwriting, incomplete prescription, and incorrect strength
2. Dose miscalculation
3. Medication reconciliation in continuity at the point of discharge medications
4. Typing error in the discharge summary
5. Failure to verify indent before finalizing
6. Look-alike and sound-alike drugs
7. Documentation after administration
8. Lack of knowledge on referring drug formulary
9. Lack of patient education
10. Timing of drug administration due to various drugs used

PDCA Analysis

Plan

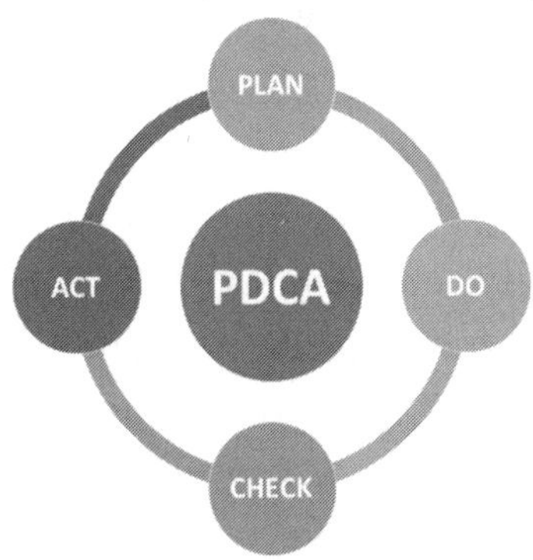

The policy and process for identification of errors was in place within the hospital, still, we thought of improving further and reducing our errors. The Drugs and Therapeutics Committee brainstormed on how the errors could be further reported/checked and minimized. The main objective of the plan was to achieve 100 per cent medication error reduction.

An implementation plan was developed that involved further stress on the strategy.

The process flow was redesigned, and the team was resensitized on how to prevent medication errors—its types, how they could be identified, and what could be done to avoid errors.

The team started functioning round the clock.

1. Look-alike and sound-alike drug list was revised and stored separately from other stock. Look-alike and sound-alike counterparts were separated by using different colour boxes (red and blue) while storing medications. Double checking was completed at the pharmacy level to prevent any medication errors.
2. Medication stored in wards/ICU was labelled: name of the drug, expiry and quantity. Imprest stock revised.
3. Medication orders were written in capital letters along with dose, route, indication and frequency.
4. Only approved abbreviations were allowed within the hospital as per the hospital policy.
5. Only use of leading zero if the number is less than one (0.1) was allowed, but use of zero after the decimal (5.0) was not allowed.
6. Prescription was redesigned to incorporate drug name, dosage, route of administration, frequency along with the doctor's signature. Verbal orders were not allowed. For any critical changes, it was expected that the staff would write a new order.

7. To scale back administration errors, two patient identifiers were used on dispensed medications as well as on patient band before medication administration.
8. Administration of some of the high-alert medications such as concentrated high-alert electrolytes, narcotics, insulin and chemotherapy drugs involved double independent checks by the nurses before administration.
9. Weekly 'med safe meetings' were scheduled with the doctors, nurses and pharmacists.

Do

The data was analysed, and the analysis depicted that the majority of the errors were prescription errors. The data was presented quarterly to the Drugs and Therapeutics Committee by the clinical pharmacologist. The decisions made by the committee were implemented and documented in the minutes of the meeting.

Corrective Action Taken:

- Medication indents were done by the pharmacist.
- The concerns were discussed with the consultants for appropriate actions.
- A double-check before administration was fully implemented.
- Regular audits were conducted to test if any patient medications were found at the bedside of the patient, and action was taken accordingly, if found.
- If any error was found, the Prescription Audit Team checked the case sheet of the patient. Further, the matter was discussed with the concerned doctor and the error was corrected.
- Auditing pharmacists were involved in educational seminars—drug club under the supervision of clinical pharmacologist.

- Tips on the safe use of medications were added to the in patient guide to bring about awareness among the patients and their families.
- Medication safety month was observed at least quarterly.

Check

- Further analysis over a period showed a downward trend in the graph.
- The obtained results were compared against the expected results from the plan.
- We achieved maximum error reduction in prescription, transcription and dispensing errors. No category D or above errors occurred. All the errors were identified because of the various checkpoints.

Act

The results were as expected, and the complete process was documented.

- The capturing of near misses improved further, by strengthening the Audit Team during attrition.
- Dispensing errors were reduced by educating the pharmacist.

The revised plan was developed to further sustain 100 per cent error reduction, especially administration errors.

Figure 8. SIPOC Diagram

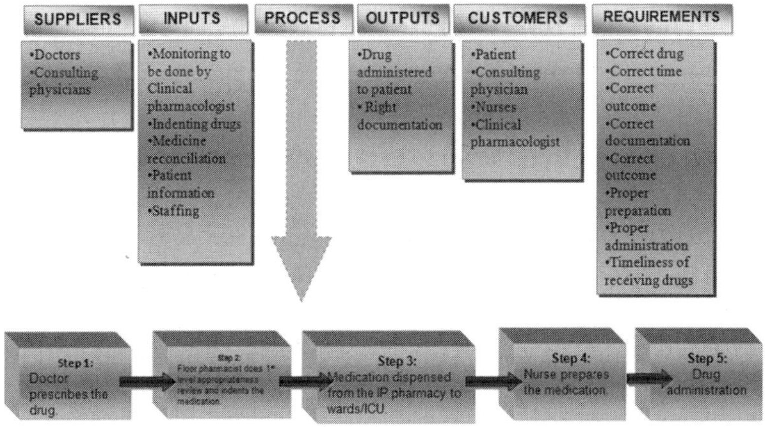

Courtesy: Apollo Hospitals

Conclusion

Today, every medication error is looked into seriously. Continuous training, engaging doctors, staff counselling and education, training handouts, and motivational activities such as Medication Safety Week and Medication Error Reduction Month have helped us to ensure that we remain a safe hospital.

References:

1. Institute For Safe Medication Practices, https://www.ismp.org/
2. European Medicines Agency, http://www.ema.europa.eu
3. L.T. Kohn, J.M. Corrigan and M.S. Donaldson, (Eds.), *To Err is Human: Building a Safer Health System* (US: Committee on Quality of Health Care in America, National Academies Press).
4. L. B. Hansen, 'Medication Errors', *American Journal of Pharmaceutical Education* (2007), Vol. 71, No. 3, p. 9.
5. A. Page (Ed.), *Keeping Patients Safe: Transforming the Work Environment of Nurses* (Washington DC: National Academies Press, 2004).
6. NCC MERP, https://www.nccmerp.org/
7. R.M. Procyshyn, et al., 'Medication errors in psychiatry: a comprehensive review', *CNS Drugs,* Vol. 24, No. 7, pp. 595–609, https://doi.org/10.2165/11533710-000000000-00000
8. 'Keeping patients safe: Institute of Medicine looks at transforming nurses' work environment', *The Quality letter for healthcare leaders* (2010), Vol. 16, No. 1.
9. M.E. Stefl, 'To Err is Human: Building a Safer Health System in 1999', *Frontiers of health services management*, Vol. 18, No. 1, pp. 1–2.
10. M.R. Cohen (eds.), *Medication Errors,* 2nd Edition (USA: American Pharmacist Association, 2007), Pharmacy Library, https://pharmacylibrary.com/doi/book/10.21019/9781582120928
.

Case Study 5

Employee Health and Safety

Safety work is today recognized as an economic necessity. It is the study of the right way to do things.

Introduction

HEALTH SERVICES REQUIRE a range of workers such as doctors, nurses, technicians, pharmacists and housekeepers in various clinical and non-clinical departments.

Workers across the healthcare settings can be easily exposed to patients; infectious materials, including contaminated body substances; medical supplies; equipment; environmental surfaces; or air.

Moreover, health services are provided in a variety of settings, i.e., small/large hospitals, outpatient clinics, inpatient rooms, birthing places, operation theatres, emergency care, specialty clinics, nursing homes, etc. The hazardous elements also include blood-borne pathogens (biological), chemicals, drugs, anaesthetic gases, lasers, workplace violence, material, ergonomics and heavy object lifting.

Several potentially hazardous chemicals include formaldehyde (used for the preservation of tissue and organs) and various other chemicals utilized in laboratories.

While trying to ensure the health of patients and the public, healthcare workers are exposed to a range of hazards to their health because of injuries (needle prick, musculoskeletal, allergens), infections (viruses, bacteria, parasites), violence, and so on. Healthcare workers have the potential to get exposed to infectious materials, including body substances, contaminated medical supplies, the environment around—including air, anaesthetic gases and radiation equipment.

A hospital's programme on staff health and safety is vital to taking care of the staff's physical and psychological state, satisfaction, productivity, and safe conditions for work.

The COVID-19 pandemic has further reinforced and made everyone realize and acknowledge the importance of staff health and safety programme for healthcare professionals. WHO gave it a renewed push by dedicating World Patient Safety Day for the year 2020 to healthcare workers, and therefore the slogan 'Health worker's safety: A Priority to Patient Safety' was identified. 'The COVID-19 pandemic has reminded all of us of the vital role health workers are playing to relieve suffering and save lives. No country, hospital or clinic can keep its patients safe unless it keeps its health workers safe,' said Dr Tedros Adhanom Ghebreyesus, WHO Director-General.

Health and Safety Hazards in Hospital Settings

Chances of hazards in health facilities are highly variable depending upon the type of the hospital. Women represent larger numbers of the health workforce that are at most risk, with an effect even on their reproductive health. Prevention of infections, injuries, and violence must all be in situ at health facilities. Healthcare workers also are the segment of society who need preventive and therapeutic guidance.

Chemical exposure can occur from sterilants, disinfectants, cleaning compounds, hazardous drugs, mercury, anaesthetic gases, latex, etc. Biological hazardous items include viruses (hepatitis B and C viruses [HBV and HCV], human immunodeficiency virus [HIV], etc.), bacteria, and parasites. Other injuries are ionizing and non-ionizing radiation. Ergonomic injuries can occur from patient handling, lifting, shifting, lifting heavy equipment, and static postures. Psychological and work organization, shift work, stress, burnout, and workplace violence are other hazards.

Pre-Employment and Annual Health Screening

All staff should be screened at the time of joining as a pre-employment health check. Also, these staff should be screened annually as well for their health maintenance. This will give the employer insights into the staff's health condition and enable them to take appropriate measures at the earliest.

Measures to Control Harmful Occupational Exposures

The hospital should identify departments most prone to harmful occupational exposures and develop strategies to handle the same for employees working in these departments. Following are the departments in the hospital requiring special attention.

Food and Beverages Staff

Routine stool examination should be done at pre-employment and every year thereafter. All food handling staff in Food and Beverages

(F&B) department should be screened for shigella, salmonella, vibrio cholerae, and other organisms in their stool during the pre-employment check-up and every year thereafter.

Typhoid vaccination should be given to F&B staff to guard them against typhoid. The dose and schedule should be followed as per the prevalent guidelines and vaccine manufacturer recommendations.

Maintenance Staff

All staff should undergo mandatory audiometry testing once a year to check for any loss of hearing while working in plant areas. All staff should be given tetanus vaccination as they are more prone to physical injuries while working.

Radiation Workers

All radiation workers are monitored for radiation exposure and safety by providing them with Thermo Luminescent Dosimeter (TLD) badges. Annual health check-ups of these staff should include a physical examination, routine blood examination, and a chest X-ray to watch their health.

Staff Working in CSSD

An annual health check-up—including physical examination, routine blood examination and a chest X-ray—is recommended to watch their health.

Laboratory Staff Working with Infectious Agents

The important element of containment is strict adherence to typical biohazard procedures and techniques. People closely involved with infectious agents or materials must be cautious about the potential hazards. They should be trained and proficient in the practices and techniques to handle such material safely.

An annual health check-up including physical examination, routine blood examination, and a chest X-ray should be done for all lab staff, especially those working in the tuberculosis division, to watch their health.

Tuberculosis (TB)

a) Laboratory technicians should have specific training for handling mycobacterium tuberculosis complex strains and must be supervised by the microbiologist. Personnel in other areas processing suspected AFB samples should take due precautions while handling such samples.

b) The health of laboratory technicians is monitored periodically. Any unexplained episodes of weight loss, fever or chronic cough should be notified to the lab in charge.

c) The laboratory should also include a procedure to regulate exposure to TB. All clinical samples for TB culture should be handled in isolation. Only designated staff should be permitted to work in the area.

Formalin Exposure

Formaldehyde is a colourless gas with a strong, pungent odour. It is commonly available in liquid form as a 40 per cent solution (generally referred to as formalin). Wherever possible, when using formaldehyde, exposure should be minimized by employing adequate engineering controls and safe working practices. Such methods include ensuring good ventilation and changing work procedures and practices. Local exhaust ventilation units (fume hoods) are installed in the grossing area in histopathology, so that the harmful vapours are exhausted. Enclosing or automating certain work procedures also reduces exposure levels.

Contagious Disease and Restrictions to the Staff

Staff should be restricted from reporting to their routine activities and should be granted a leave of absence if they suffer from contagious diseases.

Periodic Preventive Immunizations and Examinations

All employees working in the patient contact areas and other patient-related services should be compulsorily vaccinated for Hepatitis B. Following is the commonly observed practice:

- First dose on joining, second dose after one month from the first dose, and third dose after six months from first dose.
- After the third dose, in the next six to eight weeks, the titre is done. If it is >10mlU/ml then vaccination is not needed and will be valid for five years. If it is <10mlU/ml, a booster dose should be given. In case the result is negative, re-vaccination should be done.

Female employees working in the radiation area, ETO sterilization, and chemotherapy units during pregnancy should be transferred or reassigned to other areas/departments where there is no exposure to radiation or any such toxic substances.

Staff, if exposed to any infectious diseases, should be evaluated and counselled by the relevant team member (infection control head/ nursing director/medical superintendent) and a follow up should be done to ensure they are taken care of.

Workplace Violence

Workplace violence is a recognized hazard in the healthcare industry. It is any act or threat of physical violence, harassment, intimidation, or other threatening disruptive behaviour that occurs at the work site. It can affect and involve workers, clients, customers and visitors. It ranges from threats and verbal abuse to physical assaults and even homicide.

Considering the customer–client relationship to include patients, their members of the family, and visitors, this can be termed 'Client-On-Worker Violence'. Research depicts that such violence takes place quite often in emergency and during psychiatric treatment settings, waiting rooms, and geriatric settings, however, it is just not limited to those. The violence among the employees—often referred to as lateral or horizontal violence—also includes bullying and frequently manifests verbal and emotional abuse. Worker-on-worker violence is usually directed at persons viewed as being 'lower on the food chain', such as a supervisor to supervisee or doctor to nurse, although the incidences of peer-to-peer violence are also common.

How Can Workplace Violence Hazards Be Reduced?

In most workplaces where risk factors are identified, the danger of assault may be prevented or minimized if employers take appropriate precautions. One of the simplest protections employers can give their workers is to ascertain a zero-tolerance policy towards workplace violence. By assessing their worksites, hospitals can identify methods for reducing the likelihood of incidents occurring. A descriptive and well-implemented workplace violence prevention program can largely counter the incidence of workplace violence once it is well combined with engineering controls, administrative controls, and training. It is critical to ensure that workers know the policy and understand that any claims of workplace violence are investigated and remedied promptly.

Second Victims

Second victims are healthcare providers who are involved in an unanticipated adverse patient event, in a medical error and/or a patient-related injury, and become victimized in the sense that the provider is traumatized by the event. Frequently, these individuals feel personally responsible for the patient outcome. Many feel as though they have failed the patient, second guessing their clinical skills and knowledge base.

It is crucial to be informed about the second victim phenomenon and institutional response planning. They are critical steps in safeguarding the staff trauma, however, it is often experienced by clinicians and nurses after unanticipated clinical events or medical errors. When an unpleasant event occurs, the health care system with a robust culture of safety rapidly acts not only to support patients and their families, but also to guide its staff. Doing this needs leadership engagement, preparedness, and powerful infrastructure for healthcare workers' support.

Stages of Second Victim Syndrome

During the primary stage of 'chaos and accident response', the provider will experience turmoil and distraction, and might often self-chastise as an outcome of the event. During this stage, the provider may ask themselves, 'How and why did this happen?' The second stage of 'intrusive reflections' is defined as 'a period of haunted re-enactments, often with feelings of internal inadequacy and periods of self-isolation'. Within the second stage, providers may begin asking, 'How did I miss this, and was this preventable?'

During the third stage of 'restoring personal integrity' within the workplace, reputation and acceptance will be questioned by the second victim.

Questions like, 'What will others think?', 'Will I ever be trusted again?' and 'How much trouble am I in?' are pervasive during this stage.

The providers will begin to pursue support from a trusted individual like a colleague, supervisor, family, or friend.

During this stage, without a positive supportive environment, providers can be distressed to move forward from the event. The initial three stages can take place simultaneously.

'Enduring the inquisition' is the recovery process in stage four; the second victim starts to lay emphasis on the potential repercussions that can hamper job security, licensure, and future litigation. During this stage, the provider must understand what to expect and the way to get support through these stressful encounters. Stage five involves 'obtaining emotional first aid'. Peer supporters, patient safety and risk management play vital roles in ensuring the provider gets a safe space to recuperate from the event. The survivor will either thrive, survive or drop out in the final stage via 'moving on'. Once sufficient support and guidance is offered throughout the process, the provider surely thrives through professional and personal growth post the event.

How Do We Provide Support to Second Victims?

Many studies have highlighted that the management of second victims includes the love and care of providers by peer colleagues from within their speciality. However, constant support from friends, significant others, and supervisors is necessary; majority of the providers look for a support from a trusted colleague, which has driven several institutions to implement robust second victim response teams. Receiving enough help or support from a colleague from within one's specialty offers a sense of shared understanding of the complex nature of patient care. The situation for the affected provider is also normalized. Peer support teams are well-trained to offer highly beneficial emotional first aid. Within the hospital, building a strong support system largely reduces the effects of Second Victim Syndrome.

Aiming to improve the effects of Second Victim Syndrome, it is necessary to normalize mistakes and encourage discussion about adverse patient events and medical errors. Morbidity and Mortality (M&M) or Patient Safety Conferences following events during training need to be thoughtful, supportive and focused on improving patient safety and encouraging a 'just culture' rather than pointing blame at the provider.

Education and Training

Education and training of staff is significant, as this is the only tool that will help staff to deal with the situation appropriately. The education of the staff about staff health and safety programmes should start from the point of staff's induction into the system. The staff should be trained about the different types of exposures and the likely harm they might experience as an occupational hazard and ways to deal with it.

All the staff members on induction should be trained at least for general safety training such as fire safety, utility safety, general safety and security, biomedical equipment safety, bio-medical waste management, handling of sharps, facility safety, disaster response and preparedness, occupational health safety, and safety in handling hazardous materials.

There should also be annual refreshers training on environment, health and safety aspects.

Case Study: Staff Safety Event

A patient 'X' got admitted for an emergency procedure through the emergency department and was shifted to the operation theatre. On the table, during the procedure, the anaesthetist saw a vesicular lesion suggestive of chicken pox. The hospital had a process of screening patients for any infectious diseases at the time of initial assessment, but in this case, the patient was in an incubation period. Hence, the patient, too, was not aware of the condition. All due precautions were taken, and the procedure was carried out. Thereafter, the patient was shifted to an isolation room for post-operative care. From day six to day fifteen after the incident, four staff from Emergency department developed chicken pox, and subsequently, the outbreak lasted for around two weeks.

A risk assessment was carried out by the hospital to identify the influencing factors or vulnerable aspects which may cause such outbreaks in near future. Based on learnings of the risk assessment, the hospital decided to:

a) Immunize all the expected high-risk first point of contacts in case of infectious exposure.
b) Include a Varicella Zoster IgG test in the pre-employment health check. During health check, if any employee is found to be non-immune to varicella, who may be posted in areas which are expected to be the first point of contacts such as ER, OPD, etc., they were immunized.
c) Assign only Varicella Zoster Virus IgG positive staff to any patient admitted with chicken pox. Records of such staff are separately maintained by the Nursing department for their deployment, as needed.

This approach further prevented exposure in all first point contacts, along with Varicella Zoster Virus IgG test results during the pre-employment, allowing assignment of staff to ensure safety.

The hospital updated its staff health and safety policy to incorporate new policy changes, and further strengthened its processes. All the frontline workers and staff involved, including departmental heads, were trained and informed about the policy change.

References:

1. S.A. Chhabra, 'Health hazards among health care personnel', *Journal of Mahatma Gandhi Institute of Medical Sciences* (March 2016), Vol. 21, Issue 1, https://www.researchgate.net/publication/297604130_Health_hazards_among_health_care_personnel/fulltext/57ebce8308ae92a5dbd04ce4/Health-hazards-among-health-care-personnel.pdf
2. D. Susan and R.N. Scott, 'Second victim phenomenon—harsh reality', AHRQ, 1 May 2011, https://psnet.ahrq.gov/perspective/second-victim-phenomenon-harsh-reality-health-care-professions
3. S. D. Scott, et al., 'The natural history of recovery for the health care provider "second victim" after adverse patient events', AHRQ, *Quality and Safety in Health Care* (October 2009), Vol. 18, No. 5, pp. 325–330, https://psnet.ahrq.gov/issue/natural-history-recovery-healthcare-provider-second-victim-after-adverse-patient-events
4. Workplace violence, OSHA, United States Department of Labor, https://www.osha.gov/SLTC/workplaceviolence/
5. 'Second Victim Syndrome', *Emra Wellness Guide*, EMRA, https://www.emra.org/books/emra-wellness-guide/ch-8.-second-victim-syndrome/
6. M. Makary and M. Daniel, 'Medical error—the third leading cause of death in the US', *BMJ* (2016), Vol. 353.
7. L.T. Kohn, 'To Err Is Human Building a Safer Health System: A Report of the Committee on Quality of Health Care in America', Institute of Medicine, National Academy Press, https://www.scirp.org/reference/ReferencesPapers.aspx?ReferenceID=1372005
8. A.W. Wu, 'Medical error: The second victim. The doctor who makes the mistake needs help too', *British Medical Journal*, Vol. 320, No. 7237, pp. 726–727.

9. A. Waterman, et al., 'The Emotional Impact of Medical Errors on Practicing Physicians in the United States and Canada'.
10. S. Pratt and B. Jachna, 'Care of the clinician after an adverse event', *International Journal of Obstetric Anesthesia,* Vol. 24, pp. 54–63.
11. David L. Schwappach and Till A. Boluarte, 'The emotional impact of medical error involvement on physicians: a call for leadership and organisational accountability', *Swiss Medical Weekly* (January 2019), Vol. 10, No. 139, https://pubmed.ncbi.nlm.nih.gov/18951201/
12. A. White, et al., 'The Attitudes and Experiences of Trainees Regarding Disclosing Medical Errors to Patients'.
13. S. Pratt, L. Kenny, S.C. Scott and A .W. Wu, 'How to Develop a Second Victim Support Program: A Toolkit for Health Care Organizations', *The Joint Commission Journal on Quality and Patient Safety* (2012), Vol. 38, No. 5, pp. 235–40, 193.
14. S.D. Scott, et al., 'The natural history of recovery for the health care provider "second victim" after adverse patient events', *Quality and Safety in Health Care,* Vol. 18, No. 5, pp. 325–330 https://psnet.ahrq.gov/issue/natural-history-recovery-healthcare-provider-second-victim-after-adverse-patient-events
15. J. Shapiro and P. Galowitz, 'Peer Support for Clinicians: A Programmatic Approach', *Academic Medicine* (2016), Vol. 91, No. 9.
16. S.D. Scott and M.M. McCoig, 'Care at the point of impact: Insights into the second-victim experience', *Journal of Healthcare Risk Management,* Vol. 35, No. 4, Europepmc.org, https://europepmc.org/article/MED/27088770
17. S.D. Scott, et al., 'Caring for our own: deploying a system wide second victim rapid response team', *Joint Commission Journal of Quality and Patient Safety,* Vol. 36, No. 5, pp. 233-40.

18. P. Boysen, 'Just Culture: A Foundation for Balanced Accountability and Patient Safety', *Ochsner Journal* (September 2013), Vol. 13, Issue 3, https://www.ochsnerjournal.org/content/13/3/400

19. Types of Workplace Violence, Workplace Violence Prevention for Nurses (WPVHC), National Institute for Occupational Safety and Health (NIOSH), https://wwwn.cdc.gov/WPVHC/Nurses/Course/Slide/Unit1_5

Case Study 6

Anaesthesia and Surgical Care

"There are no safe anesthetic agents, there are no safe anesthetic procedures. There are only safe anesthetists."

—Robert Smith

Introduction

THE ABILITY TO provide safe and effective sedation is one of the most important proficiencies for physicians involved in paediatric emergency care. The paediatric population is more susceptible to anxiety in the acute setting and benefit greatly from sedation and analgesia. According to Joint Commission International (JCI), procedural sedation is considered as a high-risk procedure when performed outside the operating theatre.

Case Scenario

Patient J, a young two-year-old girl with a history of hydrocephalus since birth, was brought to a multispecialty hospital. She was experiencing continuous vomiting, lethargy, and her behavior was not according to her age group. The pediatric neurologist ordered MRI (Magnetic Resonance Imaging) to analyze her cerebral spinal fluid circulation.

The neurologist ordered the procedure to be performed under procedural sedation and referred to an anaesthesiologist, as patient J was not cooperative and was agitated. The anaesthesiologist reviewed her history, which was otherwise unremarkable. At home, she was not on any prescribed or over-the-counter medications; however, previously, she was on anticonvulsant medication. It was discontinued over a week before the procedure.

Upon arrival of Patient J in the radiology suite, the nurse performed a pre-sedation assessment. Her cardiac and respiratory systems were within the normal limits for her age. However, neurologic assessment of Patient J was challenging due to her decreased reflexes. The nurse noted that Patient J responded to her mother, who accompanied her to the department. Although Patient J has had previous MRIs, the anaesthesiologist discussed the procedure with the mother. He explained the use of procedural sedation to the mother, assuring her that Patient J would be comfortable and everything would be done to try and reduce her fear of separation from her mother. The anaesthesiologist obtained informed consent from the mother. When the mother asked to stay in the room with Patient J, the nurse explained that it was neither safe nor allowed.

Additional review of Patient J's chart showed that she was admitted a day before and received an antiemetic upon admission. According to her age, blood pressure was low during the admission and vital signs were as follows:

- Blood pressure, 84/68 mm Hg
- Pulse, 104 bpm
- Respiratory rate, 30 breaths/minute
- Temperature, 99.7°F

That day, her blood pressure was 92/64 mm Hg; pulse, 100; and respiratory rate, 30 breaths/minute. She had an IV line infusing 5 per cent dextrose in 0.25 per cent normal saline at a rate of 45 cc/hr. Her admission weight was approximately 11 kg. Upon questioning, her mother stated that she had lost some weight; her normal weight was about 12–13 kg additionally, she did not take anything by mouth since admission.

Anaesthetist performed pre-sedation assessment and nursing staff prepared the procedure room, equipment, and medications for Patient J. The nurse ensured that a crash cart was located in the Radiology department and checked the defibrillator for proper functioning. The oxygen set-up in the scanner was checked, as was the suction. The pulse oximeter and non-invasive blood pressure monitor were warmed up to assure that they would be ready when the sedation had to begin. Furthermore, all equipment was determined to be MR-compatible to prevent burns during the procedure.

The suggested medication for the baby girl included Midazolam 0.02 mg/kg IV or a dose of 0.5 mg/kg orally. (As Patient J had a history of vomiting, the anaesthesiologist chose to administer Midazolam via the intravenous route to ensure proper drug dosing and reduce the risk of vomiting.)

Additionally, Fentanyl 0.5 mcg/kg was kept ready for administration in the event that the Midazolam was not enough in reaching the required sedation levels. The nurse calculated the correct dose based on Patient J's weight of 11 kg. Thus, the dose of Midazolam was 0.2 mg, and the dose of Fentanyl was 5 mcg. These medications were drawn into syringes and labelled. Additionally, the nurse loaded 0.5 mg of Naloxone (based on a dose of 0.05 mg/kg); this syringe was also labelled and placed off to the side, where it was easily accessible in the event of over sedation or other complications.

Finally, the little girl was shifted into the room with the scanner and hooked up to the oxygen, pulse oximeter, and non-invasive blood pressure monitor. A pre-sedation set of vital signs were monitored that included the patient's oxygen saturation levels before and after oxygen therapy was initiated. The patient's IV was checked for patency, and another set of vital signs was obtained. At this point, the mother was asked to leave the room, and Patient J became quite agitated. The anaesthesiologist began administering the sedatives immediately to relax Patient J to prevent any further agitation.

The anaesthesiologist administered 0.2 mg of Midazolam and monitored Patient J's response to the medication. After one minute, her blood pressure was noted to fall to a systolic pressure of 84 mm Hg. Neurologically, she was less agitated and appeared to be relaxed. When her name was called, she responded appropriately. Decline in her blood pressure levels was of concern; in response to this, the anaesthesiologist increased the IV rate to 50 cc/hr. Within five minutes, her blood pressure was normalized to pre-sedation level.

The radiologist was ready to start the scan; however, Patient J continued to move on the scanner table. The radiologist requested the anaesthesiologist to administer additional medication, and the anaesthesiologist administered an additional 0.2 mg dose of Midazolam. Within two minutes, Patient J was relaxed, and the procedure started.

During the procedure, Patient J's vital signs were continuously monitored via the blood pressure monitor cycles. The nurse also observed the SPO2 levels. After ten minutes, anaesthetist noted that Patient J's pulse oximeter reading had fallen to a level of 91 per cent. The radiologist was informed, and the scan was momentarily terminated to allow the anaesthesiologist to enter the room and evaluate the patient.

Patient's respiratory rate was now 15 breaths/minute, and the pulse oximeter reading had fallen further to 90 per cent.

Noticing this, patient J's head was put into the sniffing position by the anesthesiologist to open her airway and ensure that the oxygen flow rate surged. The patient's pulse oximeter reading increased to only 91% with this maneuver. Hence, it was decided by the anesthesiologist to administer a reversal agent for the prevention of respiratory insufficiency.

It was at this point that the anaesthesiologist realized that Naloxone had been drawn as an antagonist. As the patient had only thus far received Midazolam, Naloxone would be ineffective at reversing a Benzodiazepine, as it is a narcotic antagonist. Immediately, the anaesthesiologist loaded 0.1 mg of Flumazenil and administered this through the IV line. Within two minutes, Patient J was breathing at a rate of 25 breaths/minute, her pulse oximeter reading had increased to 94 per cent saturation, and her other vital signs remained within normal limits. However, she started to move on the table and the scan could not be completed until she was sedated adequately to prevent body movement.

Patient J was allowed to stabilize for another five minutes. Radiologist requested further sedation so the scan could be completed. The remaining time to perform the scan was approximately 10 to 12 minutes. The anaesthesiologist now chose to administer 2.5 mcg of Fentanyl to Patient J. Although a dose of 5 mcg was ordered, the nurse was concerned about the risk of developing a second episode of respiratory insufficiency. After three minutes, 2.5 mcg of Fentanyl was administered. However, she remained agitated.

Throughout the administration of Fentanyl, her vital signs and oxygen saturations were constantly under the scanner and they remained within normal range. After the second dose of Fentanyl (for a total of 5 mcg), the procedure was continued and completed without further complications.

Post completion of the procedure, her mother was allowed inside the room and remained at the bedside, and the effects of the medication were allowed to wear off. Later, reversal agents were not administered. Considering the length of action of the Midazolam and Fentanyl, it was obvious that the patient would remain sedated for some more time, i.e., around 20 to 30 minutes more. Furthermore, the nurse constantly monitored the patient's vital signs and oxygen

Figure 1. Sequence of Events

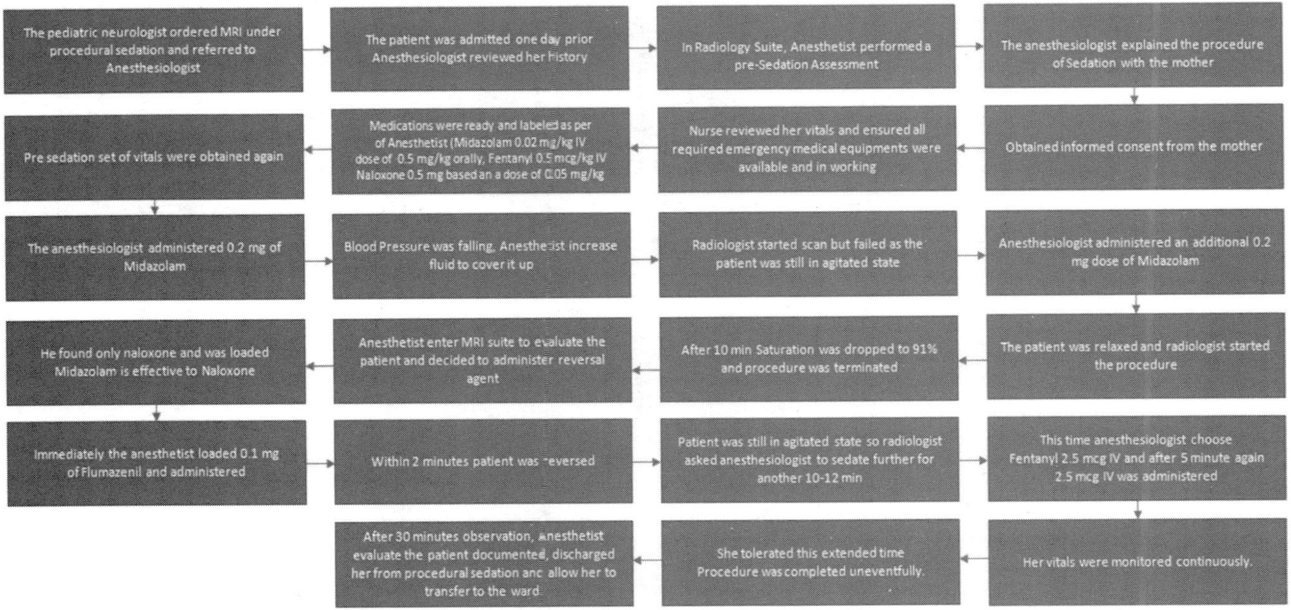

saturation levels during this recovery period; all the other parameters also remained normal.

Since Patient J was an inpatient, the recovery and discharge processes were different than for a patient who was being discharged to home. After thirty minutes, Patient J remained unconscious but opened her eyes and recognized her mother. When asked her name, she answered appropriately. At this point, the anaesthesiologist finished documenting the procedure, and she was shifted to the pediatric unit.

Figure 2. Cause-Effect Analysis

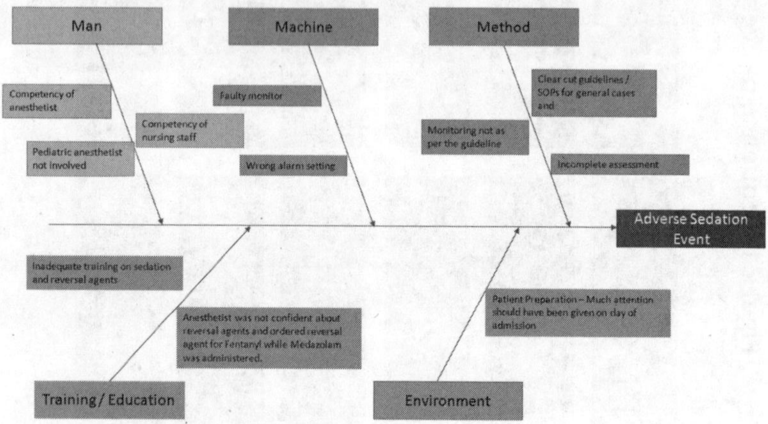

Discussion and Lessons Learnt

The anaesthesiologist caring for Patient J performed quite well. The pre-sedation monitoring was detailed; it was essential to contemplate the fact that continuous vomiting can lead to protracted volume status in children, and it could largely hamper the patient's response to prescribed medications. The anaesthesiologist recognized that the intravenous route of medication administration is much suitable than the oral route. Her history of a decreased level of consciousness could hinder oral administration. Additionally, with the patient's history of vomiting, oral drug administration could precipitate a further bout of vomiting.

Preparing the medications was challenging in this case to ensure a successful procedure. Drawing up a dose of Flumazenil in the first place could have been a better decision. The anaesthesiologist chose to prepare Naloxone, without considering that Fentanyl may not have been utilized at all. It would have been to everyone's benefit had both Naloxone and Flumazenil been prepared earlier. However, the result was positive; the patient was not harmed in any manner due to this delay.

When the radiologist nodded to go on and continue the process, the anesthesiologist gave a dose of Fentanyl that was one-half of the suggested dose, most likely depending upon the fact that Patient J had previously experienced the respiratory insufficiency. This choice was not wrong, but considering the case, it was probably inadequate as per the length of time since the initial administration of the Midazolam. Had the anaesthesiologist recognized the duration of the Midazolam, administering the full 5 mcg of Fentanyl most likely would have been safe.

However, in this case, the anesthesiologist preferred to act cautiously, and no one should find fault with this action.

Finally, the patient's recovery was uneventful as she touched her pre-sedation level of functioning and had an altered level of functioning to start with, this was a suggested and suitable process to evaluate her neurologic status. However, if the nurse had not done a commendable pre-sedation assessment, recognition of the patient's return to her pre-sedation level of functioning would have been arduous.

Conclusion

The requirement for procedural sedation and anesthesia outside the OR is constantly surging due to more use of diagnostic tools and procedural treatment methods. It is pivotal to know the functionalities and ill effects of sedatives and analgesics when choosing them, as the amount of sedation needed to enhance the patient's stability and ensure the success of the procedure may vary. Clinicians should never forget that as the degree of sedation hikes, the chances of respiratory depression and cardiovascular suppression become serious. Therefore, necessary steps and precautions should be taken by leveraging the suitable surveillance systems.

References:

1. 'Practice Guidelines for Moderate Procedural Sedation and Analgesia 2018: A report by the American Society of Anaesthesiologists Task Force on Moderate Procedural Sedation and Analgesia, the American Association of Oral and Maxillofacial Surgeons, American College of Radiology, American Dental Association, American Society of Dentist Anaesthesiologists, and Society of Interventional Radiology', *Anesthesiology* (2018), Vol. 128, pp. 437–479.
2. J.P. Cravero, et al., 'Pediatric Sedation Research Consortium. The incidence and nature of adverse events during pediatric sedation/ anesthesia with propofol for procedures outside the operating room: A report from the Pediatric Sedation Research Consortium', *Anesth Analg* (2019), Vol 108, pp. 795–804.

Case Study 7
Surgical Site Infections

'An ounce of prevention is worth a pound of cure.'

—Henry de Bracton

Introduction

PATIENTS COME TO any hospital for treatment with an expectation that they will recover from their pain and illness. It is definitely not 'right' to add on this burden another infection that the patient may acquire during or after surgery while in the hospital.

A surgical site infection (SSI) is one of those infections that may happen because of surgery-related processes in the hospital. It is a very critical indicator that is generally tracked by all healthcare organizations, and poses a major challenge to the infection control personnel due to the difficulty in capturing the data.

Post the surgery and discharge from the hospital, many patients don't follow up. Generally, significant efforts are made by healthcare organizations to strengthen the surveillance system, ensuring transparency of data and implementing effective control measures for its prevention.

We can refer to **National Health Safety Network (NHSN) for the defined surveillance periods.**

- **Superficial Incisional SSIs** are followed for procedure of all types but for a period of thirty days only. Whereas secondary incisional SSIs are followed for thirty days regardless of the surveillance period for the primary site. **Deep Incisional SSI and Organ/Space SSI** are followed for thirty days and also ninety days. The date of event occurs within thirty to ninety days after the operative procedure (where day 1 = procedure date).

Date of Event (DOE) for SSI

For a SSI, the DOE is the date when the initial element is brought to use to match the SSI infection criterion happening for the first time during the SSI surveillance period. It is necessary for the date of event to fall within the SSI surveillance period to meet predefined SSI criteria.

Timeframe for SSI Elements

As per NHSN, all elements required to meet an SSI criterion usually occur within seven to ten days, with typically no more than two to three days between elements.

Infection Present at Time of Surgery (PATOS)

The evidence of infection visualized is depicted via PATOS during the surgical procedure to which the subsequent SSI is attributed. The infection evidence should be mentioned intraoperatively and documented. It should be within the narrative portion of the operative note or report of surgery to be eligible for PATOS.

Wound Class

The seriousness of contamination of a surgical wound are assessed during surgical procedure. A person involved in the surgical procedure assigns this (for example, surgeon, circulating nurse, etc.), depending upon the wound class scheme adopted within the department. Wound classification is divided into four segments: Clean (C), Clean-Contaminated (CC), Contaminated (CO), and Dirty/Infected (D).

Superficial Incisional SSI

This involves only skin and subcutaneous tissue of the incision, along with other criteria mentioned in NHSN CDC.

Criteria

Date of event takes place within a month post any NHSN operative procedure (where day 1 = the procedure date) and involves only skin and subcutaneous tissue of the incision, and the patient has at least one of the following:

1. Purulent drainage from the superficial incision.
2. Organism(s) identified from an aseptically obtained specimen from the superficial incision or subcutaneous tissue by a culture or non-culture based microbiologic testing method, which is performed for purposes of clinical diagnosis or treatment (for example, not Active Surveillance Culture/Testing [ASC/AST]).

3. Superficial incision that is deliberately opened by a surgeon, physician* or physician designee, and culture- or non-culture-based testing of the superficial incision or subcutaneous tissue is not performed, and patient has at least one of the following signs or symptoms: localized pain or tenderness; localized swelling; erythema; or heat.
4. Diagnosis of a superficial incisional SSI by a physician* or physician designee.

There are two specific types of superficial incisional SSIs:

1. Superficial Incisional Primary (SIP): A superficial incisional SSI that is identified in the primary incision in a patient who has had an operation with one or more incisions (for example, C-section incision or chest incision for CABG).
2. Superficial Incisional Secondary (SIS): A superficial incisional SSI that is identified in the secondary incision in a patient who has had an operation with more than one incision (for example, donor site incision for CABG).

Deep Incisional SSI

This involves deep soft tissues of the incision (for example, fascial and muscle layers) along with other criteria mentioned in NHSN CDC.

Criteria

The date of event occurs within thirty to ninety days after the NHSN operative procedure (where day 1 = the procedure date) and involves deep soft tissues of the incision (for example, fascial and muscle layers), and patient has at least one of the following:

1. Purulent drainage from the deep incision.
2. A deep incision that spontaneously dehisces, or is deliberately opened or aspirated by a surgeon, physician* or physician designee, and organism(s) identified from the deep soft tissues of the incision by a culture- or non-culture based microbiologic testing method, which is performed for purposes of clinical diagnosis or treatment (for example, not Active Surveillance Culture/Testing [ASC/AST]) or culture- or non-culture based microbiologic testing method is not performed. A culture- or non-culture-based test from the deep soft tissues of the incision that has a negative finding does not meet this criterion. And the patient has at least one of the following signs or symptoms: fever (>38°C); localized pain or tenderness.
3. An abscess or other evidence of infection involving the deep incision that is detected on gross anatomical or histopathologic exam, or imaging test.

* *The term physician for the purpose of application of the NHSN SSI criteria may be interpreted to mean a surgeon, infectious disease physician, emergency physician, other physician on the case, or physician's designee (nurse practitioner or physician's assistant).*

1. Deep Incisional Primary (DIP): A deep incisional SSI that is identified in a primary incision in a patient who has had an operation with one or more incisions (for example, C-section incision or chest incision for CABG).
2. Deep Incisional Secondary (DIS): A deep incisional SSI that is identified in the secondary incision in a patient who has

had an operation with more than one incision (for example, donor site incision for CABG).

Organ/Space SSI

Organ/Space involves any body part deeper than the fascial/muscle layers and is opened or hampered during the operative process, along with other criteria submitted in NHSN CDC.

Criteria

Date of event occurs within thirty to ninety days after the NHSN operative procedure (where day 1 = the procedure date) and involves any part of the body deeper than the fascial/muscle layers that is opened or manipulated during the operative procedure.

And patient has at least one of the following:

a. Purulent drainage from a drain that is placed into the organ/space (for example, closed suction drainage system, open drain, T-tube drain, CT-guided drainage).
b. Organism(s) identified from fluid or tissue in the organ/space by a culture- or non-culture-based microbiologic testing method which is performed for purposes of clinical diagnosis or treatment (for example, not Active Surveillance Culture/Testing [ASC/AST])
c. An abscess or other evidence of infection involving the organ/space that is detected on gross anatomical or histopathologic exam, or imaging test evidence suggestive of infection, and meets at least one criterion for a specific organ/space infection site.

Note: For all these definitions, the criterion mentioned in NHSN CDC should be fulfilled before taking it as superficial, deep or organ space infection.

Tracking of SSI

Numerator and denominator are captured and calculation is done based on guidelines given in the NHSN CDC document.

Surveillance Methods

CDC SSI monitoring requires:

1. Active monitoring
2. Patient-based surveillance
3. Prospective surveillance

Concurrent and post-discharge surveillance methods should be used to detect SSIs following inpatient operative procedures and post-discharge surveillance for outpatient operative procedures.

Methods that could be adapted by hospitals:

1. SSI follow up forms are filed/attached to the patient's medical record, and patients are monitored for signs and symptoms of SSI. Day one is the day of surgery and tracking is initiated from day two. Any symptoms or signs, if seen, should be documented and escalated to the surgeon/surgical team.
2. Post discharge, follow up is done by a telephonic call to the patient. Organizations can define the interval at which these calls can be made. For example, for a thirty-day surgery, it

could be done weekly. For a 90-day surgery, it could be done weekly for one month and then bi-monthly for the next two months. These calls help in identifying the cases early on when the patient develops any signs or symptoms of SSI. If there is a concern, then the patients are asked to report to the hospital and meet the primary surgeon.

3. Patients who come back to the hospital for dressings. The staff in these areas should be trained to identify and report any ooze or pus from the surgical site. The samples should then be collected and sent to the microbiology laboratory for further evaluation. This could be followed up with detailed investigation as a part of retrospective follow up.
4. Samples received in microbiology could be retrospectively followed up for any suspected SSI by clinical microbiologists.
5. Inputs and information provided by surgeons.

Case Study

Mr A, an elderly patient, underwent craniotomy and tumour removal at a multispecialty hospital. The surgery was uneventful, and wound was healthy at the time of discharge. However, this patient presented with a surgical site infection after forty days of surgery. Pus was collected from the surgical site and was reported to be *Staph aureus*. In such an instance, it is very important for the team to conduct a root case analysis (RCA) to figure out the reasons of this infection.

RCA Methodology

First step. A meeting with the interdisciplinary team that includes the Primary Surgical Team, Operation Theatre (OT) Team and the Infection Control Team. After meeting and going through the case sheets and surgical notes, detailed analysis can be done, and the findings can then be shared with all the stakeholders.

A detailed plan of the investigation is then made. It includes, but is not limited to:

Parameters	Observation	Interventions
Maintenance		
Environmental Hygiene		
Sterility of Instruments		
Processes		
Personnel		

To make this process simpler and outcome-based, one could start with these basic questions:

1. Is it a superficial SSI, deep SSI or an organ-specific infection?
2. List of surgeries performed on that day.
3. Which OT was used?
4. Duration of the surgery.
5. When was the first event noticed? Example: Within a few days, weeks or months.
6. List out the consumables used.
7. Use of any SUD (single-use device) and its tracking data.
8. Patient factors including his comorbidities.
9. Post-operative hygiene standards and asepsis when home dressings are done.
10. Any other factors that might have been responsible for the infection.

It is again a critical step to analyse this information properly. The RCA format that is developed by the JCI is a very handy step-by-step approach to conducting RCAs. Once RCA is completed, other quality improvement tools such as FISH Bone Analysis, could be used to present a snapshot of the reasons and events.

FISH Bone Analysis is a graphical representation while working on RCA. It helps in understanding the reasons for the problem and further supports in implementing corrective and preventive measures. Use of different colour codes also help in easy interpretation.

For the above mentioned case, this was an example of the analysis.

Figure 1. Root Cause Analysis

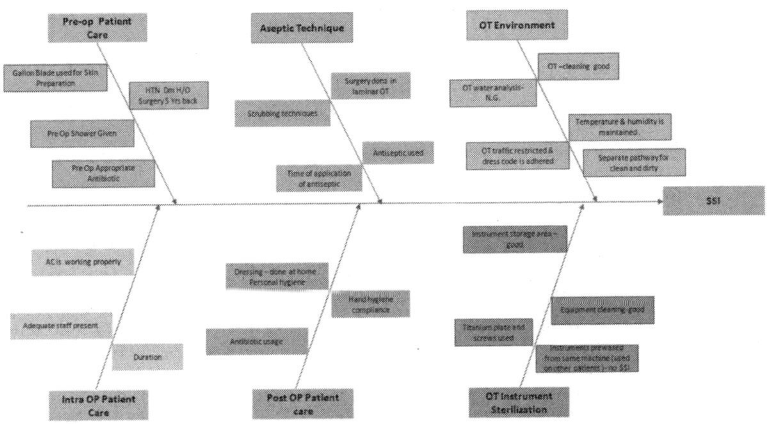

Courtesy: Apollo Hospitals

Probable Causes Attributed to the Reported SSI

1. Improper hygiene of the patient. For example, patient was scared of water entering the wound, so he did not take a bath for days (though proper education was provided on discharge).
2. Patient factors. Diabetic status of the patient could have also contributed to the infection.

3. Dressings not done aseptically. Dressing was done by the family member or some homecare services personnel, who did not follow all the precautions.

The strategy that was implemented to ensure such incidents don't happen in the future was to correct the discharge summary. Detailed instructions from the team on how to take care of a wound, when to seek consultation, personal hygiene, and taking regular bath was added to the discharge summary. This was added in a language that the patient/any layperson can understand and follow when at home.

Patient-family education has always been an integral part of SSI prevention strategies.

Learning Points

- ✓ Plan on wound care at the time of discharge to be explained clearly. Additionally, a small information leaflet on wound care could be given to the patient at the time of discharge.
- ✓ Dressings to be done aseptically. Either in a clinic or if done at home, it is preferred to be done by a nurse who is trained on infection control practices.
- ✓ Attenders need to be trained in aseptic techniques for wound care.
- ✓ Instructions to be provided on personal hygiene.
- ✓ Increased frequency of calling up the patient post discharge can help in early identification of any SSI.
- ✓ A set of standard questionnaires to be followed when calling up for SSI follow up, to get the maximum information.
- ✓ An SSI tracking group to be formed—consisting of the microbiologist, infection control nurses and the medical head —to further resolve many challenges.

Report on SSI

1. Meet the stakeholders with the final analysis once it is completed. Discuss the reasons for SSI. If a problem is identified for SSI, discuss that and initiate corrective and preventive action. If no specific reason could be identified, then based on analysis, practical recommendations can be given.
2. The above step in SSI analysis is very important, as it is vital to build confidence and trust between the surgeon and the Infection Control Team. The improvement measures could easily be implemented when there is a buy-in from management and the Surgical Team.
3. Regular audits and reviews should be conducted to ensure compliance.

Annexure 1

Place Label Here

If label not available, write Pt. Name, UHID, No. Age, Sex, Date, Name of Treating Physician

Surgical Site Infection Bundle Checklist

Date of Surgery:

Name of the Surgery

S.No.	PARAMETERS	C	N/C	REMARKS
1.	Administer prophylactic antibiotics with inb 1hr of Incision			
2.	Surgical Site Hair Removal with Clipper			
3.	Optimal glycemic control			
4.	Maintaining normothermia			
5.	Pre Op shower with soap solution / chlorhexidine			

Nurse's Signature:

Emp No. :

Remarks :

Courtesy: Apollo Hospitals

Annexure 2

Place Label Here If label not available, write Pt. Name, UHID, No. Age, Sex, Date, Name of Treating Physician

SSI TRACKING SHEET (In Patient)

(To be Tracked from PDF 2)

Name of Surgery : ______________________________ **Date of Surgery :** __________

S.No.	Components	Day 2 (Y / N)	Day 3 (Y / N)	Day 4 (Y / N)	Day 5 (Y / N)	Day 6 (Y / N)	Day 7 (Y / N)
1.	Fever (<100.4°F) for (3 reading within 24hrs)						
2.	Purulent discharge from the surgical site						
3.	Pain at surgical site >=3						
4.	Tenderness / Localized swelling						
5.	If culture send from the surgical site						
6.	Culture report received						
7.	Changes in TLC from Base line (10% Change)						
Remarks							
Signature of incharge Nurse :							
Signature of infection control nurse :							

Note: If any Two of the components are positive, Please inform ICNs and Doctor Incharges

Courtesy: Apollo Hospitals

Annexure 3

Root Cause Analysis and Action Plan Framework Template

Developed by the Joint Commission International

Sample Format for the Above-Presented Case

When did the event occur?

Date: xx/xx/xx	Day of the week: X	Time: X

Detailed Event Description Including Timeline:

Mr A, a case of parietal parasagittal meningioma, underwent surgery five years back, now presented with history of weakness on right side. CT/MRI done showed recurrent tumour. Redo of left parietal craniotomy and excision of tumour was done on date xx/xx/xx.

Diagnosis:

Recurrent left middle parasagittal meningioma

Medications:

Prophylactic antibiotic, anti-hypertensives, diabetic medicines, DVT prophylaxis

Autopsy Results:

NA

Past Medical/Psychiatric History:

- Parietal parasagittal meningioma, operated five years prior
- Hypertension
- Asthma
- Diabetic
- No history of any psychiatric illness

#	Analysis Question	Prompts	RCA Findings	Root Cause	Plan of Action
1	What was the intended process flow?	Elaborate procedure steps described via the policy, procedure, protocol, or guidelines in effect at the time of the event. Numerous processes can be infused.	Patient developed surgical site infection on craniotomy site on the scalp. Patient admitted on xx and surgery done on xx/xx/xx. Discharged 5 days later and readmitted 40 days later with low grade fever and discharge from the surgical site. Pus from surgical site: MRSA. Patient was prescribed antibiotics based on the culture reports. Shifted to OT and cleaned the site; saline wash done and 200 ml pus from the site was collected.		
2	Were there any steps in the process that did not occur as intended?	Elaborate any deviation from the intended procedure listed in Analysis Item #1 above.	Head shaving done on OT table. Galon blades were used. Clippers were not used. Site preparation as per protocol was done.		

#	Analysis Question	Prompts	RCA Findings	Root Cause	Plan of Action
3	What human factors were relevant to the outcome?	Discuss staff-related human performance factors that contributed to the event.	Doctors and nurses that were involved in patient care.		
4	How did the equipment performance affect the outcome?	Contemplate entire medical equipment and devices leveraged for patient care.	Sterile dressing sets and sterile craniotomy tray used. Cleaning and packing of sets supervised by a senior nurse. Use of titanium plate and screws was evidenced. Sterilization and process flow of the device was evaluated and found to be as per the infection control team recommendations.		

#	Analysis Question	Prompts	RCA Findings	Root Cause	Plan of Action
5	What controllable environmental factors influenced results?	What environmental factors within the organization's control affected the outcome?	OT: Neuro OT (laminar OT) Humidity: 49 per cent Temp: 22 degrees C during the surgery was noted. The environmental factors were within normal limits.		
6	What uncontrollable external factors influenced this outcome?	Identify any factors the organization cannot change that contributed to a breakdown in the internal process, for example natural disasters.	Not applicable for this case		
7	Were there any other factors that directly influenced this outcome?	List any other factors not yet discussed.	Not applicable for this case		

#	Analysis Question	Prompts	RCA Findings	Root Cause	Plan of Action
8	What are the other areas in the organization where this could happen?	List all other areas in which the potential exists for similar circumstances.	This could happen in any other theatre/patient care area. The process was evaluated in all the concerned areas.		
9	Was the staff properly qualified and currently competent for their responsibilities at the time of the event?	Include information on the following for all staff and providers involved in the event.	Yes. Employee records of all involved staff were evaluated for credentials, past history of infections, incidents, or complaints; recent appraisals; recent identified training needs; privileging; trainings and competency assessments. Senior scrub nurse assisted the case; she was also qualified and competent as per the records.		

#	Analysis Question	Prompts	RCA Findings	Root Cause	Plan of Action
10	How did actual staffing compare with ideal levels?	Include ideal staffing ratios and actual staffing ratios along with unit census at the time of the event.	Staff was adequate on that day and there was no shortage		
11	What is the plan for dealing with staffing contingencies?	Include information on what the organization does during a staffing crisis, such as call-ins, bad weather or increased patient acuity.	The staff contingency plan was found to be well implemented.		
12	Were such contingencies a factor in this event?	If alternative staff was used, describe their orientation to the area, verification of competency and environmental familiarity.	Not for this particular case.		

#	Analysis Question	Prompts	RCA Findings	Root Cause	Plan of Action
13	Did staff performance during the event meet expectations?	Describe whether staff performed as expected within or outside of the processes.	No deviations were noted while conducting this assessment.		
14	To what degree was all the necessary information available when needed? Accurate? Complete? Unambiguous?	Discuss whether patient assessments were completed, shared and accessed by members of the treatment team, to include providers, according to the organizational processes.	Knowledge of all clinical protocols were updated, and staff was aware of the same. No deviations were noted in this area as well.		

#	Analysis Question	Prompts	RCA Findings	Root Cause	Plan of Action
15	To what degree was the communication among participants adequate for this situation?	Analysis of factors related to communication should include evaluation of verbal, written, electronic communication or the lack thereof.	All touch points for communication were evaluated. No deficits were found at any touch point.		
16	Was this the appropriate physical environment for the processes being carried out for this situation?	Consider processes that proactively manage the patient care environment.	No deviations were noted here.		
17	What systems are in place to identify environmental risks?	Identify environmental risk assessments.	Weekly rounds were conducted by the infection control nurse. Additionally, surveillance for OT, monthly culture swabs and air counts from OT were found to be satisfactory.		

#	Analysis Question	Prompts	RCA Findings	Root Cause	Plan of Action
18	What emergency and failure-mode responses have been planned and tested?	Describe variances in expected process due to an actual emergency or failure mode response in connection to the event.	No deviations were noted here.		
19	How does the organization's culture support risk reduction?	How does the overall culture encourage change, suggestions and warnings from staff regarding risky situations or problematic areas?	There was a constant surveillance and promotion of high degree of SSI prevention steps by the organization (monthly swabs and air counts). Sterilization protocols, infrastructure support, trainings and tracking.		

#	Analysis Question	Prompts	RCA Findings	Root Cause	Plan of Action
20	What are the barriers to communication of potential risk factors?	Describe specific barriers to effective communication among caregivers that have been identified by the organization.	No deviations were noted here.		
21	How is the prevention of adverse outcomes communicated as a high priority?	Describe the organization's adverse outcome procedures and how leadership plays a role within those procedures.	Monthly infection control meetings were conducted, and any deviations were discussed. This was evident from the minutes of the meeting.		
22	How can orientation and in-service training be revised to reduce the risk of such events in the future?	Describe how orientation and ongoing education needs of the staff are evaluated, and discuss its relevance to event.	In OT, all healthcare workers were trained and assessed at periodic intervals. Trainings also included surgical handwashing and aseptic precautions compliance.		

#	Analysis Question	Prompts	RCA Findings	Root Cause	Plan of Action
23	Was available technology used as intended?		No deviations were noted here.		
24	How might technology be introduced or redesigned to reduce risk in the future?	Describe any future plans for implementation or redesign.	Implants and mesh sterilization/ reuse/process flow was also found to be in place.		

Action Plan	Organization Plan of Action Risk Reduction Strategies	Position/Title Responsible Party	Method: Policy, Education, Audit, Observation and Implementation
For each of the findings identified in the analysis as needing an action, indicate the planned action expected, implementation date and associated measure of effectiveness.	Action Item #1: Identification of high-risk patients with co-morbid factors. Make an additional effort to discuss outcomes and special post-operative care with the family.	Surgical Team	

Action Plan	Organization Plan of Action Risk Reduction Strategies	Position/Title Responsible Party	Method: Policy, Education, Audit, Observation and Implementation
	Action Item #2: The process on educating patients/ families on post-discharge dressings at home with complete asepsis needed improvement. Discharge advice to be more specific and to include wound care points.	Surgical Team	
	Action Item #3: Discharge summary specifying the follow up by patients after how many days and to consult in case if any symptoms needed improvisation.	Surgical Team and Medical Head	
	Action Item #4: Patient hygiene. At the time of discharge, patients need to be counselled about personal hygiene. Pre-operative shower is already included in SSI bundle checklist. Needs to be adhered to.	Surgical Team and Infection Control Team	

References:

1. CDC NHSN Guidelines, https://www.cdc.gov/nhsn/pdfs/pscmanual/pcsmanual_current.pdf
2. Infection prevention and control manual, Health Systems Virginia, Knowledge Link, UVA Health, https://www.healthsystem.virginia.edu/docs/manuals/policies/ic_manual
3. *JCI Accreditation Standards for Hospitals*, 7th Edition, Joint Commission International https://store.jointcommissioninternational.org/jci-accreditation-standards-for-hospitals-7th-edition/
4. Healthcare-Associated Infections (HAIs) CDC, https://www.cdc.gov/hai/ssi/ssi.html
5. *Surgical Site Infections*, Hopkins Medicine, https://www.hopkinsmedicine.org/health/conditions-and-diseases/surgical-site-infections
6. Surgical site infection, WHO, https://www.who.int/teams/integrated-health-services/infection-prevention-control/surgical-site-infection
7. C. Owens and K. Stoessel, 'Surgical site infections: epidemiology, microbiology and prevention'.
8. Surgical Site Infection, Teach Me Surgery, https://teachmesurgery.com/perioperative/skin/surgical-site-infections/
9. 'Surgical wound infection – treatment', *MedlinePlus Medical Encyclopedia*, https://medlineplus.gov/ency/article/007645.htm .
10. R. Foster, C. Amundsen and G. Webster, 'Complications of Vaginal Surgery' (2008), Duke University.

11. S. Berríos-Torres, et al., 'Centers for Disease Control and Prevention Guideline for the Prevention of Surgical Site Infection', *JAMA Surg* (August 2017), Vol. 152, No. 8, pp. 784-791.

12. 'Surgical Site Infections: prevention and treatment', Nice.org, https://www.nice.org.uk/guidance/ng125/resources/surgical-site-infections-prevention-and-treatment-pdf-66141660564421

Case Study 8

Pause the Pressure Injury

A collaborative effort by multidisciplinary team members, supported by interventions, is leading to a significant reduction in the occurrence of hospital-acquired pressure injuries.

Superman. Yes, even he was not spared by the pressure ulcers. The late actor Christopher Reeve died at the age of fifty-two due to the complications associated with infected pressure ulcers.

Introduction

ALTHOUGH COLLABORATIVE EFFORTS by health organizations have considerably reduced hospital-acquired pressure injury (HAPI) rates, they are yet to be eliminated. A study in a hospital revealed that there was a significant rise in the number of cases of pressure ulcers during a particular year, stating an incidence of eighteen cases.

Upon reviewing various literature and medical journals, it became evident that pressure injury is one of the prominent causes leading to prolonged patient hospital stay, cost of treatment and mortality.

Assessment of Problem and Analysis of its Causes

Retrospective analysis of the case records of patients' existing pressure injuries—along with literature and best practices review—was conducted. Inpatient episodes of pressure injury were reviewed retrospectively for the patients hospitalized in the given year when the incidences were high.

Case Presentation

The month-wise cases were presented in the below-mentioned data matrix, with a total of eighteen cases in Year 1. The coherent and comprehensive trend analysis was completed for the same.

Figure 1.0 Year 1 Pressure Ulcers Trend

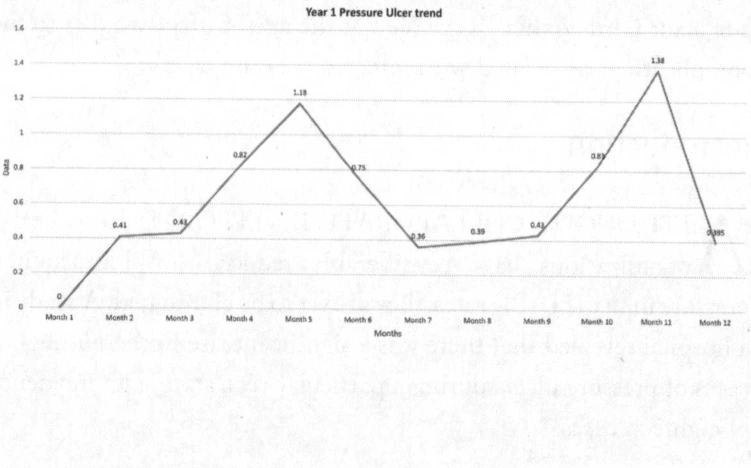

Year 1 **Fig.1.0**	**INDICATOR**			**NUMERATOR**			**DENOMINATOR**			**FORMULA**			
	Incidence of hospital associated pressure ulcers after admission (bed sores per thousand patient days)			Number of patients who develop new /worsening of pressure ulcer			Total number of patient days			Percentage = (N/D) x 1000			
Month	1	2	3	4	5	6	7	8	9	10	11	12	
Benchmark	1%												
Target	0%			0%			0%			0%			
Numerator	0	1	1	2	3	2	1	1	1	2	3	1	
Denominator	2095	2416	2286	2417	2537	2650	2713	2521	2306	2399	2167	2526	
Result	**0.00**	**0.41**	**0.43**	**0.82**	**1.18**	**0.750**	**0.36**	**0.39**	**0.43**	**0.83**	**1.38**	**0.395**	

Trend Analysis (Year 1, Q1)	Trend Analysis (Year 1, Q2)	Trend Analysis (Year 1, Q3)	Trend Analysis (Year 1, Q4)
Increasing Trend	Increased as compared to Q1	Decreased as compared to Q2	Increased as compared to Q3
Root Cause	**Root Cause**	**Root Cause**	**Root Cause**
Negligence of nursing staff dry, skin texture	Hyperproteinemia leading to fluid leakage, Poor Skin Texture	Position restricted as patient was on high PEEP prolonged stay	Position restricted as patient was on high PEEP poor skin texture

Tools Used: Various quality tools were applied, from problem analytics to problem solving. These were:

a. A3 problem-solving toolkit, including fishbone diagram (Figure 1.1)
b. Audit and data collection
c. Knowledge enhancement and skills training of staff on prevention of pressure ulcers
    - On-the-job training by ICN/Nurse educator to staff
    - Training and implementation of the PUSH Tool (Pressure Ulcer Scale for Healing)
    - Training and implementation of Pressure Injury Pathway
    - Training of staff on techniques of Pressure Ulcer Prevention

Figure 1.1. A3 Problem-Solving Toolkit

A 3 PROBLEM SOLVING

PROBLEM — DEFINATION

Title: Pressure Injury Analysis	Start Date: Year 1		Estimated Completion Date: Year 3	
Problem Description	**Problem Category**			
High number of Pressure Injury/Ulcers cases in the Financial year 1.	Quality	Yes	Waste and efficiency	Yes
	Cost	Yes	Health and Safety	Yes
	Customer Satisfaction	Yes	Other	Brand image
Goal	**Expected Benefits**			
To Reduce the number of incidences of Pressure Ulcer to **Zero within Three** years. (Year 3)	**Reduced pressure ulcer increased patient care & safety within the organization.**			

CAUSE ANALYSIS

Cause And Effect And 5 Whys

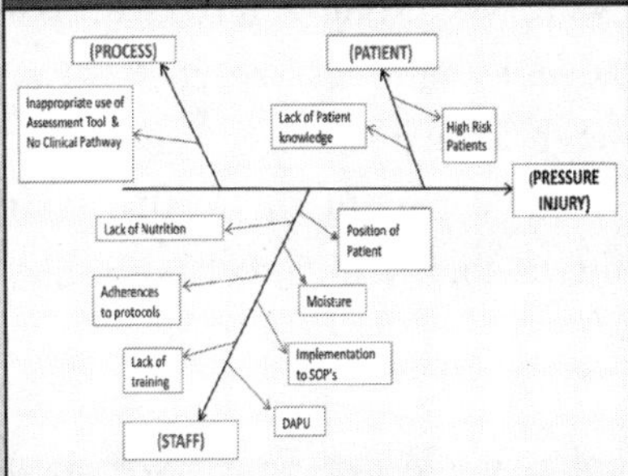

Cause Analysis summary (Prioritize in order of Importance)

Daily Assessment of patient is important for prevention of pressure injury which can be easily done by correct implementation of assessment tools **(PUSH and BARDEN Tool).**
SOP's provide healthcare staff with the standards of care and processes to be followed by all staff caring for patients Improper implementation of SOP's increases the risk of pressure ulceration.
Higher Temperature and Irregular monitoring, Improper usage of devices used by staff in patient care can lead to device associated pressure ulcer.
Moisture breaks down the outer layer of the skin (epidermis) and hence lead to People need enough **fluids, calories, protein, vitamins and minerals** in their daily diet to maintain healthy skin and prevent the breakdown of tissues.
Health care providers must have proper Knowledge about assessment of Patient , prevention of pressure Injury and clinical pathway for pressure Ulcer and Hence proper Training of staff is important.

COUNTER MEASURES

Corrective And Quick Wins	Team Members	
Priority	**Name**	**Roles**
Control of moisture from perspiration while urinary and faecal incontinence	Nursing Staff	To remove the device causing Pressure Ulcer
Devices Causing DAPU should be checked and handled properly with care	Nursing Staff	To control moisture also check for the equal pressure distribution
Nutritional assessment and supplementation of nutrients if required	Dietitian	To provide proper nutrition counseling to the patient
Use of support surface to address pressure redistribution (both bed and chair)	Quality Department	To track compliance and analysis
Repositioning (offloading) and turning schedules	Nursing Staff	To change the position of the patient on a regular bases
Daily skin assessment	Nursing Staff	To do skin assessment on a regular bases
Risk assessment tool (BARDEN and PUSH tool)	Nursing Staff	Assessment of patient according to PUSH tool and
Patient and family education about pressure ulcer	Nursing Educator	To educate the patient and Family, competency
Categorization of patients upon the risk matrix	Nursing Staff	Pressure ulcer Risk assessment and planning care based

Implementation Plan

Activity	Who?	Start Date	Status
Tanning for Staff on prevention and causes of Pressure Injury	Nursing Educator	Every Month	Implimented
Implementation of pressure injury pathway.	NS, ICN	Every Month	Implemented
Implementation of PUSH Tool	NS, Nursing Staff	Every Month	Implemented
Audit and regular monitoring is conducted on a regular bases	ICN	Every Month	Implemented
Targeting reduction in pressure injuries at hospital	Quality ,NS	Every Month	Implemented
Conducting campaigns for focused approach to bring down the numbers and increase the level of patient care	Quality ,NS, Nursing educator	Every Month	Implemented

RESULT

Result Summary(Including benefits obtained)	Further Plan
All the Possible causes for pressure ulcer where analyzed and counter measures where taken which helped to reduce the number of Pressure Injury to 89.33%, satisfactory level.	**Sustancence and further improvement of the work done by continous efforts to decrease the pressure ulcer rate further.**

Strategy for the Change

A Quality Circle was formed to reduce the number of incidents. It included the Quality Team (Regional and Unit level), head of medical services, head of nursing services, infection control officer, infection control nurse, intensivist and nursing staff.

1. Structuring Staff Training

Inputs on best practices from the various subject matter experts, including clinicians and other clinical staff, were taken. Classroom and on-the-job trainings were accordingly provided. Based on the inputs from the various subject-matter experts, best practices training was structured through a curriculum and imparted to the staff. These trainings were made a part of the regular on-the-job training programme. The methodology included both classroom-based and bedside training.

- Risk Assessment Tool (e.g., Water Low, Norton, Braden Tools)
    - Daily skin assessment
    - Repositioning (offloading) and turning schedules
    - Use of support surface to address pressure redistribution (both bed and chair)
    - Control of moisture from perspiration, and urinary and faecal incontinence
    - Nutritional assessment and supplementation when appropriate
    - Education of patient and/or family

2. Implementation of the Toolkit 'Zero is Hero'

The toolkit provided by the Apollo Corporate Quality Team to prevent pressure ulcers was implemented.

3. Clinical Pathway

A clinical pathway to monitor compliances for pressure ulcers prevention was developed by the clinicians.

Result

During Year 1, the unit had eighteen incidences of pressure ulcers that is 1.5 incidences per month (Figure 1.0). Year 2 had only one incidence of pressure ulcers, that is 0.2 incidence per month (Figure 1.2). Year 3 also had only one incidence of pressure ulcers, or 0.2 incidence per month (Figure 1.3). The focus is now to continue the sustenance of outcomes and work towards becoming a HAPU-free hospital.

Figure 1.2: Year 2 Pressure Ulcers Trend

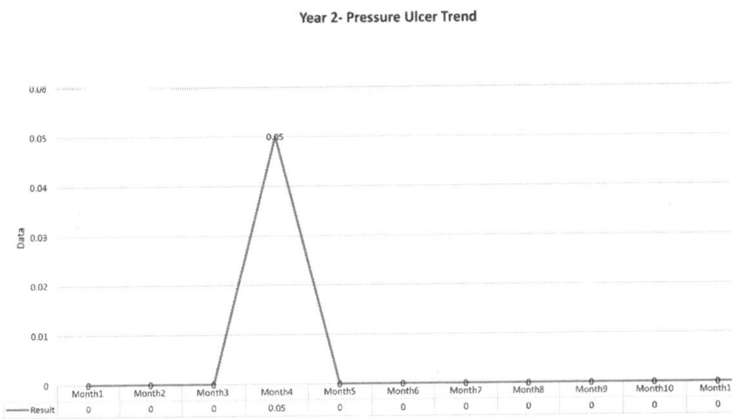

Year 2 Figure 1.2	Indicator	Numerator	Denominator	Formula
	Incidence of HAPU after admission (bed sores per thousand patient days)	Number of patients who develop new/ worsening of pressure ulcers	Total number of patient days	Percentage = (N/D) x 1000

Month	1	2	3	4	5	6	7	8	9	10	11	12
Benchmark	1%											
Target	0%	0%		0%			0%			0%		
Numerator	0	0	0	1	0	0	0	0	0	0	0	0
Denominator	2306	2231	2270	2152	2152	2451	2599	2495	2610	2327	2426	2319
Result	0	0	0	0.05	0	0	0	0	0	0	0	0

Figure 1.3: Year 3 Pressure Ulcers Trend

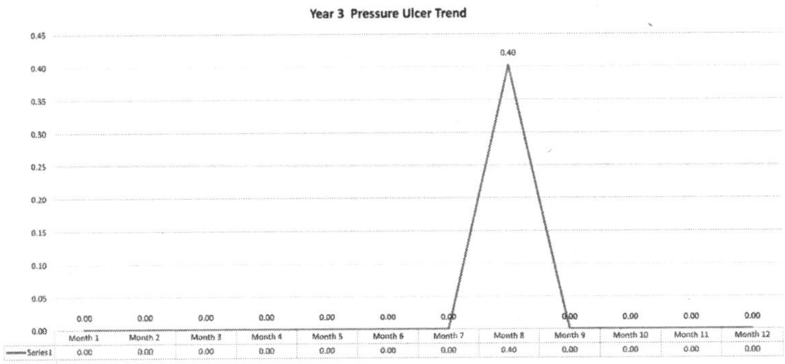

Figure 2. Comparative Data on HAPU over Three Years

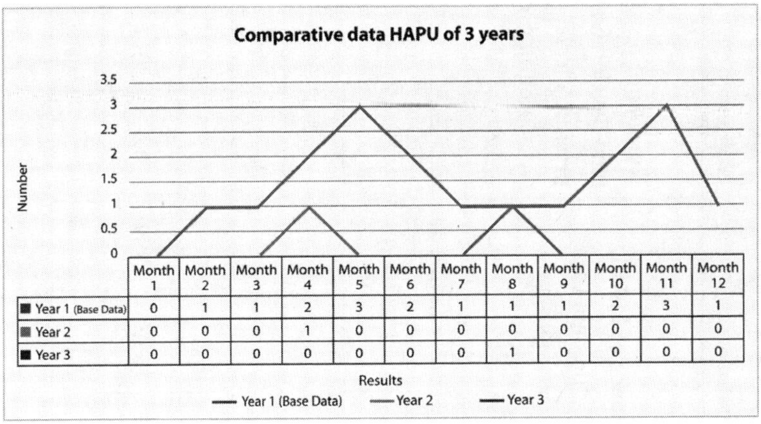

Year 3 **Figure 1.3**	**Indicator**			**Numerator**			**Denominator**			**Formula**		
	Incidence of HAPU after admission (bed sores per thousand patient days)			Number of patients who develop new/ pressure ulcers worsening of pressure ulcers			Total number of patient days			Percentage = (N/D) x 1000		
Month	1	2	3	4	5	6	7	8	9	10	11	12
Benchmark	1%											
Target	0%			0%			0%			0%		
Numerator	0	0	0	0	0	0	0	1	0	0	0	0
Denominator	1197	1639	1889	2142	2014	1976	2808	2489	654	2450	677	823
Result	0	0	0	0	0	0	0	0.0402	0	0	0	0

Figure 3. Glimpse of Training on Prevention of Pressure Injuries

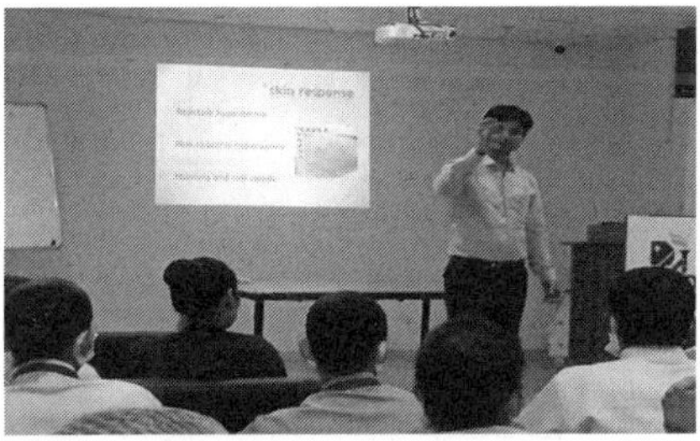

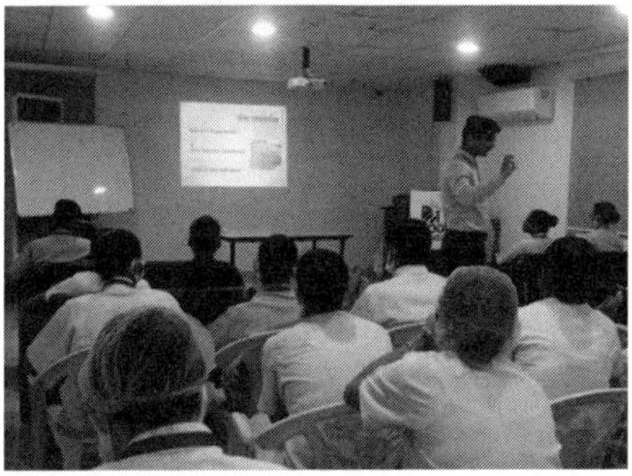

Courtesy: Apollo Hospitals

Figure 4. Clinical Pathway Monthly Audit Tracker [Sample]

			RISK ASSESSMENT						STANDARD CARE								NUTRITION				POSITIONING AND MOBILIZATION			MONITORING AND TRAINING	
Sr.No	Date	IP NO	Skin assessment on admission & on every shift.	Head to toe assessment on focus areas (eg occiput, shoulder, elbows, sacrum, heels)	Risk assessment tool value <18	Patient have pressure injury & history Awair ICN.	Skin abnormality finding informed to family and educate them.	Document the skin assessment & Braden - scoring.	Keep skin clean and dry	Apply moisturizing lotion to dry areas	Clean skin promptly after episodes of incontinence	Use skin cleansers that are pH balanced	Skin preparation by 3M cavilon transparent dressing	Provide Pressure area care system	Avoid positioning the patient on an area of pressure injury	Minimise friction & shearing damage	Reference registered dietician	Assessed the patient's weight regularly	Provided supplemental nutrition as indicated	Maintain adequate oral, enteral and parenteral intake	Reposition on atleast every 2 hourly, If not contraindicated	Scheduled frequency of turning	Provide Pressure area care device system	Monitor the prevalence & incidence of pressure injuries	Educate & train all members of the interdisciplinary team
			Observation (Yes/ No)	Observation (Yes/ No)	Observation (Yes/ No)	Observation (Yes/ No)	Observation (Yes/ No)	Observation (Yes/ No)	Observation (Yes/ No)	Observation (Yes/ No)	Observation (Yes/ No)	Observation (Yes/ No)	Observation (Yes/ No)	Observation (Yes/ No)	Observation (Yes/ No)	Observation (Yes/ No)	Observation (Yes/ No)	Observation (Yes/ No)	Observation (Yes/ No)	Observation (Yes/ No)	Observation (Yes/ No)	Observation (Yes/ No)	Observation (Yes/ No)	Observation (Yes/ No)	Observation (Yes/ No)

Figure 5. Skin Assessment Tool Used Nursing Care Plan and Interventions Guide

SKIN ASSESSMENT TOOL USED

ELEMENT OF A COMPREHENSIVE SKIN ASSESSMENT

Background: This sheet summarizes the elements of a correct comprehensive skin assessment. You could, for example, integrate them into your documentation system or use this sheet for staff training. Reference: Developed by Boston University Research Team

SKIN TEMPERATURE

Most clinician use the back rather than palm of their hand to assess the temperature of the patient's skin. Remember that increased skin temperature can be sign of fever or impending skin problems such as a stage 1 pressure ulcer or a diabetic foot about to ulcerate.

- Touch the skin to evaluate if it is warm or cool.
- Compare symmetrical body parts for difference in skin temperature.

SKIN COLOR

- Ensure that there is adequate light.
- Use an additional light source such as a penlight to illuminate hard to see the skin areas such as heels and sacrum.
- Know the person's normal skin tone so that you can evaluate the changes.
- Look for differences in colour between comparable body parts such as left and right leg.
- Depress any discoloured area to see if they are blanchable or non-blanchable
- Look for redness or darker skin tone, which indicate infection or increased pressure.
- Look for paleness flushing or cyanosis.
- Remember that the changes in coloration may be particularly difficult to see in darkly pigmented skin.

SKIN MOISTURE

- Touch the skin to see if the skin is wet or dry, or has the right balance of moisture.
- Remember that the dry skin or xerosis may also appear scaly or lighter in colour.
- Check if the skin is oily.
- Note that macerated skin from too much moisture may also appear lighter or feel soft or boggy.
- Also look for water droplets on the skin, is the skin clammy?
- Determine whether these changes are localised or generalised.

SKIN TURGOR

- To assess skin turgor, take your fingers and pinch the skin near the clavicle or the forearm so that the skin lifts up from the underlying structure then let the skin go.
- If the skin quickly returns to place, this is normal skin turgor finding.
- If the skin does not return to place, but stays up this is called tenting and is an abnormal skin turgor finding.
- Poor turgor is sometimes found in person who are older, dehydrated or oedematous or have connective tissue disease.

SKIN INTEGRITY

- Look to see if the skin is intact without any cracks or openings
- Determine whether the skin is thick or thin
- Identify the signs of pruritis, such as excoriation from scratching
- Determine whether any lesion is raised or flat
- Identify whether the skin is bruised
- Note any disruption in the skin If the skin discolouration is found, the type of skin injury will need to be identified. Since there are many different aetiologies of skin wounds and ulcers, differential diagnosis of the skin problem will to be determined. For example, is it a skin tear, pressure ulcer, or moisture-associated skin damage or injury?

NURSING CARE PLAN & INTERVENTIONS GUIDE

Braden Category	Braden Score : 1	Braden Score : 2	Braden Score : 3	Braden Score : 4
Sensory Perception	**Completely limited** • Skin assessment and inspection q shift. Pay attention to heels. • Elevate heels and use protectors. • Consider specialty mattress or bed. • Use pillows between knees and bony prominences to avoid direct contact.	**Very limited** • Skin assessment and inspection q shift. Pay attention to heels. • Elevate heels and use protection. • Consider specialty mattress or bed.	**Slightly limited** • Skin assessment and inspection q shift. Pay attention to heels. • Elevate heels and use protectors	**No limited** • Encourage patient to report pain over bony prominences. • Check heels daily.
Moisture	**Constantly Moist** • Skin assessment and inspection q shift. • Use moisture barrier ointments (protective skin barriers). • Moisturize dry unbroken skin. • Avoid hot water. Use mild soap and soft cloths or packaged cleanser wipes. • Check incontinence pads frequently (q 2-3h) and changes as needed. • Apply condom catheter if appropriate. • If stool incontinence, consider bowel training and toileting after meals or rectal tubes if appropriate. • Consider low air loss bed	**Moist** • Use moisture barrier ointments (protective barriers). • Moisturize dry unbroken skin. • Avoid hot water. Use mild soap and soft cloths or packaged cleanser wipes. • Check incontinence pads frequently (q 2-3h). • Avoid use of diapers but if necessary, check frequently (q 2-3h) and change as needed. • If stool incontinence, consider bowel training and toiletting after meals. • Consider low air loss bed	**Occasionally Moist** • Use moisture barrier ointments (protective skin barriers). • Moisturize dry unbroken skin. • Avoid hot water. Use mild soap and soft cloths or packaged cleanser wipes. • Check incontinence pads frequently. • Avoid of diapers but if necessary, check frequently (q 2-3 h) and change as needed. • Encourage patient to report any other moisture problem (such as under breasts). • If stool incontinence, consider bowel training and toileting after meals.	**Rarely Moist** • Encourage patient to use lotion to prevent skin cracks. • Encourage patient to report any moisture problem (such as under breasts).

Activity	**Bedfast** • Skin assessment and the inspection q shift. • Position prone if appropriate or elevate head of head no more than • Position with pillow to elevate pressure points off the bed. • Consider specialty bed. • Elevate heels off bed/or use heel protectors. • Consider physical therapy consult for conditioning and W/C assessment. • Turn /reposition q 1-2 h • Post turning schedule. • Teach or do frequent small shifts of body weight.	**Chairfast** • Consider specialty chair pad • Consider postural alignment, weight distribution, balance, stability and pressure relief when positioning individuals in chair or wheelchair. • Instruct patient to reposition q 15 minutes when in chair • Stand every hour • Pad bony prominences with foam wedges, rolled blankets or towels • Consider physical therapy consult for conditioning and W/C assessment.	**Walks occasionally** • Provide structured mobility plan. • Consider chair cushion • consider physical therapy consult.	**Walks frequently** • Encourage ambulating outside their room at least bid • Check skin daily • Monitor balance and endurance
Mobility	**Completely immobile** • Skin assessment and inspection q shifts • Turn /reposition q 1-2 hours • Post turning schedule. • Tech or do frequent small shifts of body weight • Elevate heels • Consider specialty bed	**Very limited** • Skin assessment and inspection q shift • Turn/reposition 1-2 hours. • Post turning schedule • Tech or do frequent small shifts of body weight • Elevate heels • Consider specialty bed.	**Slightly limited** • Check the skin daily • Turn/reposition frequently • Teach frequent small shifts of small weight. • PT consult for strengthening/conditioning. • Gait belt for assistance	**No limitation** • Encourage ambulating outside their room at least bid • Check skin daily • No intervention needed
Nutrition	**Very poor** • Nutrition consult • Skin assessment and inspection q shift. • Offer nutrition supplements & water • Encourage family to bring favorite food • Monitor nutritional intake • If NPO>24 hours	**Probably inadequate** • Nutrition consult • Offer nutrition supplements and water. • Encourage family to bring fav food. • Monitor nutritional intake • Small frequent meals. • If NPO >24 hours discuss plan with MD. • Record dietary intake and I&O ,if appropriate.	**Adequate** • Monitor nutritional intake • If NPO >24 hours discuss plan with MD. • Record dietary intake and I&O ,if appropriate.	**Excellent** • Out bed for all meals. • Provide food of choice • offer nutrition supplements and water • If NPO >24 hours discuss plan with MD. • Record dietary intake
Friction and shear	**Problem** • Skin assessment and inspection q shift • Minimum of 2 people + draw sheet to pull patient up in bed • Keep bed linens clean, dryand wrinkle free • Apply elbow/heel protectors to intact skin over elbows and heels • Elevated head of bed 30 degrees or less.	**Potential problem** • Keep bed linen dry, clean and wrinkle free • Avoid massaging pressure points. • Apply transparent dressing or elbow/heel protectors to intact skin over elbow and heels	**No apparent problem** • Keep bed linen dry, clean and wrinkle free	

Figure 7: Pressure Ulcers Assessment Flowchart

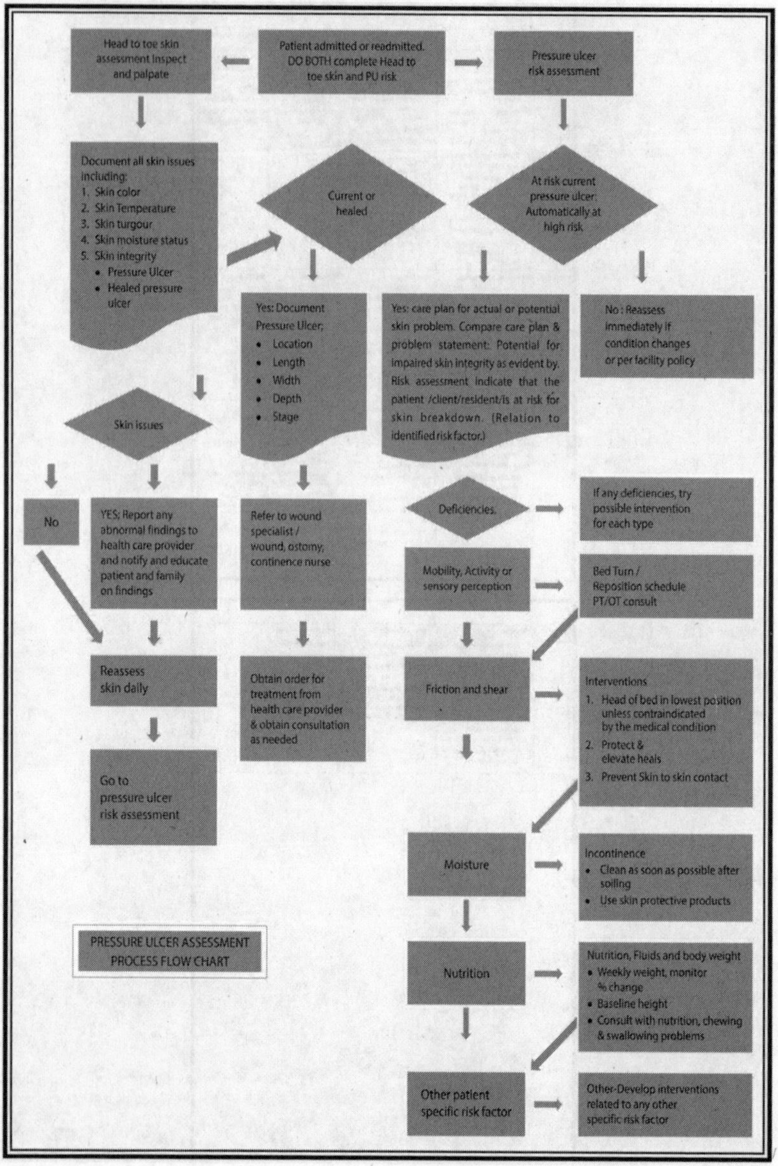

Lessons Learnt

- Daily assessment of patient is important for prevention of pressure injuries, which can easily be ensured by correct implementation of assessment tools (PUSH and BRADEN tool).
- The protocols laid down guide the healthcare staff in performing the essential procedures and during patient care, to reduce the risk pressure ulceration.
- Training and regular staff sensitization has lowered the incidences of HAPU in our hospital.
- A structured approach, using a patient safety toolkit and a clinical pathway for HAPU prevention, has helped our staff refine patient care improvement and processes.

Conclusion

The incidence of pressure ulcers reduced by 88 per cent in our hospital during the course of this three-year focused project. We managed to go from eighteen HAPU incidences per year to only one HAPU incidence per year. The use of pathways, toolkits and trainings for HAPU prevention were instrumental in achieving this outcome. Additionally, the patient and family education and training through educational pamphlets and demonstrations were undertaken for pressure ulcers prevention by the staff at the time of discharge. This helped us complete the continuum of care.

References:

1. J. Bisbee, 'Pressure Injuries in the Healthcare Setting: Even Superman Is Not Immune', *Patient Safety*, Vol. 2 No. 1, pp. 80–83, https://doi.org/10.33940/HAPI/2020.3.6
2. L. Demarré, A. Van Lancker, et al., 'The cost of prevention and treatment of pressure ulcers: A systematic review', *International Journal of Nursing Studies* (2015), Vol. 52 No. 11, pp. 1754-74. doi: 10.1016/j.ijnurstu.2015.06.006
3. S. Zaidi and S. Sharma, *Pressure Ulcer* (StatPearls Publishing, 2022), https://www.ncbi.nlm.nih.gov/books/NBK553107
4. *Pressure Ulcers (Pressure Sores)*, National Health Service (NHS), https://www.nhs.uk/conditions/pressure-sores/
5. Shpresa Syla, Gadaf Rexhepi, 'Quality Circles: what do they mean and how to implement them?', *International Journal of Academic Research in Business and Social Sciences* (December 2013), Vol. 3, No. 12, https://www.researchgate.net/publication/269813121_Quality_Circles_what_do_they_mean_andhow_to_implement_them
6. Joseph A DeFeo, *The Juran Trilogy: Quality Planning,* 15 April 2019, https://www.juran.com/blog/the-juran-trilogy-quality-planning/
7. 'How to care for pressure sores: MedlinePlus Medical Encyclopedia', MedilinePlus, https://medlineplus.gov/ency/patientinstructions/000740.htm
8. Bedsores, Johns Hopkins Medicine, https://www.hopkinsmedicine.org/health/conditions-and-diseases/bedsores.
9. 'What Are the Stages of Pressure Sores?', WebMD, https://www.webmd.com/skin-problems-and-treatments/pressure-sores-4-stages

10. 'Pressure ulcers symptoms and treatments', NHS Inform, https://www.nhsinform.scot/illnesses-and-conditions/skin-hair-and-nails/pressure-ulcers

11. J. Kottner, et al., 'Pressure ulcer/injury classification today: An international perspective', *Journal of Tissue Viability* (August 2020), Vol. 29, No. 3, pp. 197–203, doi: 10.1016/j.jtv.2020.04.003.

12. Dan Berlowitz, et al., 'Preventing Pressure Ulcers in Hospitals', *AHRQ*, https://www.ahrq.gov/sites/default/files/publications/files/putoolkit.pdf.

13. Janette M. Bisbee, 'Hospital Improvement Innovation Network (HIIN) Pressure Injury Prevention Project', https://www.haponline.org/Portals/0/docs/Downloads/HEN/Pressure-Injury-Prevention-Project-2019-Update-Infographic-Final.pdf

CASE STUDY 9

Apollo Safety Development Model: Building a Culture of Safety at Apollo Specialty Hospitals

Introduction

PATIENT SAFETY HAS emerged as a critical component of healthcare quality. As healthcare organizations continually strive to enhance patient safety, there's a growing recognition of the importance of building a culture of safety. Achieving a culture of safety requires an understanding of the values, beliefs and norms about what's important in a company, and what attitudes and behaviours associated with patient safety are expected and appropriate.

Safety culture encompasses the attitude held within a workplace—from the leadership to the frontline staff. This includes how open healthcare workers are to discussing patient questions of safety and concerns with their colleagues and their leaders; how safe they feel about speaking out if they think that a patient is in danger; how serious they think the organizational leadership is about patient safety; and the way they think they work as a team.

Background

The Leadership Team at Apollo Specialty Hospitals specifies that leaders must create a culture of safety and quality throughout the organization. The principles of performance for this standard are that leaders regularly evaluate the culture of safety and quality using valid and reliable tools on safe practices. Measurement, reviews, feedback and intervention suggest that 'healthcare organizations must measure their culture, provide feedback to the leadership and staff, and undertake interventions which will reduce the patient safety risk'. Other safety initiatives depend upon the existence of a workplace culture that's intrinsically motivated to enhance/ reduce errors and complications, instead of by external factors like accreditation requirements.

Keeping this in mind, it was necessary to make a baseline, grasp where we are coming from, and trace what proportion of progress we've made. Hence, it is was critical that we survey all stakeholders by employing a validated and reliable tool. A comprehensive survey questionnaire of around forty-five touchpoints was designed, inspired by AHRQ's Safety Culture Survey tool. The questionnaire broadly encompassed twelve areas of patient safety culture:

1. Communication openness
2. Feedback and communication about the error
3. Frequency of events reported
4. Hand-offs and transitions
5. Management support for patient safety
6. Non-punitive response to error

7. Organizational learning—continuous improvement
8. Overall perceptions of patient safety
9. Staffing
10. Supervisor/manager expectations and actions promoting safety
11. Teamwork across units
12. Teamwork within units

With this drive, the culture of safety survey using the AHRQ tool was conducted online, in August–September of Year 1. Results of the survey showed that safety culture varied not just between different hospitals, but also between departments/clinical units/wards, levels of care and roles. While the leadership team was positive towards a patient safe environment at the hospitals, there have been specific problems and hazards identified by the frontline staff.

This indicated that the uniform dissemination and inculcation of a 'culture of safety' within the organization was the immediate need of the hour, which led to the design of the Apollo Safety Development Model.

Following were the tangible and intangible goals envisaged from the project:

- Acknowledgement of the high-risk nature of the hospital's activities, and therefore, the determination to attain consistently safe operations. A target for an average patient safety score of 80 against a baseline of 60.
- A blame-free environment, where individuals are ready to report errors or near misses without worrying about reprimand or punishment. Increase the overall number of

incidences reported from 8 to 10 per month, to over 50 per month.

- Encouragement of collaboration across ranks and disciplines to hunt solutions to patient safety problems. Average overall grade for the departments of 4 out of 5.
- Organizational commitment of resources to deal with safety concerns.

Figure 1. Tangible and Intangible Goals for a Safety Development Model

Methods

To address the problem at hand, a multipronged approach was needed to be incorporated. This was to deal with multiple issues at multiple levels and form a wholesome culture of safety within the hospital. To form an enduring environment or culture in a corporation, it's necessary that employees at every level—i.e., from the leadership team to the frontline staff—were involved within the project. It is vital to see the safety culture not as a one-time fix or some simple steps to boost quality. It's the recognition that this can be a journey, and there are many steps the organization must take to make it successful. And this may be achieved only if the leadership promotes safety at every level—together with a decent team structure—where staff members are supportive and vigilant if patient safety is not exercised.

The programme was innovative with respect to the overall model, which had multiple aspects, taken from well-known safety and workplace management principles such as 5S, Kanban boards, and Committees. These principles were restructured to simplify them, and implemented with better understanding and awareness among the employees. Better understanding leads to better compliance with the safety principles, eventually leading to a safer environment for both patients and employees.

The Apollo Safety Development Model incorporated the following stages:

1. Leadership
    - Leadership Safety Rounds
    - Committee Meetings
2. Teamwork
    - Daily Safety Huddles
    - Buddy Programme
3. Effective Behavioural Change
    - Star Department
    - Q4E Toolkits
    - Departmental Checklists
4. Evidence Based

- SSC with 'Voice Over'
- High-Alert Drug Check

5. Just Culture
    - Rewards and Recognition
6. Communication
    - Safety Leaders
    - Nursing Kanban Board
    - Apollo Educational Video
    - Online Incident Reporting
7. Learning
    - Safety Fair
    - Code Blue Mock Drill Day
    - Infection Control Week
    - Fire Safety Week

A central executive core committee was developed, which was responsible for conceptualizing the project and designing its framework. The committee, led by the Quality Team, included teams from various departments of Operations, IT, Medical Services, Human Resources, Finance, Projects and Maintenance. The purpose of the committee was to design a comprehensive programme, which would cover all the aspects of a safety culture in the hospital. The online incident reporting portal and SSC with voiceover were created with the help of the IT team. The operations team supported the implementation of the project on the ground. Individual departments at various locations on the ground contributed to the project in terms of implementation of the programme and regular training and reporting. Overall, the project became an example of true teamwork across the organization.

Figure 2. Apollo Safety Development Model

Apollo Safety Development Model

Transforming the Culture of Safety

1. **Leadership**
   - Leadership Safety Rounds
   - Committee Meetings
2. **Teamwork**
   - Daily Safety Huddles
   - Buddy Program
3. **Effective Behavioral Change**
   - Star Department
   - Q4E Toolkits
   - Departmental Checklists
4. **Evidence Based**
   - SSC with 'Voice Over'
   - High Alert Drug Check
5. **Just Culture**
   - Rewards & Recognition
6. **Communication**
   - Safety Leaders
   - Nursing Kanban Board
   - Apollo Educational Video
   - Online Incident Reporting
7. **Learning**
   - Safety Fair
   - Code Blue Mock Drill Day
   - Infection Control Week
   - Fire Safety Week

Leadership Safety Rounds: 'Safety Rounds' were conducted and documented by the hospital head every month. Safety issues and potential risks were identified for timely mitigation. Designated a 'Patient Safety Officer' in every unit for effective closure of all the identified issues.

Figure 3. Leadership Safety Rounds in Progress

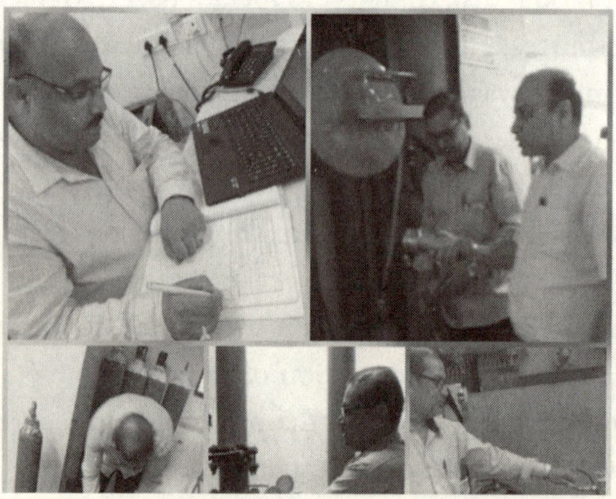

Committee Meetings: Three mandatory committees were formed in all the units, i.e., Quality Steering, Safety and Infection Prevention, and Control Committees. All the HODs, including physicians and consultants, are part of these committees, which meet periodically to take decisions on critical issues.

Figure 4. A Committee Meeting in Progress

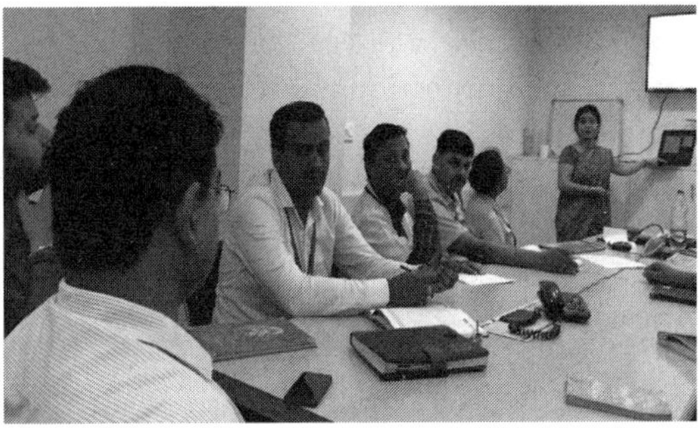

Daily Safety Huddles: This involves the entire team along with the administration, where the staff is encouraged to speak up about the issues in their respective areas or departments. This practice gives a spirit of collegiality, collaboration and cooperation to exist among the staff by empowering the employees.

Figure 5. Staff Sharing their Experiences in One of the 'Daily Huddles'

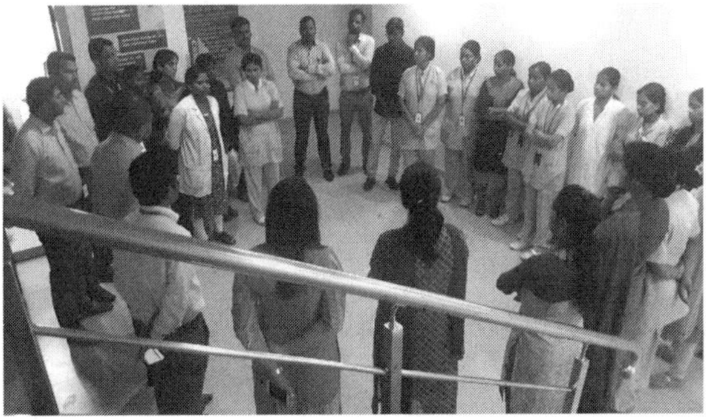

Buddy Programme: This approach is for new recruitments. A buddy is assigned to the new employee, who is part of the hospital team for a minimum period and gives an orientation to their respective department and the hospital. This helps in imbibing the culture of the hospital from the moment they join.

Star Department: Based on the 5S principle of workplace organization that has been turned into a quarterly competition, a trophy is awarded to the winning department as the 'Star Department' for motivation. Helps in infection control and safety.

Q4E (Quality for Excellence) Toolkits: Focused approach towards a critical parameter to improve the outcomes. A dedicated team is formed to formulate the toolkit that designs the resource tool for implementation to tackle the issue. On successful implementation, the toolkit is standardized across all units.

SSC with 'Voiceover': The standard WHO checklist for surgical safety has been implemented uniformly across all the hospitals with a process of voiceover during timeout, which mandates the participation of all the stakeholders and compliance to the IPSG.

Figure 6. Voiceover Process in Progress

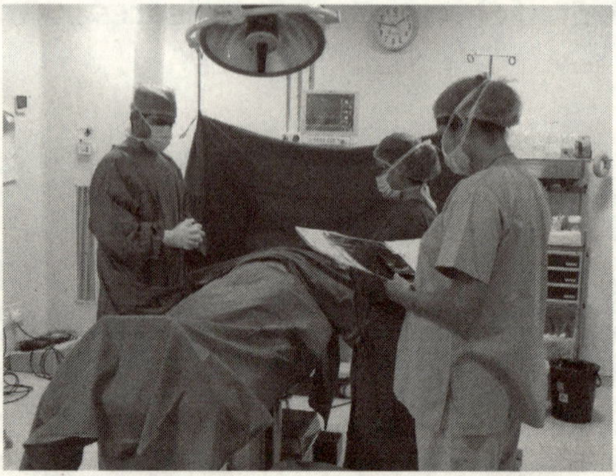

Medication Safety: High-alert medications are counterchecked during administration as well as double-checked and signed by the pharmacist while dispensing. This way, every high-alert drug is documented and has to pass through two levels of monitoring—thus reducing medication errors.

Just Culture: A culture that recognizes errors as system failures rather than individual failures, ensuring employee accountability with a non-punitive approach. Employees identifying and raising incidents are appreciated in the monthly Rewards and Recognition Programme for further motivation.

Figure 7. One of the R&R Programmes Conducted

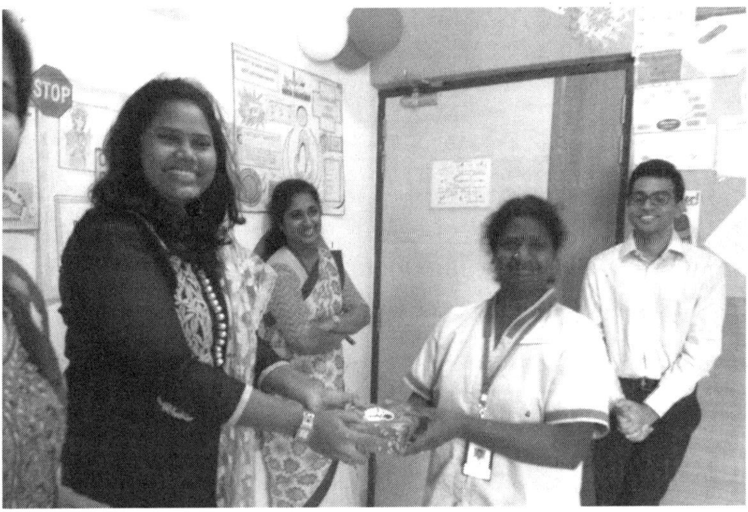

Communication: An in-house online incident-reporting software was developed, making the system more convenient and accessible, leading to better compliance. The in-house software also helped in direct intervention by HODs centrally. Automated daily reminders and alerts are sent to HODs for swift closures. Stakeholders can also directly track the status and closure of different incidents. Other communication improvement methods included Designated Safety Leaders, Nursing Kanban Boards and Apollo Educational Videos.

Figure 8. Incident Reporting Portal Page

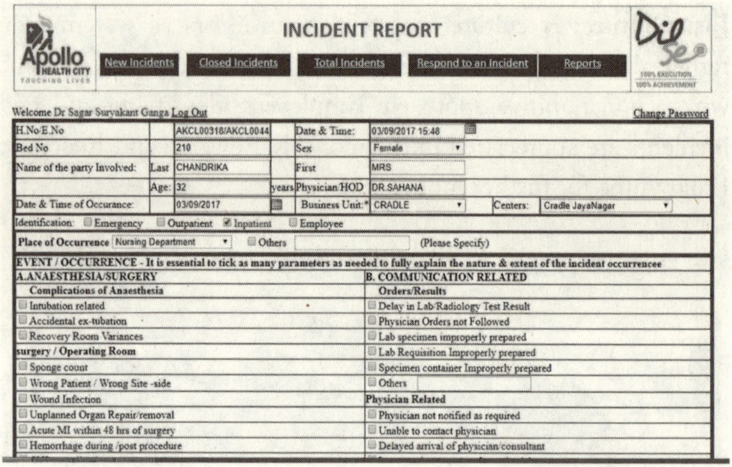
INCIDENT REPORT

New Incidents | Closed Incidents | Total Incidents | Respond to an Incident | Reports

Welcome Dr Sagar Suryakant Ganga Log Out — Change Password

H.No/E.No: AKCL00318/AKCL0044 — Date & Time: 03/09/2017 15:48
Bed No: 210 — Sex: Female
Name of the party Involved: Last CHANDRIKA — First MRS
Age: 32 years — Physician/HOD: DR.SAHANA
Date & Time of Occurance: 03/09/2017 — Business Unit:* CRADLE — Centers: Cradle JayaNagar
Identification: Emergency, Outpatient, Inpatient, Employee
Place of Occurrence: Nursing Department — Others (Please Specify)

EVENT / OCCURRENCE - It is essential to tick as many parameters as needed to fully explain the nature & extent of the incident occurrencee

A.ANAESTHESIA/SURGERY	B. COMMUNICATION RELATED
Complications of Anaesthesia	Orders/Results
Intubation related	Delay in Lab/Radiology Test Result
Accidental ex-tubation	Physician Orders not Followed
Recovery Room Variances	Lab specimen improperly prepared
surgery / Operating Room	Lab Requisition Improperly prepared
Sponge count	Specimen container Improperly prepared
Wrong Patient / Wrong Site -side	Others
Wound Infection	Physician Related
Unplanned Organ Repair/removal	Physician not notified as required
Acute MI within 48 hrs of surgery	Unable to contact physician
Hemorrhage during /post procedure	Delayed arrival of physician/consultant

Courtesy: Apollo Hospitals

Figure 9. Provision for Documenting Quality Analysis

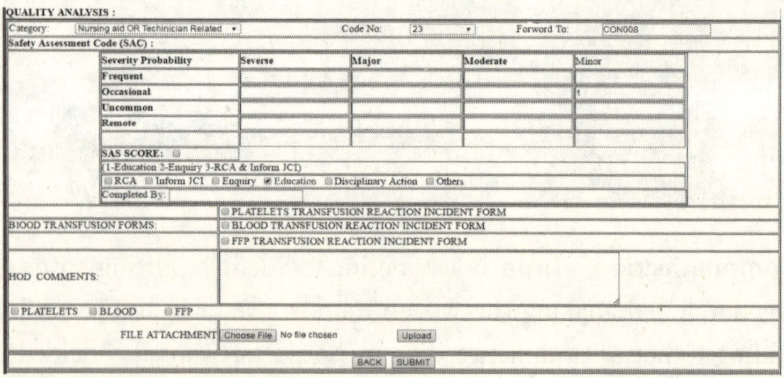
QUALITY ANALYSIS :
Category: Nursing aid OR Techinician Related — Code No: 23 — Forword To: CON008
Safety Assessment Code (SAC) :

Severity Probability	Severse	Major	Moderate	Minor
Frequent				
Occasional				1
Uncommon				
Remote				

SAS SCORE:
(1-Education 2-Enquiry 3-RCA & Inform JCI)
RCA, Inform JCI, Enquiry, Education, Disciplinary Action, Others
Completed By:

BIOOD TRANSFUSION FORMS: PLATELETS TRANSFUSION REACTION INCIDENT FORM; BLOOD TRANSFUSION REACTION INCIDENT FORM; FFP TRANSFUSION REACTION INCIDENT FORM

HOD COMMENTS:

PLATELETS, BLOOD, FFP

FILE ATTACHMENT: Choose File No file chosen — Upload

BACK | SUBMIT

Courtesy: Apollo Hospitals

Learning: Knowledge needs to be imparted in innovative ways to make it more effective and sustainable. Staff were trained in various aspects of Patient Safety through Infection Control Week, Safety Fair, Fire Safety Week, Code Blue Mock Drill Day, etc. The innovative methods included skits, quizzes, dance, etc., apart from the regular lectures and on-the-job training.

Figure 10. Staff Education Methods

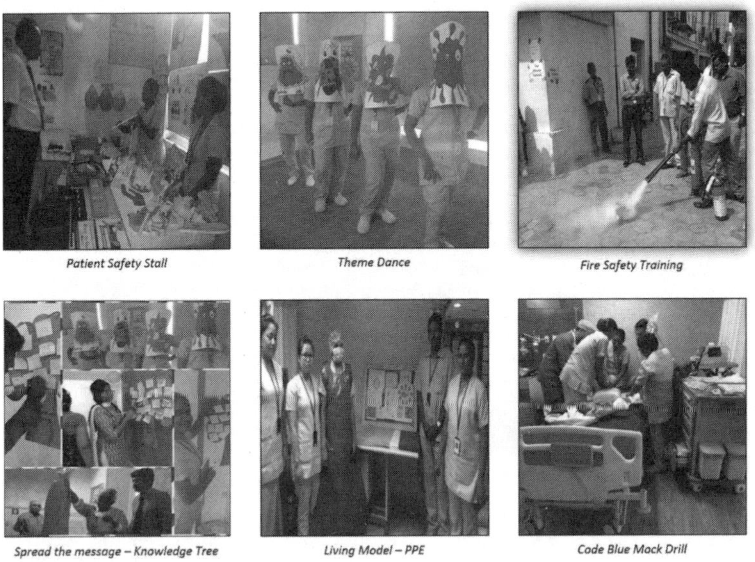

Patient Safety Stall — *Theme Dance* — *Fire Safety Training*

Spread the message – Knowledge Tree — *Living Model – PPE* — *Code Blue Mock Drill*

Courtesy: Apollo Hospitals

Results

In the next round of the online Safety Culture Survey conducted in March of Year 2, the participation of the employees increased by around 31 per cent, which itself was an indication of the rising awareness among employees about the importance of safety at the hospitals. The results of the survey showed that the improvement methods implemented had a tremendous impact on the culture of the organization. Overall, there was a substantial improvement in the perception, knowledge and execution of the safety-related activities.

Table 1. Safety Culture Survey Comparison: September Year 1 vs March Year 2

Parameter	Aug–Sep 'Y1	Mar 'Y2
Average Patient Safety Score (out of 100)	59.2	87
Grade for Overall Safety at the Unit (out of 5)	2.46	4.24
Awareness about Incident Reporting (in percentage)	68.8	89.2

Figure 11.

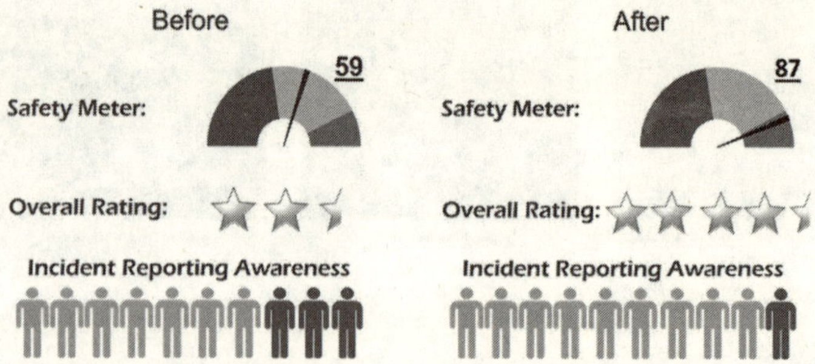

Courtesy: Apollo Hospitals

Incident reporting improved remarkably with the implementation of the above interventions. The number of incidents reported peaked in between, with a gradual decline subsequently as the preventive actions for the root causes were implemented.

Figure 12. Total Number of Incidents Reported

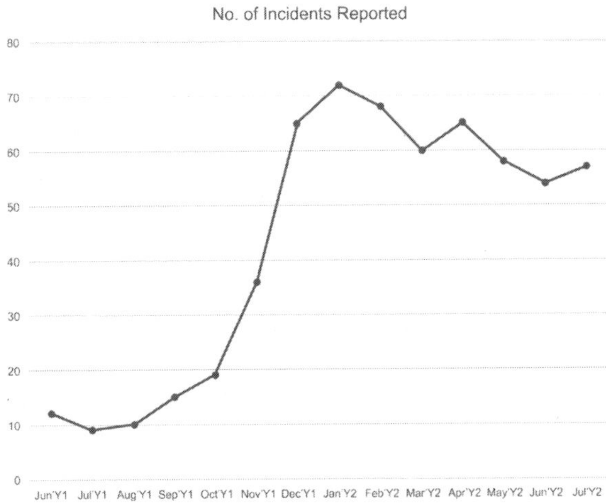

Conclusion

A multipronged approach with a balanced mix of small persistent steps, along with the use of technology and innovation, is important to inculcate a culture within the organization. Additionally, motivating the staff in various ways also goes a long way in reinforcing this newly developed culture. Statistically, numbers indicated the success of the Apollo Safety Development Model. The ultimate goal was patient safety, which was achieved as in the subsequent survey results. Substantial improvement in facility and process safety led to increased employee satisfaction. Streamlined processes helped in improving overall patient satisfaction. Ground staff got a sense of involvement, accountability and responsibility towards safety initiatives and eventually became responsible for further improvement of their respective processes. The project also fostered teamwork through different activities.

References:

1. Our Standards, Joint Commission, https://www.jointcommission.org/accreditation-and-certification/health-care-settings/hospital/learn/our-standards/.
2. 'National Quality & Health Service Standards: Guide for Hospitals', Australian Commission on Safety & Quality in Healthcare, https://www.safetyandquality.gov.au/.
3. 'Functions of the Victorian Surgical Consultative Council', Health VIC Government, https://www.health.vic.gov.au/quality-safety-service/functions-of-the-victorian-surgical-consultative-council
4. 'ACORN Standards', Australian College of Operating Room Nurses, https://www.acorn.org.au/
5. 'Hospital Survey on Patient Safety Culture', AHRQ, http://www.ahrq.gov/sops/quality-patient-safety/patientsafetyculture/hospital/index.html
6. Hospital SOPS Translation Information, AHRQ, https://www.ahrq.gov/sops/international/hospital/translators.html
7. A. Nacioglu, 'As a critical behavior to improve quality and patient safety in health care: speaking up!', https://safetyinhealth.biomedcentral.com/articles/10.1186/s40886-016-0021-x
8. T. Bisbey, 'Safety Culture: An Integration of Existing Models and a Framework for Understanding Its Development', *Human Factors* (February 2021), Vol. 63 No. 1, pp. 88–110.
9. M.D Cooper, 'Towards a model of safety culture', *Safety Science* (2000), Vol. 36, https://www.behavioral safety.com/articles/Towards_a_model_of_safety_culture.pdf
10. S. Kirk, et al., 'Patient safety culture in primary care: developing a theoretical framework for practical use', *Quality and Safety in Health Care* (August 2007), Vol. 16, No. 4, pp. 313–20.

11. R. Hughes, 'Tools and Strategies for Quality Improvement and Patient Safety', NCBI, https://www.ncbi.nlm.nih.gov/books/NBK2682/
12. S. Singer, 'Relationship of Safety Climate and Safety Performance in Hospitals', Health Service Research (April 2009), Vol 44, pp. 399–421.
13. National Patient Safety Goals, Joint Commission, https://www.jointcommission.org/standards/national-patient-safety-goals/

Case Study 10

The Quality for Excellence (Q4E) Programme

'In today's era of volatility, there is no other way but to re-invent. The only sustainable advantage you can have over others is agility, that's it. Because nothing else is sustainable, everything else you create, somebody else will replicate.'

—Jeff Bezos

Introduction

THE ABILITY TO monitor the efficacy of treatment decisions and patient outcomes will further the power to boost patient safety. Ultimately, 'quality healthcare depends on the provision of quality data'—a statement that summarizes the importance of appropriate data collection and measurement.

Apollo is committed to providing the safest and highest quality of care to patients. We measure our performance against our own rigorous standards and also compare the outcomes of our care with top medical centres worldwide—in our effort to continually improve the care we provide.

Apollo Health and Lifestyle Ltd. manages the wide network of Apollo Clinics, Apollo Cradles and Apollo Spectra Hospitals spread across India. Apollo Clinics are primary healthcare setups, along with facilities such as health checks and specialist consultations; Apollo Cradles are women and children hospitals; and Apollo Spectra Hospitals are short-stay surgery centres. Unlike in the case of standalone hospitals, our setup—spanning multiple locations and formats—created a problematic situation, which made it difficult to monitor the outcome measures. At the same time, the situation gave us an opportunity to standardize the processes and aim for continual quality improvement across all the units—to provide uniform care to the patients. There was a requirement for a robust model across the wide range of Apollo centres to monitor the performances in terms of structure, processes and outcomes; standardize the protocols; and improve and evaluate against international benchmarks.

Objectives

The Q4E Program provided an all-round solution for all the aforementioned problems. The essential goals or targets of the project were:

1. Standardize the data collection and monitoring of quality indicators or outcome measures across the network of Apollo Clinics, Cradles and Spectra Hospitals.
2. Continuous improvement in critical areas like compliance to incident reporting, reduction in reporting errors, and increase in patient and employee satisfaction among others.
3. External assessment/evaluation to measure the amount of implementation, validation of data collection process,

continuous quality improvement, and to recognize best practices.

4. Award and Recognition for centers with the best compliance and innovative practices towards quality improvement.

Figure 1. Aspects of Q4E App

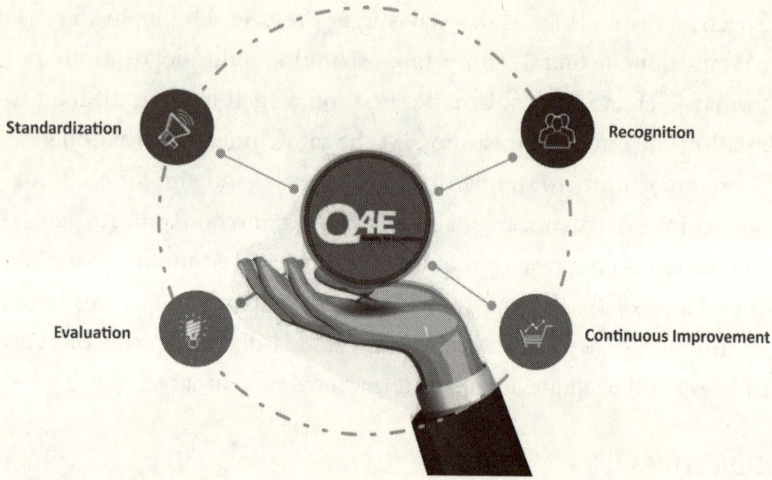

Implementation

A central executive core committee was developed, which was liable for conceptualizing the project and designing its framework. The committee, led by the Quality Team, included teams from various departments of Operations, IT, Medical Services, Human Resources, Finance, Projects and Maintenance. The aim of the committee was to form a comprehensive programme that covers all the aspects of healthcare setup management. An online dashboard was created with the assistance of the IT team. The operations team supported the implementation of the project on the ground. Individual departments at varied locations on the ground contributed to the project in terms of implementation of the programme and monthly data collection for their respective parameters. Overall, the project was a real teamwork across the organization.

The Q4E Program is a comprehensive annual cyclical project, which might be outlined with a five-stage approach, as seen in Figure 2.

Figure 2. Implementation of Q4E App

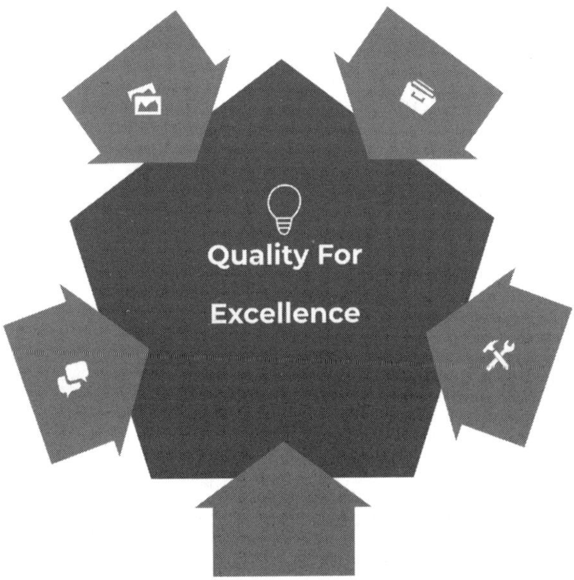

The team executed the programme with the subsequent steps within the same order:

1. The concept was created, and objectives and targets were outlined by the executive core committee.
2. A set of twenty standard parameters, for every business unit, were listed down and defined.

3. An online dashboard was created for these indicators.
4. End users, i.e., the staff at the units, was trained.
5. Pilot testing done at some select centres across business units.
6. Data from the pilot study was analysed, issues/concerns were identified, and modifications were made accordingly.
7. The project extended to all the business units pan India.
8. Monthly data collection and reporting by the units along with action-taken report for low-scoring parameters.
9. Data validation and analysis by the quality team.
10. External assessment/validation through Q4E Survey.
11. Annual Q4E Award presented to the best performing centres across all business units.
12. Programme revised at the end of the financial year based on the trends and requirement.

Online Q4E Dashboard

The twenty measurable indicators cover various categories such as:

- process;
- satisfaction (patient and employee);
- volume;
- clinical outcomes; and
- consultant connect.

Q4E has an online dashboard, wherein each unit collects and uploads the data for the defined indicators.

Figure 3. Screenshots of the Online Q4E Dashboards

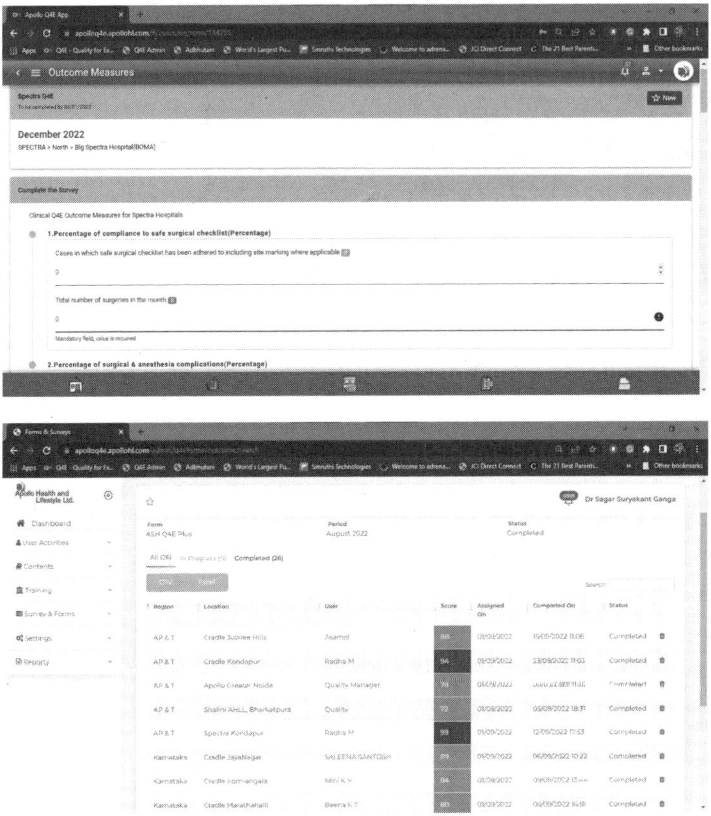

Action Taken Reports

Units fill the ATR automatically generated for low-scoring parameters based on the data uploaded to the dashboard. This helps in focusing on the low-scoring areas, developing an improvement plan, and assigning responsibilities and timelines for achieving the same.

Figure 4. An ATR Format

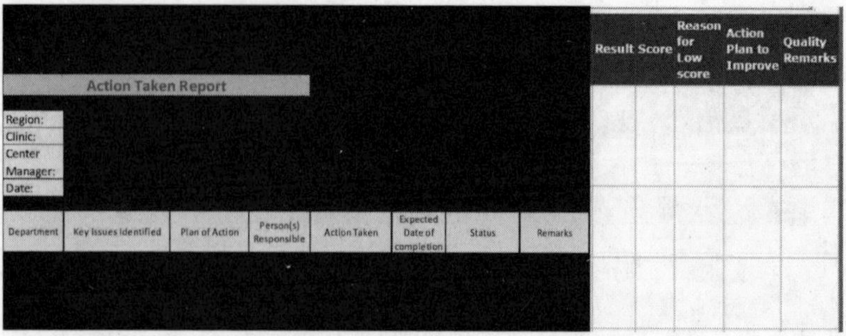

External Assessments/Evaluations

- Conducted every six months.
- Conducted by external surveyors from the main Apollo Hospitals.
- Standard checklist used.
- Used as a tool for validating the dashboard data and ATR, and the overall quality audit.

Figure 5. The Unit-Wise Monthly Dashboard Format

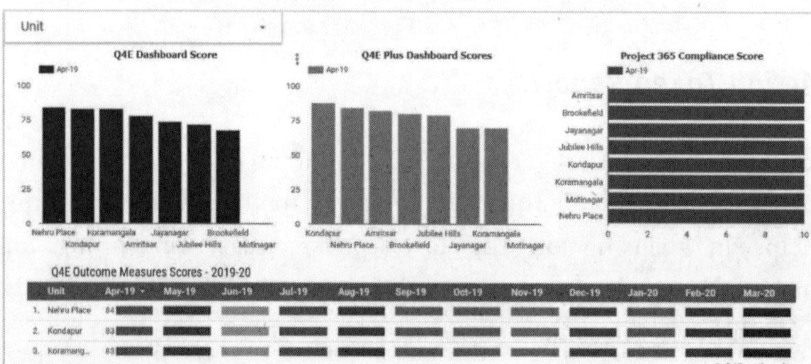

Q4E Award:

- Recognition and appreciation for sustenance.
- Best performing unit in terms of quality, i.e., Q4E scores, implementation of improvements and external surveys, are recognized.
- Trophy during the Founder's Day celebrations, and cash incentive for each staff of the centre.

Figure 6. Q4E Award Being Presented to the Winning Centres by the Managing Director during the Founder's Day Celebrations

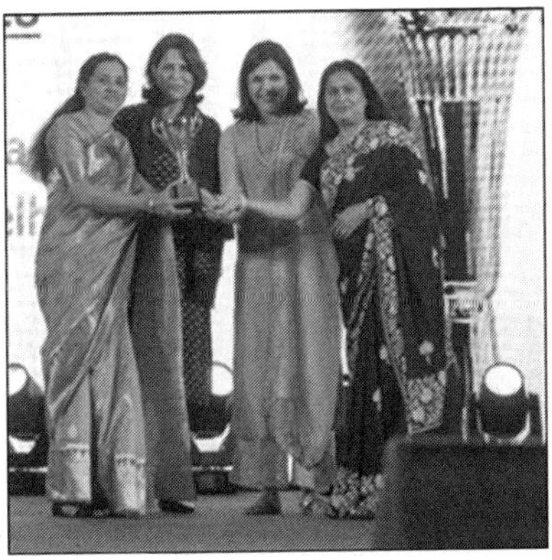

Courtesy: Apollo Hospitals

Results

The results/outcomes of the project were measured through different methods such as self-assessment and reporting by the units, automatic data capture from the MIS, data validation by the central quality team, and evaluation of on-the-ground implementation by external Q4E Surveys.

The biggest quantifiable information regarding the success of the project was the improvement of the average Q4E dashboard score from a baseline of 60 to 84, which was much ahead of the outlined target of 75 (a significant improvement of 40 per cent).

Figure 7. Q4E Dashboard

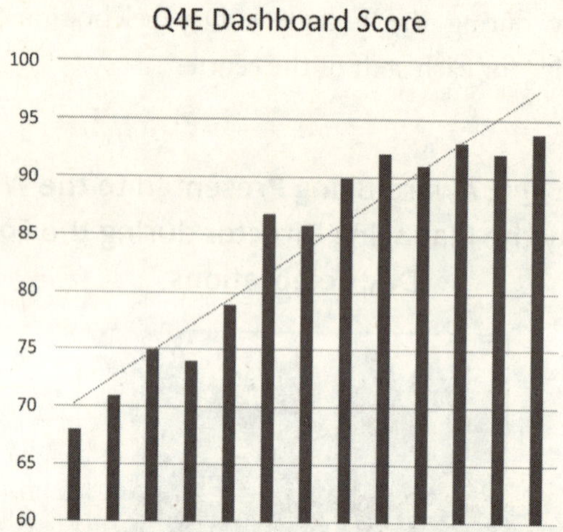

Parameter	Baseline	Month 01	Month 02	Month 03	Month 04	Month 05	Month 06	Month 07	Month 08	Month 09	Month 10	Month 11	Month 12	Month 13	Avg. Score	% Im-provement
Q4E Dashboard Score	60	68	71	75	74	79	87	86	90	92	91	93	92	94	84	40

Net promoter score, indicating the patient satisfaction rate, improved from less than 40 to 82, against a target of 75 (105 per cent improvement over the baseline). This is a clear indicator that the project—with its multidirectional approach—has improved the quality of care and service, eventually improving patient satisfaction.

Figure 8. Q4E Impact–Patient Experience

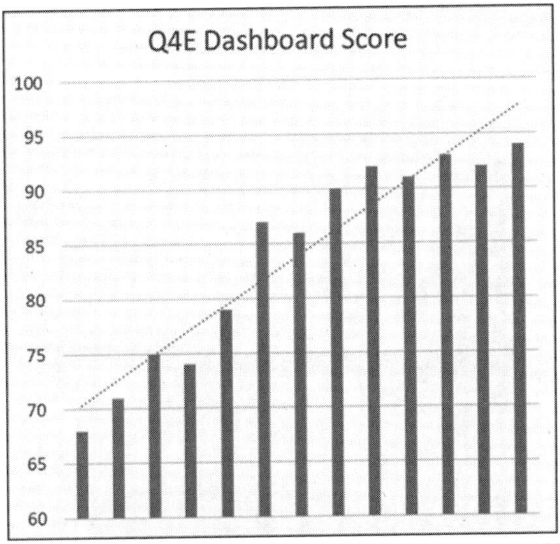

Parameter	Baseline	Month 01	Month 02	Month 03	Month 04	Month 05	Month 06	Month 07	Month 08	Month 09	Month 10	Month 11	Month 12	Month 13	Avg. Score	% Improve-ment
Net Promoter Score	40	52	58	65	71	75	79	86	89	93	92	94	97	97	82	105

Courtesy: Apollo Hospitals

Nosocomial infection rates came down to 0.35 per cent from 5.6 per cent against a target of ~0.

Figure 9. Q4E Impact–Nosocomial Infection Rates

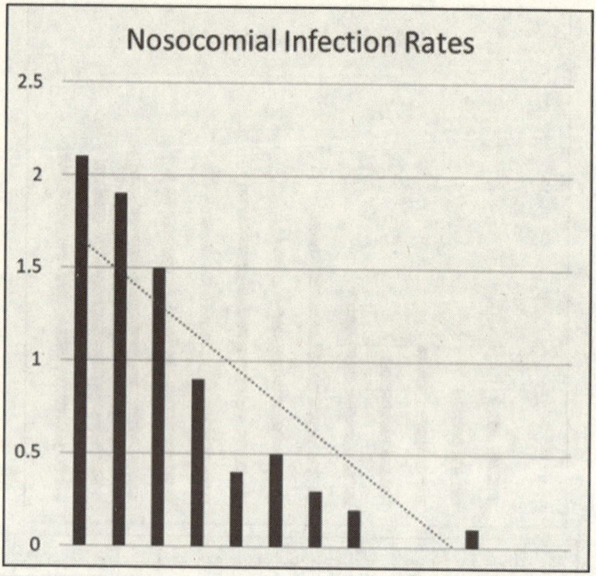

Parameter	Baseline	Month 01	Month 02	Month 03	Month 04	Month 05	Month 06	Month 07	Month 08	Month 09	Month 10	Month 11	Month 12	Month 13	Avg. Score	% Improvement
Nosocomial Infection Rates	5.6	2.1	1.9	1.5	0.9	0.4	0.5	0.3	0.2	0	0	0.1	0	0	0.35	-93.75

Courtesy: Apollo Hospitals

The average number of incidents reported per month improved from 1 to 4, against a target of 5.

Figure 10. Q4E Impact–Incident Reporting

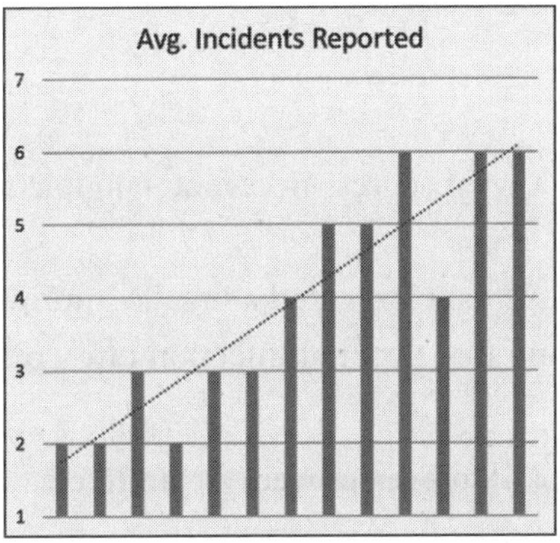

Parameter	Baseline	Month 01	Month 02	Month 03	Month 04	Month 05	Month 06	Month 07	Month 08	Month 09	Month 10	Month 11	Month 12	Month 13	Avg. Score	% Im-provement
Avg. Incidents Reported	1	2	2	3	2	3	3	4	5	5	6	4	6	6	4	300

Courtesy: Apollo Hospitals

The average Q4E Survey scores improved from less than 70 to 86, against a target of 85 (i.e., an improvement of 23 per cent).

Figure 11. Q4E Survey Score

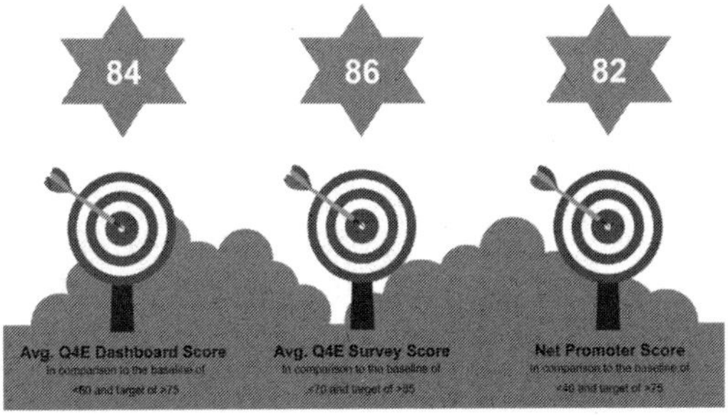

Courtesy: Apollo Hospitals

These numbers also indicate that the biggest beneficiary of this project was undoubtedly the patients of the hospitals.

Conclusion

The project was a great success in several tangible ways:

- Quantifiable data indicated a drastic improvement in patient satisfaction rates, hospital infection rates, process compliance rates, etc.
- Operationally, processes were streamlined.
- Ground staff got a sense of involvement, accountability and responsibility as they were involved in the data collection process, and were eventually responsible for the improvement of their respective processes.
- Substantial improvement in patient safety, and patient and employee satisfaction.
- The project also fostered teamwork and activity, which started from data collection, outcome analysis and implementation for improvement.

The following steps are being taken to sustain the improvements achieved and to move further ahead:

- Continual trainings for all the staff on data collection, importance and relevance of each indicator, especially a two-hour induction on the programme for every new employee who joins the organization.
- ATRs enable focus on solutions to overcome certain low-scoring parameters, leading to continuous quality improvement and sharing of best practices.

- Recognition/appreciation in the form of Q4E Awards gives the teams a sense of motivation to take ownership towards quality improvement.
- The Q4E Programme is dynamic in terms of the revision of the quality indicators annually. The outcome measures are modified according to the requirement or improvement trend post analysis.

Overall, the project was very well received by all the units and their staff. Feedback was taken from the board member and CEO to the staff nurse working in a clinic, and everybody appreciated the project in different ways. Dr Arun Rai, Board Member, noted, 'Quality and Patient Safety should always be the top priority of any healthcare organization, and this project ensures we stick to our priorities.' Mr Chandrashekhar, CEO, said, 'Merit is always the only measure to succeed, and this program helps to assess the merit of the centres in an objective manner.' Sr Noel, a staff nurse from Apollo Spectra Jaipur, shared this feedback, 'We learnt a lot of new things through Q4E. It also helps us in understanding where can we improve.'

The project has also received various national and international accolades, such as the Gold Award in Clinical Services by Hospital Management Asia, Recognition by the International Society for Quality (ISQua) as a 'Leading for Quality' Project, Certificate of Merit from Project Evaluation and Research Programme by Frost & Sullivan, Best Healthcare Project from CMO Asia Awards, and Healthcare Project of the Year from Express Healthcare Achievers and Leaders Award.

In Gratitude

WHAT HAVE WE learnt over the years is that every time we implement a process, it prevents errors, reduces risk, and helps to save lives. We have worked relentlessly across the Apollo ecosystem to level up the patient safety standards continuously. This has resulted in setting the right measures, monitoring and sustaining good practices, improving outcomes, and reducing duplications.

The idea of this book is to share what we have learnt and to disseminate the knowledge and concepts. We have conducted International Health Dialogue over the last ten years with a focus on patient safety and transforming health with information technology. Now along with this book, we are opening a forum where healthcare professionals could discuss quality and share best practices while also being a part of the Patient Safety Club. This will further improve the patient safety and quality environment in India.

I am personally very grateful to everyone who enabled this and my sincerest love to every team member at Apollo. Thank you to every smile, every step and every life touched. Finally, a big thanks to our inspiration—Dr Prathap C. Reddy, my father, mentor, guide and chairman on his 90th birthday. Because of your purity of thought and vision, we will continue to grow and spread the patient safety environment in our country.

Such is the banyan tree that you have planted and because your mission is for India and your vision is for good health across the world, we dedicate this book to the good health of humanity.

Sangita Reddy,
Joint Managing Director, Apollo Hospitals

Chapter Contributors

Sangita Reddy

Dr Hari Prasad Kovelamudi, MBBS, MD (Anaesthesiology), FCEM (Hon), FIFEM

Dr Anupam Sibal, MD, FIMSA, FIAP, FRCP (Glasgow), FRCP (London), FRCPCH, FAAP

Gaurav Loria, MBA, MHM, Lean Six Sigma Master Black Belt

Yogamaya Nayak, MHM, Lean Six Sigma Green Belt

Capt. (Dr) Usha Banerjee PhD, BSC Nursing (AFMC, Pune)

Dr Rohini Sridhar, MD, DNB, FRCPA (Haematology)

Major (Dr) Sanjay Dalsania, MBBS, MBA, PhD

V. Balaji, MHSM, Master Black Belt Six Sigma

Soma Das, MHM

Rekha Chakrabarti, MHA, Lean Six Sigma Black Belt

Pritindira Kaur, MBA, Lean Six Sigma Black Belt

Satish Kumar, MBA, PGD QM and AHO, PGDHHM, PGD in HRD

Dr Ratna Mani, MD (Micro), PGID (Infectious Diseases), AMPH (ISB)

Dr Mohammed Ziauddin Member Secretary, IEC-CS & BMR, MBBS, MD (Pharmacology)

Akash Tiwari, PGCPM (IIM, Indore), MBA (HR & OPS), PCBSc (Nursing), DHM

Bhumika Desai, MHA

Shaik Mukram Mohiuddin, BSc (Nursing), Master of Business Administration (MBA)

Dr Sagar S Ganga, BDS, MBA

Batul Nayani, MHHM

Dr Prem Nanakram Chawla, MBA (Hospital Administration), PGDHHM, BAMS, D. Pharmacy

Neha Panchal, BE (Mechanical), Graphic Designer

Aamrin Pagare, MBA

Dr Arpita Malani, MBBS, MBA (Hospital Administration)

Himani Sharma, MBA (Hospital Administration)

Abhilash Pillai, AMP (IIM), Executive Programme in Business Management IIM, BCG Leadership Development, BSc

Dr Sushil Jain, MBBS, MBA (Hospital Administration)

Juned Siddiqie, PGDM in Hospital Management, PGDCR (ACRP), BSc, BT

Namita Barik, GNM, Infection Control Advance Certification

Vamshi Krishna Jannam, PGD (Hospital & Healthcare Management), B Pharmacy

Ramya Mulpuri, MBA in Hospital and Health Systems Management, MSc Nursing

Karike Sandhya Rani, MSc Nursing OBG, MSc Professional Practice (Nursing) UK, PGDSBA.

Akash Sharma, PGDM (Hospital and Health Management)

30 Years *of*

HarperCollins *Publishers* India

At HarperCollins, we believe in telling the best stories and finding the widest possible readership for our books in every format possible. We started publishing 30 years ago; a great deal has changed since then, but what has remained constant is the passion with which our authors write their books, the love with which readers receive them, and the sheer joy and excitement that we as publishers feel in being a part of the publishing process.

Over the years, we've had the pleasure of publishing some of the finest writing from the subcontinent and around the world, and some of the biggest bestsellers in India's publishing history. Our books and authors have won a phenomenal range of awards, and we ourselves have been named Publisher of the Year the greatest number of times. But nothing has meant more to us than the fact that millions of people have read the books we published, and somewhere, a book of ours might have made a difference.

As we step into our fourth decade, we go back to that one word – a word which has been a driving force for us all these years.

Read.

Harper Collins · 4th · HARPER PERENNIAL · HARPER BUSINESS · HARPER BLACK · हार्पर हिन्दी

HarperCollins *Children'sBooks* · HARPER DESIGN · HARPER VANTAGE · Harper Sport

The Quality Mind Map

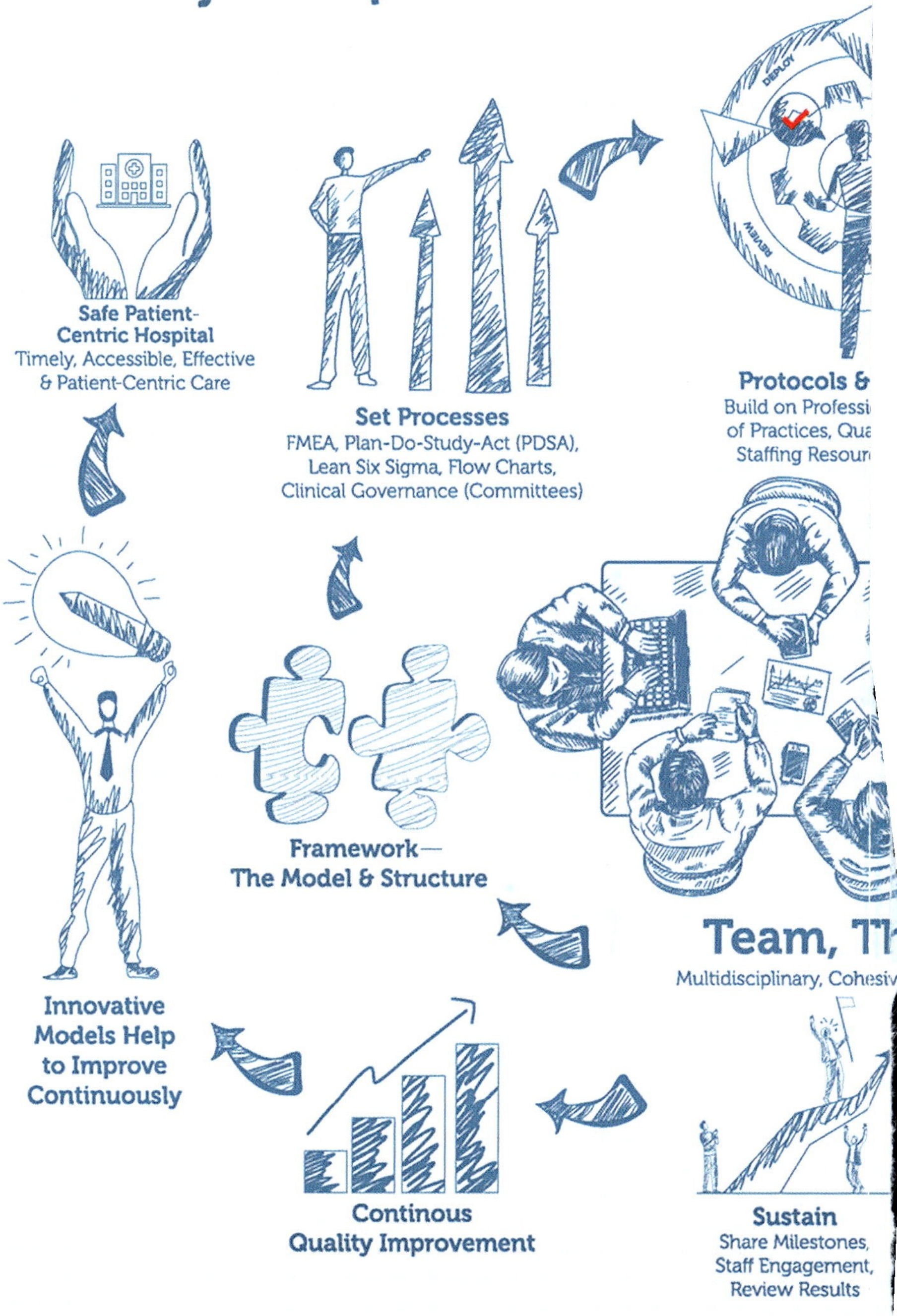

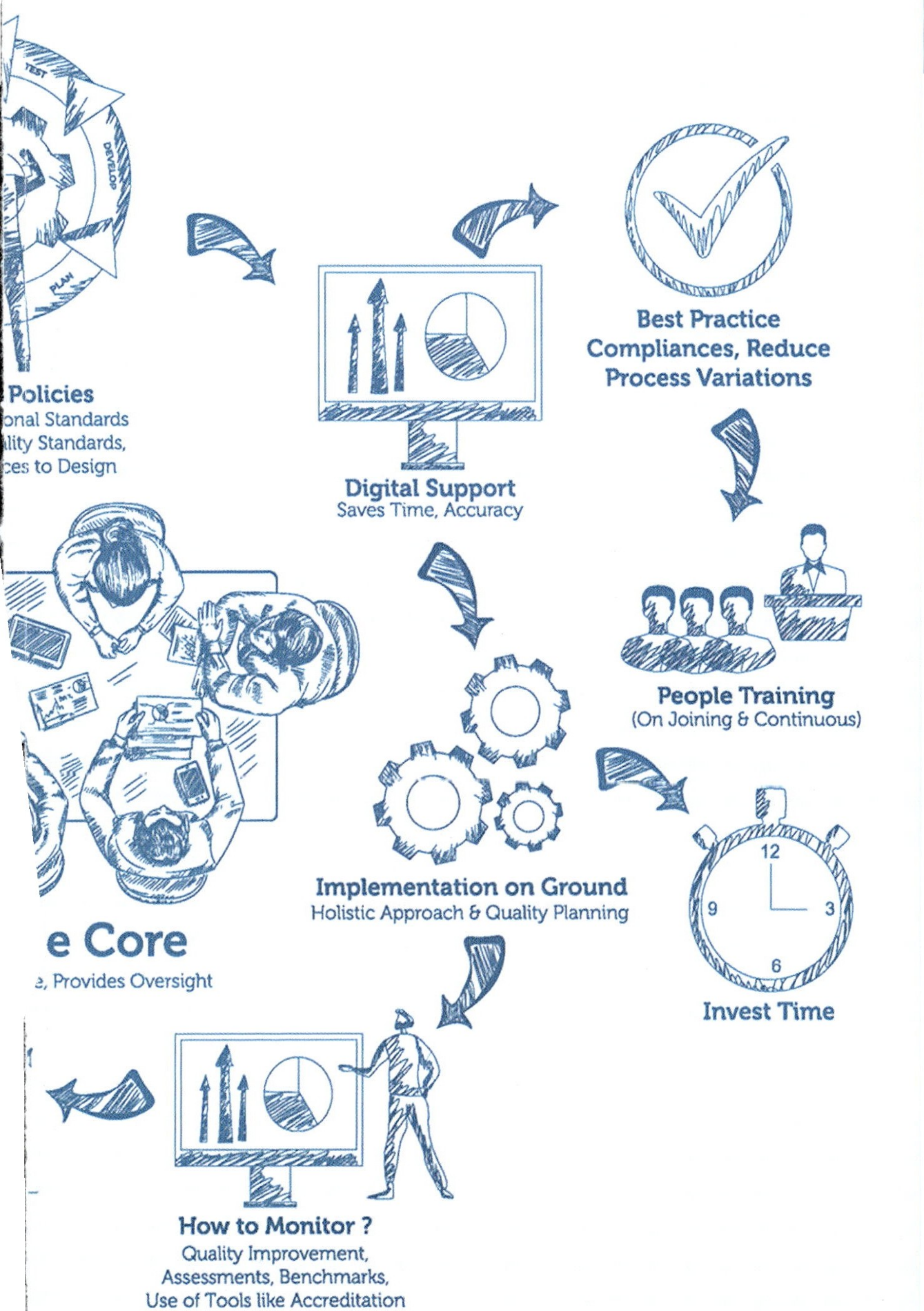

Courtesy: Apollo Hospitals